D1577495

Applied
Dental Materials

Applied
Dental Materials

John N. Anderson

M.D.S., L.D.S.(Sheffield)

Professor of Dental Prosthetics, University of Dundee.
Consultant in Dental Prosthetics,
Tayside Health Board, Scotland.
Dean of Dentistry, University of Dundee.
Formerly Lecturer in Dental Mechanics and Prosthetics
in the Universities of Sheffield, Durham and Birmingham.
External Examiner in Dental Prosthetics,
Universities of Baghdad, Birmingham, Bristol, Liverpool,
Malaya (Kuala Lumpur), Newcastle upon Tyne
and Royal College of Surgeons in Ireland.
Author of *Immediate and Replacement Dentures.*

Fifth Edition

Blackwell Scientific Publications
OXFORD LONDON EDINBURGH MELBOURNE

© 1965, 1972, 1976, by Blackwell Scientific Publications
Osney Mead, Oxford, England
8 John Street, London, W1, England
9 Forrest Road, Edinburgh, Scotland

First published February 1956
Second edition June 1961
Reprinted January 1965
Third edition September 1967
Fourth edition April 1972
Fifth edition August 1976

British Library Cataloguing in Publication Data
Anderson, John Neil
    Applied dental materials. – 5th ed.
    Bibl. – Index.
    ISBN 0–632–00028–7
    1. Title
    617.6'95   RK652.5
    Dental materials

Printed in Great Britain by
Billing & Sons Limited,
Guildford, London and Worcester
and bound at Kemp Hall Bindery

Contents

Preface   vii

Acknowledgements   ix

1 Introduction   1

Section A.   General properties of materials

2 Structure and properties of materials   6
3 Determining properties   19
4 The application of these properties to dentistry   37

Section B.   Cast and wrought metals

5 Grain structure. Metallography   44
6 Deformation of metals. Softening heat treatment   52
7 Alloys. Hardening heat treatment   58
8 Gold. Yellow and white gold alloys   71
9 Base metal casting alloys   90
10 Alloys for metal/ceramic structures   102
11 Steels   110
12 Wrought base metal alloys. Stainless steels   114
13 Tungsten carbide   122
14 Die and counterdie alloys. Fusible alloys   125
15 Soldering and welding   128
16 Electrodeposition. Electrolytic polishing. Corrosion   142

Section C.   Dental precision casting

17 Waxes and similar thermoplastic materials   154
18 Casting investment materials   162
19 Variables in casting techniques. Defects in castings   175

Section D.   General non-metallic materials

20 Gypsum products   190
21 Non-elastic impression materials   205
22 Elastic impression materials. Hydrocolloids   216
23 Elastic impression materials. Elastomers   233
24 Non-metallic denture base materials. Heat-cure PMMA   245
25 Self-cure acrylic denture bases   271
26 Flexible materials   277
27 Alginate mould seal   281
28 Acrylic teeth, acrylic crowns, temporary crown and bridge
    materials   283
29 Abrasives and polishing agents. Denture cleansers   291
30 Dental porcelain   303
31 Materials for implants   313
32 Materials for dies   321

Section E.   Filling materials

33 Introduction   326
34 Dental amalgams   329
35 Non-metallitc filling materials. Lining and luting cements   351
36 Silicate, silicophosphate and ionomer cements   373
37 Polymeric filling materials   387

    Appendix   409
    Further reading   416
    Index   417

Preface

Information about dental materials was once gained by trial, but mainly by error. Our present knowledge, however, rests firmly on a broad basis of scientific investigation.

A complete discussion of the large volume of research which has been carried out, however, is of interest mainly to other dental research workers, to the physicist or chemist, or to the student or practitioner who is pursuing a particular line of thought. To the general practitioner and the student who, one day, will achieve this status, much of the research work is conflicting in results, and is not easily interpreted in terms of everyday practice.

This book is therefore intended as a guide to the everyday manipulation of materials, rather than a scientific treatise upon their properties. It is intended both as a text-book for students, and also as a reference book to which dental practitioners and their technicians will turn when difficulties arise in the manipulation of materials, or when practical information upon their use is required.

The scope of the book has been purposely limited, as I feel that dental education is already sufficiently complex without burdening the student with a large mass of academic knowledge of dental materials which has little or no application. Although some of the text may still be considered to be academic in character, an attempt has been made to keep the information of a practical nature.

An argument may well be put forward that Applied Dental Materials is really part of dental technology, prosthetics, or conservation. But this is not a book giving details of techniques. Any reference to practical details which have been given are those which affect the properties of the material. The details of manipulation are not complete, as it is anticipated that instruction in other dental subjects in which the materials are used will accompany or even precede the teaching in dental materials.

While writing this book, reference has been made to numerous texts, and to the literature. The text is based on published work available in Scotland up to October 1975.

A book on dental materials is seldom, if ever, read from cover to cover. Moreover, the sequence in which experience of handling materials is gained differs in the various teaching establishments. The materials have, therefore, been grouped together under headings which should enable them to be readily found in the text.

JOHN N. ANDERSON
Dundee, 1975

Acknowledgements

Due to the large increase in recent years in the volume of publications on the properties of dental materials, I found it necessary to take the helpful advice of a number of experts in this field. Dr D. C. Tidy, Lecturer in Dental Materials Science in the University of Manchester, and Mr F. F. Lyon of the Department of Dental Prosthetics of this University have both read the entire manuscript and made very many helpful suggestions to try to ensure that this edition was up to date. Professor M. Braden of the London Hospital Dental School gave particular help on the many chapters which deal with polymers. Dr D. R. Beech, Senior Physicist, Australian Dental Standards Laboratory, and Mr J. A. Hobkirk, Eastman Dental Hospital, commented upon the chapters on polymeric filling materials and materials for implants respectively. I am most grateful for the advice and help of these gentlemen. They, however, are not responsible for any errors which remain in the text.

The accuracy and speed of Mrs M. G. High's typing have again contributed greatly to the preparation of the manuscript. My thanks are also due to my wife for typing, proof reading and indexing.

Chapter 1
Introduction

The materials used in dentistry may be divided into two main groups. In the first group are those materials which are selected for use because they possess certain physical properties, and have little or no chemical action upon living tissues. Indeed, one of the major requirements of this group of materials is that they shall be as chemically inert as possible when used in the mouth. The second group comprises those drugs and medicaments which are used primarily for their effect on living tissues. This book deals only with the first group. For information on the properties and manipulation of drugs and medicaments, reference should be made to text-books on materia medica and pharmacology.

Some of the relatively inert materials show a chemical reaction when used in the mouth. This reaction is frequently undesirable and a discussion of such unwanted effects finds its place in a book on the first group of dental materials.

In the fields of both prosthetic and conservative dentistry a great deal of the success which is achieved by the dental surgeon in his practical treatment of the patient depends upon the correct manipulation of the materials which he uses. His skill in the use of instruments plays an equal, if not greater part in his work, but skill and knowledgeable manipulation of materials must go hand in hand in order to produce the desired final result. For example, the life of a filling within a tooth depends not only on the shape of the cavity which is prepared, but also upon the properties of the filling material which is placed within it. These properties vary widely according to the care which the operator or his chairside assistant uses in the preparation of the filling material, and also on the conditions under which the filling is placed in the cavity. An error at either stage of manipulation can affect the properties of the resultant filling. Similarly, in the construction of a denture or other appliance, both the dentist and his technician can bring about success only by the intelligent manipulation of the various materials which are used.

Therefore, the correct use of dental materials must have as its foundation a knowledge of the material itself, and also of the changes in its properties which take place under varying conditions of manipulation.

The properties of the material as purchased depend upon the skill and care which have been exercised during its manufacture and subsequent storage. The dental surgeon or his technician can produce the best results only when he has access to suitable materials. It is essential, therefore, that the materials purchased conform to certain specifications, so that with correct manipulation they will produce satisfactory results.

In Great Britain, the British Standards Institution has formulated dental standard specifications, and arranges for the testing of materials on application by manufacturers. In addition, the Department of Health and Social Security issues a list of acceptable dental materials for use within the National Health Service. Each manufacturer is expected to test his products to ensure that they meet the British Standard Specification and the Department tests samples purchased on the open market as an additional safeguard.

In the United States of America, the Council on Dental Materials and Devices, sponsored by the American Dental Association, formulates specifications for dental materials. On application by a manufacturer, the Council tests samples of his materials purchased on the open market. If approved, the product appears on the list of certified materials and devices. If subsequently it is found to be not up to standard, then it is removed from the list.

The Standards Association of Australia defines specifications and the Australian Dental Association through its Standards Committee publishes an accredited list of materials and works in a manner similar to that of the Americans.

Many other countries have laid down their own standards for dental materials.

There exists an international organization for standardization (ISO) which has a technical committee, ISO/TC 106 Dentistry, whose purpose is to formulate dental specifications on an international basis. It is hoped that eventually there will be world-wide acceptance of the same standards with perhaps variations to cover different climatic conditions. A list of specifications appears in the appendix.

Specifications help to guard the dental profession against the activities of the less scrupulous manufacturers who make over-optimistic claims for their products, and who also place new materials in the hands of the profession without previous adequate testing. Specifications also help to improve the general standard of materials available.

If the dentist purchases only certified materials, he has a safeguard against high-pressure salesmanship of inferior products. Specifications do not exist, however, for all dental materials as they are by no means easy to formulate.

Perhaps one of the greatest difficulties in assessing the value of a material which has no specification arises because the manufacturer does not offer any scientific information about his product. Indeed, some manufacturers cloud their products in secrecy and do not encourage persons seeking information. Nor do they give precise details as to how their products should be manipulated. These remarks fortunately do not apply to the whole of the dental trade, and some manufacturers supply excellent details of the properties of their materials, together with precise instructions on how to use them.

Since specifications do not exist for all materials, it is necessary that the dental surgeon and his technician shall be able to assess the suitability of a material from the information given by the manufacturer.

The study of dental materials requires a previous knowledge of physics and chemistry, both organic and inorganic. It borrows from many applied sciences, including engineering, metallurgy and ceramics, and in its final application to the patient, owes much to the arts.

The properties of materials is one of the few dental subjects in which research can be carried out in a laboratory. No research into dental materials is complete, however, until its findings have been proved in clinical practice, though a close estimate of the behaviour of a material in the mouth can be gained from laboratory studies.

A great amount of literature exists as the result of this research. Indeed, almost a quarter of recent dental literature is related to dental materials research.

Section A
General properties of materials

Chapter 2
Structure and properties of materials

Many of the dental materials in use today are manipulated by the dentist in a plastic or semi-liquid state. In this condition, they are formed to the required shape, and then by a physical change or a chemical reaction, they become a solid. Any consideration of the physical and chemical properties of dental materials deals, therefore, with these materials in two states. First in the manipulative condition, and secondly as a material carrying out its intended purpose.

The suitability of a dental material depends to the greater extent upon its properties in the finished or solid condition, though the ease and accuracy with which it can be manipulated are important also.

RELATION OF STRUCTURE AND PROPERTIES

The detailed internal structure of solids and liquids affects the way in which they react to the environment in which they are placed. An understanding of the forces which hold the atoms or molecules of materials in a certain relation and which resist changes of shape of that material is therefore important.

Liquids

In a liquid, there is little or no ordered arrangement of atoms. In fact, irregularity and indefinition of structure is an essential feature of the liquid state. Short-term relations do exist, however, which try to ensure that each atom has a similar number of more closely related neighbours. The atoms are attracted to each other within the liquid, whilst those at its free boundaries are attracted more by the same atoms within the liquid than to the air. Hence the production of a boundary between the atmosphere and the surface of the liquid.

Within a liquid, the thermal energy is sufficient to keep the atoms in constant relative motion. Change in atomic relations, i.e. flow, takes place readily.

Solids

Solids, on the other hand, have internal structures which vary from a haphazard arrangement, usually called amorphous, to a highly regular or crystalline pattern. For example, glass has an amorphous structure, whilst all solid metals have a regular, well-defined atomic structure.

There is no sharp dividing line between these two classes of substance, and a crystalline material nearly always contains a few defects where the atoms are not regularly arranged, while an amorphous material frequently contains regions where a portion of its atoms or molecules conform to some regular pattern.

The forces of attraction between atoms or molecules may be divided into strong or primary bonds and weaker, secondary bonds.

Primary bonding forces

Ionic bonds

Some atoms readily give up their valence electrons and so become ions with a positive charge, whilst others accept these electrons to complete their outer electron shell and so become negatively charged ions (Fig. 1). Both atoms are then more stable and less reactive.

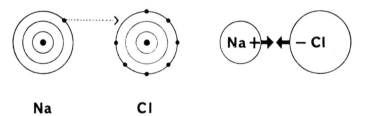

Na   **Cl**

Fig. 1. Ionic bond A transfer of an electron from Na to Cl forms positive and negative ions. These are mutually attracted by coulombic forces

Covalent bonds

Atoms whose outer orbitals are only partly filled may become more stable by sharing electrons with other atoms and so becoming a molecule. For example, two chlorine atoms may share a pair of electrons, thus completing their outer shells of eight electrons and so become a more stable chlorine molecule (Fig. 2). The covalent bond is the most frequent bond in chemistry and it is also a strong one.

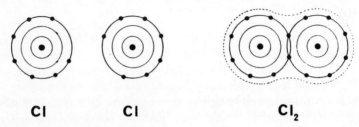

CI   CI CI_2

Fig. 2. Covalent bond. Sharing of outer shell electrons to form a chlorine molecule

Metallic bonds

A third form of bonding exists peculiar to metals. The valence electrons from each metallic atom no longer belong to any particular atom, but form an 'electron cloud'. The positive ions formed by the loss of these electrons and the electron cloud itself produce strong forces of attraction bonding the metal together. In general, metal atoms which have only a few loosely held valence electrons are more metallic in their bonding. Atoms such as Na, K, Cu, Ag, Au, have high electrical and thermal conductivity since their valence electrons are very mobile. As the number of valence electrons increases, the bonding becomes less metallic and more covalent, e.g. Fe, Ni, W, Ti. Tin exists in two forms of bonding, one mostly metallic and the other mostly covalent.

Secondary bonding forces

There are other, weaker forces joining molecules together. These are dipole bonds, and hydrogen bonds or bridges. They are often known collectively as *van der Waals'* forces.

Permanent dipole bonds

These intermolecular forces arise from an electrical imbalance in some molecules. The electron-sharing processes of primary bonds do not always produce two electrically balanced partners within the molecule.

One may have a slight negative charge and the other a slight positive one. Thus, each end of the dipole may attract the oppositely charged end of another dipole (Fig. 3).

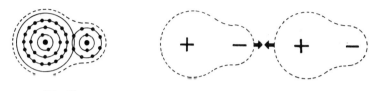

ZnO

Fig. 3. Permanent dipole bond. The *centre* of positive charge does not coincide with the *centre* of negative charge due to electrical imbalance

Fluctuating dipole bonds

Electrons move round their nuclei. Within a molecule this movement of electrons can produce a situation where there are more electrons on one side of the nucleus than on the other. One end of the molecule is at one instant slightly positive and shortly after slightly negative. This fluctuating charge may interact with adjoining molecules to produce a weak attraction.

Hydrogen bonds

These may be considered to be a special type of stronger dipole bond. They occur between molecules when a hydrogen atom is at one end or at the end of an 'offshoot'. The one electron belonging to this hydrogen atom is only loosely held. If the adjacent atom of the molecule is strongly electronegative it may attract the hydrogen's electron, thus leaving the hydrogen virtually as a positive ion. This can bond to other dipoles with a force almost as strong as an ionic bond.

ATOMIC PACKING

The arrangement of a large number of atoms in a solid is dependent upon the type of interatomic bonds present. Ionic, metallic and fluctuating dipole bonds are generally non-directional, whilst covalent and permanent dipole bonds are directional. Atoms joined together by directional bonds pack in a way which satisfies the bond angle. On the other hand, atoms joined together by non-directional bonds can be considered to behave as tightly packed rigid spheres. The arrangement of such spheres follows certain geometric rules but is obviously also affected by the relative sizes of the different atoms being packed together.

Non-directional bonding

The anions and cations in ionic bonding are usually of different sizes and pack in such a way so that each cation tends to be surrounded by the largest number of anions. A typical example is NaCl where the ions pack in a simple three-dimensional cubic arrangement (Fig. 4).

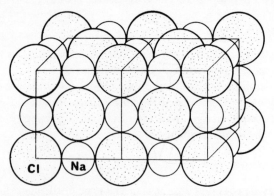

Fig. 4.   Simple cubic structure of NaCl

Atoms of equal size pack in several different ways producing a greater or lesser degree of density. Two very dense arrangements observed in metallic structures are close-packed hexagonal (cph) and face-centred cubic (fcc) arrangements (Fig. 5, a, b). In both of these arrangements, each atom is surrounded by twelve other atoms, this being the maximum number of equally sized atoms which can be accommodated. A less closely packed structure seen in about one-third of the metals is a body-centred cubic (bcc) (Fig. 5c). Here each atom has only eight neighbouring atoms in contact and the structure is therefore less dense.

Directionally bonded atoms

When the bonds are directionally orientated at certain angles, the

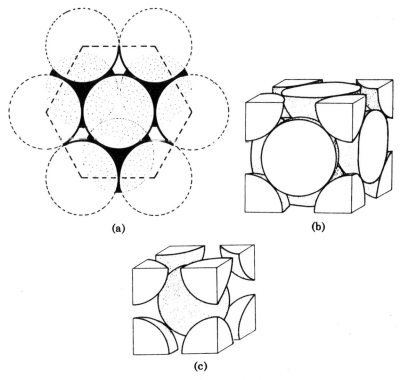

Fig. 5. (a) Close packing of atoms in layers. The atoms in one layer lie in the 'holes' of the adjacent layer. The close-packed hexagonal arrangement is indicated by the dotted line and consists of one layer of three atoms (shaded) between two layers of atoms (unshaded). (b) Face-centred cubic packing. (c) Body-centred packing.

spatial relation is controlled by the bond angles and a large number of less closely packed arrangements is therefore possible. Of course, both primary and secondary bonds may occur together in the one solid. For example, atoms may be bonded together by primary bonds to form molecules and these molecules joined together by secondary directional or non-directional bonds. The joining together of molecules into long chains is the basis of structure of many polymers both natural and synthetic.

Crystal structure

The three-dimensional pattern of the atoms in space is called its crystal structure. The regularity with which atoms are packed in solids arises from the possibilities of packing the atoms together and limitations imposed by directional bonding. It will be appreciated that the more dense the packing, the less is the energy of the solid. Crystal structures are generally described on the basis of an idealized geometric concept called a *space-lattice*. A space-lattice is a three-dimensional array of points of infinite extent in which every point has surroundings identical with that of every other point. Thus we speak of the unit cell of a face-centred cubic, close-packed hexagonal and body-centred cubic lattice of metals (Fig. 6). Ionic crystals, such as those of NaCl or SiO_2 are formed by the packing together of anions and cations so as to maintain electrical neutrality but without inducing strong repulsion between ions of similar charge. Molecular crystals occur when the regularity of a molecular chain allows close packing with neighbouring chains. Then a crystal structure is apparent. This might be local or it might be spread through a considerable extent of the solid. Generally speaking, it is the simpler molecules which crystallize more readily than the complex ones, though there are some polymers which are chemically complex but still have a symmetrical structure so that they can crystallize.

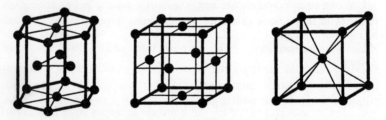

Fig. 6. Types of space-lattice. Close-packed hexagonal, face-centred cubic, body-centred cubic

Polymers

Polymers consist of simple or complex molecules which are joined together to form large molecules or *macromolecules*. One macromolecule consists of at least 5000 molecules and may contain as many as 50,000,000. Macromolecules or polymers are produced from single molecules or *monomers* by two main processes known as condensation polymerization and addition polymerization.

Condensation polymerization

Condensation is the chemical union of unlike molecules resulting in a larger molecule, together with the loss of some simple radical such as water. The new large molecule may form a long carbon chain as in Fig. 7.

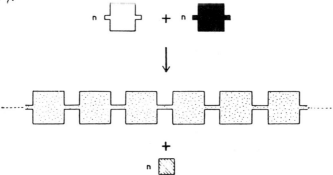

Fig. 7. Condensation polymerization

In other polymers, condensation continues into three dimensions so that a complex molecular network is formed.

Condensation reactions are not reversible and the polymer cannot easily be changed back to the monomers from which it arose.

Addition polymerization

Polymers are also made by the union of molecules of the same compound. From a single monomer a polymer is formed with the same empirical formula but with a greater molecular weight (Fig. 8).

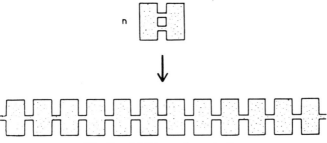

Fig. 8. Addition polymerization

Molecules with an unsaturated double bond undergo this type of polymerization to form long chains. The chains may be single or may show branching.

Addition polymerization is reversible and depolymerization will produce the monomer again.

Copolymerization

On mixing monomers which will polymerize together either by condensation or by addition, mixed molecular chains can be made (Fig. 9a).

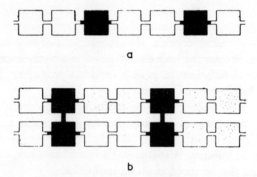

Fig. 9.   Copolymerization. (a) Random copolymer. (b) Cross-linked copolymer

The copolymer molecules may occur randomly, or in blocks along the length of the chain. These are called *random* or *block* copolymers. Alternatively the copolymer may be grafted on to the side of the chain, producing a *graft* copolymer. Simple copolymerization may bring about only small changes in the properties of a polymer. But, by suitable selection of monomers, cross-linking can also be achieved (Fig. 9b).

A whole series of copolymers can be made which vary not only with the properties of the constituents, but also with the degree and type of copolymerization and cross-linking which is achieved.

Effect of structure on properties

Any solid responds initially to an applied force by elastic deformation of the interatomic or intermolecular bonds. This is followed, on the application of a larger force, by a permanent change in relation of the atoms or molecules, and therefore a change in shape of the solid.

In metals and alloys, the dense packing produces materials which are heavy and have a high melting point. There is little directional bonding and a change of shape is possible when the applied force overcomes the elasticity of the intermetallic bonds. In a face-centred cubic lattice metal there are a number of possible planes and directions in which atoms can slide over each other. Such a lattice is typical of the metals Ag, Au, Cu which can be made into a new shape by bending or swaging without fracture. The body-centred cubic lattice is a little more rigid, while the close-packed hexagonal lattice is relatively difficult to distort (e.g. Mg, Cd, Zn).

The ions which make up ionic crystals have alternate charges on them and these restrict the number of planes of movement which are available. In covalent crystals, the directional bonding resists plastic deformation. Fracture of both these types of structure occurs when the applied force is sufficient to cause a crack to propagate through the crystal in a brittle type of fracture.

Polymers vary widely both in structure and properties. A three-dimensional network of primary bonds gives a hard and brittle material. This type of polymer is often called *thermo-hardening* or *thermo-set* as in industry heat is applied to cure it. Thermo-hardening polymers can also be cured at room temperature.

When linear polymers are held together by entanglement of their chains, or by branching, secondary bonds are present and flow is much easier. In a linear polymer, adjacent chains are attracted to each other by secondary or van der Waals' forces. The higher the molecular weight of the polymer the greater these forces will be, and the more they will resist a change in relation of the chains. These forces can be overcome by the increased vibration of molecules at a higher temperature. Then, on the application of a stress, the chains slide over each other and the material is plastic. Linear polymers are therefore *thermo-plastic* and can be softened by heat and then moulded or extruded in a new shape.

In some linear polymers, the chains lie irregularly together and the material deforms under a small stress. In addition, water or a solvent is able to enter between the chains and push them farther apart. This softens the polymer as it enables the chains to slide more easily over each other when a stress is applied. In other linear polymers, the chains lie neatly and closely together and the molecules may take up a regular relation with those of adjacent chains. Thus, a degree of crystallinity is evident and resistance to distortion or solution is improved.

Molecular chains are not usually straight, but are kinked in a random manner. The first effect of a stress is to straighten out the 'kinks'. Since longer chains are more entangled with each other, the material will resist distortion to a greater extent. The elastic properties of long tortuous polymer chains are best shown in the elastic polymers or 'elastomers'. Their chains are very long and coiled, and are joined together every 100 to 300 molecules by a cross-linkage. Therefore, the structure can be elastically extended while the few cross-linkages prevent rupture of the material. A branched chain also reduces deformation of the polymer, as it acts in a manner similar to that of a single cross-linkage.

The properties of polymers are also affected by the addition of a plasticizer. This acts as an internal lubricant between the chains and enables them to slip over each other more readily. It increases the flexibility of the polymer, but by forcing the chains apart, increases its solubility and lowers its softening point.

STRESS AND STRAIN

Stress

The force applied to a material in an attempt to change its shape is called the load. Any external force applied to a material sets up within it an equal and opposite force. Since in a state of equilibrium the stress within the material is equal and opposite to the load, it is more convenient to measure the force applied.

The value for stress is obtained by measuring the external force which is applied and recording this in terms of force per unit area. The direction of the force must be known, and the area of application is then taken as the cross-section of the material in a plane at right-angles to the line of the force.

Whilst force is commonly given in kilograms, pounds, tons, etc., it is more accurately the product of a mass and its acceleration. Since gravity differs slightly throughout the world, a mass of 1 kg exerts a different weight or force in different places. The variation is only slight on the earth's surface, but movement away from the earth produces a marked reduction in gravity. In order to overcome this variation, force should preferably be defined as mass times its acceleration due to gravity at the place where it is being applied. In the international system of units (SI) the unit of force is called the Newton (N). On the earth's surface:

$$1 \text{ kg-wt} = 1 \text{ kg} \times 9 \cdot 81 \text{ m/s}^2 \text{ (acceleration due to gravity)}$$
$$= 9 \cdot 81 \text{ N (approx.)}$$

Whilst this unit is being used in some parts of the world, its acceptance is not yet universal. However, conversion of the values given in this text to metric units is relatively simple when accuracy is not essential. Values in MN/m^2 or, as used in this text, N/mm^2 are approximately ten times values in kg/mm^2.

Strain

This is measured by the change in shape of the material. Strain is expressed as the ratio of the dimensional change to the original dimension, and is usually measured along the line of the stress which produces it.

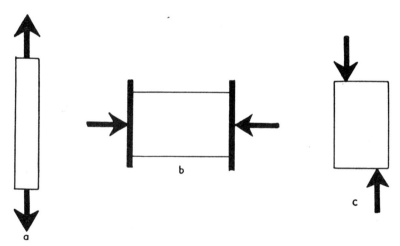

Fig. 10.   Types of stress. (a) Tensile (b) Compressive (c) Shear

Types of stress and strain

A load can be applied to a material in many different ways, but for simplicity we will consider only three of these.

If a stretching force is applied to both ends of the material, a tensile stress is set up, and the lengthening of the material is a tensile strain.

On reversing the direction of both forces the material is compressed and a compressive stress is set up. The reduction in length is a compressive strain.

The third type is a shear stress. This is set up by the application of loads in opposite directions which do not directly oppose each other. The same type of stress is set up between the inner and outer layers of a material when it is twisted.

Although these three examples are given as different types of stress and strain, a little thought will show that in none of the examples given are the types of stress set up in the material the same throughout its bulk. For instance, in a piece of wire under a tensile stress, some of the atoms slide over an adjacent layer so that the wire can increase in length. This is due to a shear stress.

Chapter 3
Determining properties

When testing dental materials an attempt is made to measure only one aspect of the suitability of a material at a time. In this way, the investigator can get a value for that property of the material, and then pass on to a further property.

A full account of the properties of a material consists, therefore, of a list of its reactions when subjected to a number of limited conditions.

The properties usually investigated may be divided into three groups:

Group 1 Tensile strength
Compressive strength
Elasticity
Ductility and malleability
Transverse strength
Impact strength
Fatigue strength
Tear or rupture strength
Hardness
Abrasion resistance
Flow or creep

Group 2 Thermal expansion or contraction
Conduction of heat and electricity
Specific heat
Density
Thermal diffusivity

Group 3 Ease of manipulation
Expansion or contraction upon setting (chemical)
Surface properties
Permanence of shape and colour
Effect on living tissues and organisms

The properties in the first group have been investigated, some of them for many years, by metallurgists and engineers in the study of metals. In many cases the method of testing as used by the engineer has been adapted for dental testing, usually by a reduction in the size of the specimen. It is always preferable to test the properties of a dental material in a bulk similar to that used in normal dental practice. The manipulation of materials in bulk to form large test specimens will not necessarily produce the same properties as are to be found in small dental constructions of the same material.

The second group are physical properties which may be found for metallic and non-metallic materials.

The third group consists of properties which are of particular interest in the application of all materials to the exacting requirements of dentistry.

It is seldom necessary to record the behaviour of any one material when subjected to all these tests. Some of the tests find a greater application in the study of metals, while others reveal the important properties of non-metallic materials.

Group 1

Tensile strength

Tensile strength is the resistance of a material to a tensile or stretching force. A test specimen in the form of a wire, flat strip or rod, is made from the material by the normal dental procedure (Fig. 11). This

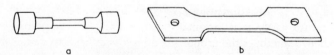

Fig. 11. Tensile test specimens. (a) Cast. (b) Flat sheet

specimen is held at both ends in a testing machine, and an initial load applied. The load is then increased by equal amounts at regular intervals of time, and both the load and the elongation of the specimen are measured. By plotting the stress (related to the original cross-section) against the strain, a tensile stress–strain curve is obtained (Fig. 12).

The first portion of each curve is a straight line, and denotes the

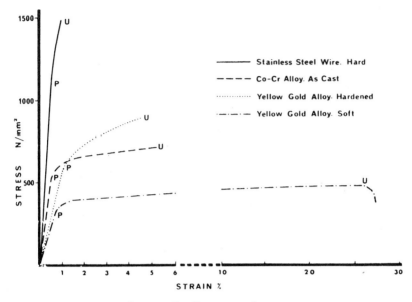

Fig. 12. Tensile stress–strain curves

fact that the strain increases linearly with stress. At the point P, the lines begin to curve, and this point is therefore the limit of load which can be applied to keep the strain proportional to the stress. It is called the *proportional limit* (PL). Up to this load (or, to be more precise, a slightly higher point called the *elastic limit*), the material is deformed elastically, and if the load is removed at any time the specimen will return to its original dimensions. Beyond this point, the specimen will only return partly to its original dimension and will be permanently stretched. Sometimes the proportional limit is difficult to define and a *proof strength* is defined as the stress necessary to produce a certain degree of permanent strain (usually 0·2 per cent). The proof strength is therefore slightly higher than the proportional limit. The maximum stress which is resisted by the material is at the point U, this is the *ultimate tensile strength* (UTS). After this point, the specimen fractures.

An indication of other properties can be gained from the tensile test. The ductility of a metal is indicated by its percentage elongation and also by the reduction in cross-sectional area at the time of fracture. Percentage elongation is obtained by reassembling the two portions and relating the new length to that of the original specimen.

When a specimen is broken in the tensile testing machine, it must break near the middle of its length or the results will not be accurate. Quite often specimens are made with a centre portion which is of the correct cross-section for testing, but with thicker end pieces which are gripped by the jaws of the testing machine.

Tensile strength of brittle materials which are difficult to grip in tension may be determined by the diametral or Brazilian method. A disc or rod of the material is compressed along a diameter producing a tensile stress at right angles to this (Fig. 13).

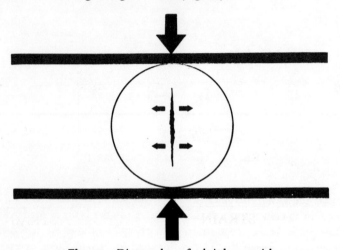

Fig. 13. Diametral test for brittle materials

Elasticity

The first part of a stress–strain curve up to the proportional limit is a straight line. Therefore, if we divide any figure for stress by its appropriate strain, we shall get a constant result. This constant for the material is known as its *modulus of elasticity*. When confined to tensile and compressive stresses, it is known as *Young's modulus*.

Since the strain is the divisor in the equation:

$$\text{Modulus of elasticity} = \frac{\text{Stress}}{\text{Strain}}$$

the greater the strain for a given stress, the less will be the modulus of elasticity. Therefore, a material which stretches elastically or flexes easily will have a lower modulus than a 'stiffer' material. From Fig. 9, it will be noticed that a stainless steel wire and cobalt–chromium alloy are both stiffer than a yellow gold alloy.

The term *resilience* is often used to try to describe the springiness of a material. The correct definition of this term is, however: 'The amount of energy absorbed by a structure when it is stressed below its proportional limit.' A resilient body, therefore, has a high elastic modulus and a high proportional limit. The amount of energy stored in a stressed material at its proportional limit is indicated by the area under the curve *up to the PL*. In Fig. 14a, alloy X is more resilient than Y.

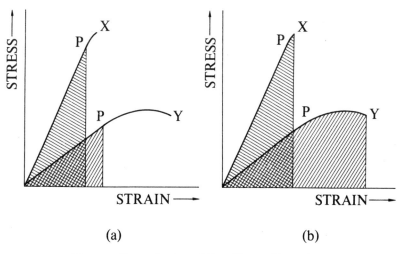

Fig. 14. Determination of (a) resilience. (b) toughness

On the other hand, the material with high resilience initially followed by a capacity for plastic flow, is described as *tough* since it absorbs a great deal of energy before fracture. The amount of energy absorbed is related to the *total* area under the stress–strain curve. In Fig. 14b, alloy Y is very much tougher than X. A material with little plastic flow is *brittle*.

Flexibility indicates a property of allowing large deflections with light loads. A flexible structure has a low modulus of elasticity but a high proportional limit.

Bulk modulus is the ratio between a three-dimensional stress and the change in volume produced. In an elastic body under longitudinal stress, *Poisson's ratio* indicates the relation of the strain at right angles to the stress, to the strain parallel to the stress.

Anelasticity

Not all materials recover immediately from a stress below the PL. Whilst the return to original shape is rapid in the case of metals and ceramics, the recovery of polymers and other structures formed from large molecules is often much slower. These materials may take several seconds or several hours to recover completely. The degree of recovery at a period of time after stressing provides a measure of the *anelastic* behaviour. Since the material behaves partly like a viscous liquid and partly like an elastic solid, its behaviour is generally termed *viscoelastic*. A small degree of viscoelastic behaviour can be detected in many apparently elastic or fluid materials. The classification of materials as elastic or plastic is rather dependent upon the accuracy with which the stress/strain/time relationship is measured.

Compressive strength

A similar stress–strain curve is obtained when a material is compressed instead of stretched. Cylindrical specimens, slightly greater in length than in diameter, are made of the material to be tested and the ends of the specimen are made flat and square to the axis of the cylinder. This specimen is compressed between the flat plates of a testing machine. The applied stress is plotted against reduction in length and the maximum load before fracture recorded.

Ductility and malleability

When a metal or alloy is required in the form of a wire, a round bar of it is made by casting or by rolling between biconcave rollers. This round bar is then drawn through a series of holes of decreasing sizes until the wire is of the correct diameter. The capacity of a metal to undergo this process without breaking is a measure of its ductility. If a metal or alloy can be hammered or rolled into thin sheets without breaking, it is said to be malleable.

As already noted, when conducting a tensile test, the percentage elongation and reduction in area may be calculated. The greater the percentage elongation and reduction of area, the greater is the ductility and malleability.

Transverse strength

For some dental materials, the transverse or flexure strength test gives a better indication of their mechanical properties than does a simple tensile or compressive test. Tensile, compressive and transverse strengths of a material do, however, bear some relationship to one another. A transverse test specimen is made in the shape of a flat strip or bar. This is placed in the machine so that it rests on two supports, one near each end (Fig. 15). The specimen is then loaded in the middle, and the load increased at regular intervals of time until the specimen breaks. The deflection is recorded after each increment, and is plotted against the load. Comparative results are usually obtained by testing different dental materials under the same conditions.

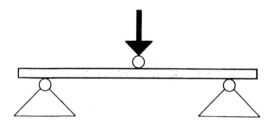

Fig. 15. Transverse test

Impact strength

Some materials will resist a large force when it is applied gradually in tension or compression, but will break easily if subjected to a sudden blow.

The impact testing machine is designed to deliver a blow to the specimen, and to measure and record the amount of energy which has been used in fracturing it. Impact testing measures the 'toughness' of a material and determines whether it is liable to ductile or brittle failure. On ductile failure, energy is absorbed by plastic deformation of the specimen as it breaks. Brittle materials show no plastic flow and the energy absorbed by the fracture is low.

The results of impact strength are comparative, and all specimens must be of the same shape and tested on the same machine before comparisons can be made.

Fatigue strength

All the above methods of testing apply an increasing load to the specimen until it breaks. Failure of materials, however, often follows the repeated application of relatively small stresses below the proportional limit. Local plastic deformation may then produce fatigue failure as a crack gradually propagates through the material. Fatigue life depends upon the amount of stress applied. Usually the length of fatigue life increases as the stress decreases, though some materials show an endurance limit below which fatigue life is indefinite. Stress concentration at sharp corners or notches in a structure of complicated shape, may impose high stresses in one small area, thus reducing the fatigue life locally.

This type of test is therefore of considerable importance when testing dental materials.

The testing machine consists of some mechanical means of applying and removing a load at frequent intervals and a counting mechanism to note the number of stress cycles. The counting mechanism is usually designed to stop the machine when the specimen breaks. It will be appreciated that this test may take hours or even weeks to perform.

As with impact testing, results are comparable only when specimen dimensions and conditions of testing remain identical.

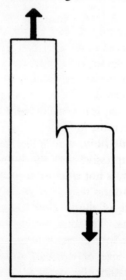

Fig. 16. Tear test using trouser-leg specimen

Tear or rupture strength

In the previous tests, the energy expended is that required to deform the entire specimen. When a material tears, however, the application of energy is concentrated in one small area. Such a situation can be achieved when testing flexible materials such as rubbers by using a trouser-leg specimen (Fig. 16). The legs are pulled apart in opposite directions, thus propagating a tear. The load across the cleavage surface is measured together with the rate of propagation of the tear, and the tear energy calculated. It is important that this test is carried out under controlled temperature conditions and if comparisons are to be made, that the specimens are similar.

Hardness

This may be defined as resistance to penetration or scratching. Since there is no direct relation between the hardness recorded by these two methods, hardness is defined according to the method testing, i.e.

Indentation hardness (Brinell, Vickers, Rockwell, Knoop).
Scratch hardness (Moh's scale, Microcharacter).

Indentation hardness

Hardness is most commonly defined in terms of the response of the material to a load localized in a very small area. A stress is applied by indenters of various shapes for certain periods of time. A large indentation indicates a soft material and a small indentation a hard one. Whilst hardness values can be worked out in relation to the stress and the size of the indentation, it is usual to refer to tables.

The similarity between the indentation hardness test and a localized compressive test indicates how, with some metals and alloys, indentation hardness and compressive and tensile properties bear a definite relation. This, however, is not true for all materials.

With the Brinell hardness testing machine, a hardened steel ball is pressed into the surface of the specimen under a known load for a definite period of time. The diameter of indentation produced is measured by means of a low-power microscope with a calibrated eyepiece. Since both the size of the ball and the load applied vary, depending upon the material being tested, a Brinell hardness number (BHN) should preferably indicate the ball diameter and the load used.

There are several disadvantages in this type of hardness testing. First, an elastic material will give a hardness number which is too high, as the indentation will 'recover' and become smaller on removing the load. Secondly, a brittle material such as tooth enamel will shatter and crumble. A third disadvantage is that when very hard materials are tested, some distortion of the steel ball takes place with resulting inaccuracy of the hardness value.

These difficulties are partly overcome by the Vickers hardness machine, which employs a diamond in the shape of a square-based pyramid, instead of a steel ball. This cuts the material rather than squashes it and gives an indentation with two diagonal axes which are both measured and averaged to give a hardness number (Fig. 17).

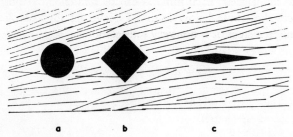

a   b   c

Fig. 17. Indentations produced by hardness testing machines. (a) Brinell. (b) Vickers. (c) Knoop

The figures for BHN and VHN show a linear relation up to the number of 400, after which the Brinell test gives progressively lower values due to distortion of the indenter.

The Rockwell machine measures the difference in penetration of an indenter under a 10 kg (98·1 N) 'minor' load and then a heavier 'major' load. Two scales are used. For readings on the B scale, a $\frac{1}{16}$-inch ball and a 100 kg (981 N) 'major' load is used, and for the C scale, a 120° cone diamond point with a 150 kg (1471 N) 'major' load.

A fourth machine for testing hardness is the Knoop indenter. This machine, like the Vickers, has a diamond indenter, but one axis of the diamond pyramid is much longer than the other. The advantage of using this type of indenter is that the material being tested is cut along the long axis of the diamond, and is then pushed aside along the short axis. In this way, elastic recovery takes place on the sides of the pyramid and does not affect the length of the long axis of the indentation. This length is measured and KHN obtained from tables. A further advantage of the Knoop indenter is that it can be used for measuring the hardness of brittle materials such as tooth enamel.

When testing the hardness of small specimens or of thin materials, the depth, and therefore the size of the indentation, must be limited. Microhardness testing employs diamond indenters of the Vickers or Knoop type under low loads followed by accurate measurement of the indentation produced. This technique is also suitable for detecting changes in hardness over short lengths of a specimen.

Scratch hardness
Moh's scale, used by the mineralogist, ranges from talc, the softest, to diamond, the hardest. Each mineral can be scratched by those above it and scratches those below it in the scale. As the complete scale shows only ten steps, it is not very satisfactory.

Table 1. Hardness numbers

These are Brinell Hardness Numbers except where stated

Hardened carbon steel	700–850 VHN
Porcelain (fused)	415 VHN
Stainless steel (cold worked)	350
Cobalt–chromium alloys	270–370
Yellow wrought gold alloys (work hardened)	250–350
Tooth enamel	270–380 KHN
Yellow cast gold alloys (hardened)	260
Stainless steel (soft)	180
Hard inlay golds	90–140
White golds (as cast)	150
Mild steel (non heat treated)	130
Medium inlay golds	70–100
Amalgam	90
Tooth dentine	60–70
Silicate cement	58
Soft inlay golds	40–75
Gold foil restoration	20–60
Zinc phosphate cement	36
Composite filling	25–35
Aluminium	18–35
Pure gold	18–30
Acrylic polymer (heat-cure)	18–22
Acrylic polymer (self-cure)	16–18
Vinyl denture base	14–20

To give a more accurate comparison, an instrument known as the 'Microcharacter' tester can be used on metals and hard materials. A diamond point is drawn across the polished surface of the material under a known load, and from the depth and width of the scratch, a hardness number is calculated.

Abrasion resistance

This is not proportional to indentation hardness. Some hard materials abrade easily, whilst other softer materials resist wear.

Abrasion resistance can be measured by applying a rotating abrasive wheel to the specimen under a constant load for a given time and measuring the depth of cut.

In other methods the specimen is pressed against a rotating abrasive disc or is moved backwards and forwards over a suitable abrasive surface. In either case lubricants may be used to control the temperature and modify the abrasive effect. The amount of material lost from the specimens by wear is determined by measurement or by weighing. Identical tests for comparison are carried out on other materials. Meaningful values of abrasion resistance are hard to obtain. It is essential to simulate service conditions closely.

Flow or creep

When a material changes shape slowly under the influence of an external load, or under its own weight, it is said to exhibit creep or flow. Flow is a property usually attributed to the amorphous state as in this type of structure the forces of attraction between atoms are not as great as in crystalline structures. Wax and plastics change shape readily under a light load, particularly when heat is applied.

Nearly all materials, however, show some permanent change of shape even when they are apparently behaving elastically. Conversely, many viscous fluids show some elasticity to small forces or to forces quickly applied. Flow of materials is very much a function of load, time and temperature. For example, pitch or tar is brittle under impact at certain temperatures, yet, without heat, will flow in time under its own weight. A glass tube placed against the wall will gradually bend and become permanently curved at room temperature.

Many methods exist for determining viscous flow. For dental applications the time and loading should be similar to the conditions which will occur either during manipulation or during the life of the structure. It is often convenient to measure flow under a compressive force. A simple method is to note the reduction in height of a cylindrical specimen over a period of time.

Group 2

Thermal expansion or contraction

The higher melting point metals show an approximately linear expansion with rise in temperature and a similar contraction on cooling over relatively small ranges of temperature. It is often assumed, however, that metals and alloys have a constant linear coefficient of expansion. Ceramic materials in general show a lower thermal expansion, whilst polymers and waxes expand to a greater extent.

Changes in dimension as a result of change of phase, e.g. liquid to solid, are large, though not all are accompanied by a reduction in volume on solidification. Perhaps the best example is the expansion of water as it freezes.

Difficulties arise in measuring the expansion of materials at elevated temperatures, as the specimen must be enclosed within a furnace. The linear expansion of the specimen can still be measured, however, if rods of invar or fused quartz are inserted through the walls of the furnace to touch either end of the specimen.

Table 2. Average coefficients of linear expansion per °C between 20 and 50°C $\times 10^6$

Inlay wax	250–500
Other waxes	200–700
Silicone elastomer	100–220
Polyether elastomer	150–170
Polysulphide elastomer	100–150
PMMA	80–82
Composite filling	25–35
Amalgam	22–28
Gold alloy	12–16
Stainless steel	11–13
Plaster of Paris	10–15
Co–Cr alloys	9–12
Tooth substance	8–11
Silicate cement	7–8
Porcelain	6–8
Invar	0·9
Fused quartz	0·5

Conduction of heat and electricity

The coefficient of thermal conductivity indicates the quantity of heat passing through a material as a result of a temperature gradient. In the same way, the electrical resistance of a material indicates the amount of electricity which will flow as a result of a potential difference.

Specific heat

This indicates the quantity of heat needed to raise the temperature of a mass of the substance.

Density

The density of material is its mass per unit volume. Density varies with the amount of impurity present within the material, or the presence of air in porous materials.

Table 3. Melting point and density of metals

	M.P. (°C)	Density (g)/cm^3
Al	660	2·70
Sb	630	6·68
Cd	321	8·64
Cr	1890	7·20
Co	1495	8·90
Cu	1083	8·92
Ga	30	5·90
Au	1063	19·30
In	156	7·30
Ir	2454	22·40
Fe	1535	7·86
Pb	327	11·34
Hg	−39	13·55
Mo	2620	10·20
Ni	1455	8·90
Pd	1549	11·97
Pt	1774	21·45
Ag	961	10·50
Ta	2996	16·60
Sn	232	7·28
Zn	419	7·14

Thermal diffusivity

This indicates the speed with which a temperature change will spread through an object when one surface is heated. It is calculated from the formula

$$\frac{\text{thermal conductivity}}{\text{specific heat} \times \text{density}}$$

Thus a material with a high specific heat and a high density requires a lot of heat energy to bring about a large rise in its temperature, and therefore has a low thermal diffusivity. Such a material changes its temperature slowly.

Group 3

Ease of manipulation

The final test of any material is its use under normal working conditions. Very careful control over the properties of a material can be exercised while it is being tested under research laboratory conditions. These conditions do not necessarily apply in the dental surgery or workshop. Variations in properties frequently arise due to the limitations imposed on techniques by the fact of having to work in the cramped and humid space of the oral cavity. In the dental workshop personal variations in technique arise. It is essential to find out to what extent these small variations affect the final properties of the material.

Clinical trial is perhaps most important in the testing of a filling material. Only after a period of several years can the true value of a filling or denture material be assessed. Frequently new materials are made available to the profession before they have undergone sufficient clinical testing. The dentist using these materials is therefore carrying out clinical tests. In using the material he must exercise strict control over his technique and should record details of his manipulation so that the results seen in a few years can be correctly interpreted.

Expansion or contraction on setting (chemical)

The measurement of dimensional changes of a material on setting, or when subjected to conditions of varying humidity after setting, presents a problem, as it is desirable that any change in dimension can occur freely. A simple method of measuring expansion or contraction is to record changes in the length of a specimen by means of a micrometer gauge. Instead of measuring the specimen directly, markers can be embedded in it, and the alteration in the distance between these noted. To reduce friction the specimen may be held in a smooth, highly polished and greased metal trough. Another method for avoiding the restraining influence of a container is to float the specimen on a mercury bath. In this way, friction between the specimen and its support is greatly reduced, and there is little restriction of any change in shape.

When the alteration in dimension of a complex shape is being investigated, it is usual to test the specimen for accuracy of fit on to a metal or other hard model which is maintained at a constant temperature. This method gives a purely comparative result.

Surface properties

On many occasions in dentistry we wish to join two or more materials together. When two dissimilar materials join by chemical bonds, *adhesion* is said to occur and an *adhesive joint* is produced. If there is no chemical bonding but only mechanical interlocking, then there is no adhesion, only *attachment*. The surface energy of the *adherend* (the substance to which the adhesive is applied) and of the *adhesive* affect the quality of the bond. An adherend with high free surface energy more readily adsorbs an adhesive on its surface than one with low surface energy. Conversely a liquid adhesive with low surface energy wets a surface more readily. The greater the affinity or degree of adsorption between adherend and adhesive the smaller the interfacial energy and the better the wetting.

Wettability between an adhesive and an adherend is measured by the contact angle between the two when a drop of the adhesive is placed on the surface of the adherend (Fig. 18). The lower the contact

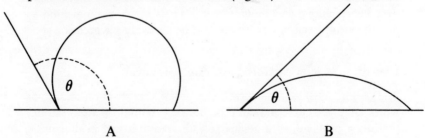

Fig. 18.   Contact angle. (A) Non-wetting. (B) Wetting

angle, the better the surface wetting. A contact angle greater than 90°, as in A, indicates non-wetting. Less than 90° (B) indicates wetting, whilst a zero angle indicates that the adhesive will flow and spread over the adherend. Wetting is also influenced by the presence of debris and by surface roughness and surface contamination.

The strength of the joint produced may be measured under tensile or shear stress by a variety of methods. In general, the thicker the adhesive layer, the weaker the joint. Adhesives which are tough usually form stronger joints than those which are brittle. The quality of the joint is affected by the dimensional stability of the adhesive. Shrinkage or swelling of the adhesive may cause a breakdown in the adhesion at the interface and thus weaken the joint.

Permanence of shape and colour

Loss of shape may also be due to solution of a material in the oral fluids. The conditions in the mouth vary quite widely, depending upon the type of food which is being eaten. Moreover, such conditions are difficult to reproduce outside the mouth. However, varying degrees of humidity, temperature, acidity and alkalinity can be produced in a sealed container and the loss of weight of an enclosed specimen can be determined.

Corrosion of metals in the mouth is frequently accompanied by the passage of small electric currents. These may be measured and their effect on living tissues determined.

To test the colour stability of materials they are usually exposed to ultraviolet light for some hours, thus speeding up the effects of normal exposure to daylight. Changes in colour or translucency after exposure to various solutions may also be noted.

Effect on living tissues and organisms

It is important that none of the dental materials which remain in contact with the living tissues for long periods of time has an irritant or toxic effect. Tests of new materials may be carried out by feeding animals with the new material, or by placing specimens of it upon or in the skin, or in relation to other organs. Whilst the result of such tests gives a good indication of lack of toxicity, it is not always possible to estimate the degree of irritation which might occur in humans.

The method is also limited to solid materials. Testing of powders, liquids and materials which flow readily is difficult. Tissue culture methods in which the effect of the material on growing cells is noted, are generally more sensitive, but are more difficult to carry out. In addition, whilst they reveal initial toxicity, they are not suitable for showing the effects of degradation products which arise over a relatively long period of time. Careful clinical testing with frequent examination is therefore essential, subsequent to animal testing, before a new material can be accepted for general dental use.

The effect of the material upon bacteria or fungi is also of importance. Tests are carried out by trying to grow cultures in the presence of materials, or alternatively to grow and identify bacteria or fungi in or upon materials which have been in the mouth.

Chapter 4

The application of these properties to dentistry

In the design of metal and non-metal constructions in the engineering and building worlds, the shape and material for each component can be decided in relation to the load it has to carry. The maximum stress which will be applied to each component can be calculated with some degree of accuracy, as most engineering designs conform to a pattern of straight lines together with curves of known radius. Usually the engineer calculates the forces mathematically and then increases this figure by a proportion known as the 'safety factor'. From this final figure he can decide upon the material to be used and the thickness in which it must be employed.

When the dentist is designing a structure which is to be placed in the mouth or in some cases fabricated *in situ*, he is at a serious disadvantage, because of two factors. First, the forces which will be applied to his construction in use are difficult to estimate and in some cases unknown, and secondly, the shape and section of most dental structures are so complex that the problem of working out mathematically the stress applied to each part is difficult.

When dealing with a material which is not used in the mouth but in the laboratory, the forces to which it is subjected can be determined with greater accuracy. For example, dimensions have been recommended for component parts of partial dentures. Similarly, a figure for the compressive strength of plaster or stone enables the operator to decide how much pressure he can safely apply to a mould when packing it full of acrylic dough.

It is necessary, therefore, to look at these physical and chemical properties and discuss how they can be interpreted and applied to dental constructions.

The fact that an alloy has a certain proportional limit under tensile stress does not mean very much to the dentist unless he knows, by experience, that when this alloy is used in a certain section, it will withstand a certain type of use within the mouth. What is important is that if he purchases a different alloy, he wants to be assured that this has the same or better properties than that which he used previously. The figure given for the proportional limit of a known material is one against which the properties of any new material must be compared. The value for ultimate tensile strength is not very useful in service since before failure, permanent deformation will have taken place and this is usually unacceptable. The effects of incorrect manipulation on the properties of a material should also be known to the dentist.

Besides giving a good general indication as to whether a material will tolerate strong forces, that is, whether it will withstand the relatively large chewing forces applied in the mouth, the tensile test gives other valuable information. The proportional limit together with the modulus of elasticity show how the material will behave when a force is applied to it. When a material is selected to produce a rigid structure in the mouth, it should be capable of receiving a large stress without a great distortion. For instance, a filling must not alter shape within the tooth when the patient bites on it, or the tooth will break and the filling will become loose. In other words, a material which is to be rigid in the mouth must have a high modulus of elasticity coupled with a high proportional limit.

On the other hand, a small orthodontic spring requires somewhat different properties. Such a spring is designed to gently push a misplaced tooth into line, and a material with a low modulus of elasticity, but with a high proportional limit is required. A spring with such properties is flexible and can be bent elastically through a large angle without using a large force. When used in the mouth, the converse of this statement is more important, that is the spring will apply a small force over a large range of movement so that it will move a tooth a long way without constant adjustment of the tension. The deflection of a structure such as a clasp varies not only with the modulus of elasticity of the alloy used, but also with its dimensions as follows:

$$\text{Deflection} \propto \text{length}^3$$

$$\text{Deflection} \propto \frac{1}{\text{breadth}}$$

$$\text{Deflection} \propto \frac{1}{\text{thickness}^3}$$

To make a spring, however, a material which can be bent fairly easily to the desired shape is required. That is, it must have a low proof stress and be ductile. If the ductility of the metal is too low, it will fracture while being bent to the required shape. Yet if the proof stress is too low, the finished spring will soon lose its shape when a light force is applied to it. In a further chapter, it will be seen that a workable material is frequently more elastic after it has been conformed to the required shape, due to an alteration in its structure.

Transverse strength tests are particularly applicable to materials which are used for denture construction, since a similar type of stress is applied to an upper denture during mastication. The test indicates whether the denture material will stand up to this stress and also shows the amount of flexion of the denture which may occur. It is desirable that a denture should not alter its shape under biting force as it will damage the supporting bone and gum tissues.

Sometimes the patient will drop a denture on the floor while cleaning it, and although this can hardly be called a dental stress, it is preferable that the material of which the denture is constructed will withstand this impact force. Similarly, if the jaws close suddenly upon a piece of metal or bone which has been introduced accidentally with a mouthful of food, the stress applied is much greater than that normally used in mastication. The impact strength of all materials used for dentures or for fillings must be sufficiently high to prevent breakage in these circumstances.

During normal mastication, the patient crushes the food between the upper and lower teeth some fifteen to forty times for every mouthful of solid food that is taken. This amounts to a large number of applied stresses with their resulting strains in a filling or denture whose life may extend over many years. The fatigue resistance of the material used is therefore of the greatest importance. Fatigue strength bears little relationship to the other properties of a non-metallic material. For example, it is possible for a denture base material to be satisfactory in all other properties, and yet dentures constructed from it fracture repeatedly from fatigue failure.

The hardness of a metal frequently bears some relationship to its proportional limit. For non-metals this relationship does not apply so readily, and a separate indentation hardness or abrasion test is necessary. A high abrasive resistance is necessary to reduce wear and so give the appliance or restoration a long life. In some circumstances, however, a hard surface can be a disadvantage during fabrication. For example, the Co–Cr alloys resist abrasion very well indeed, but they are difficult to grind and polish ready for the mouth.

If a material flows readily under stress, it will not be very suitable for a permanent structure in the mouth. The surface of a filling consists of a series of carefully shaped cusps and fissures. This detailed shape must be maintained throughout the life of the filling. On the other hand, flow is an essential property of all impression materials when they are first inserted in the mouth. Unless an impression material flows freely it will not record the detail over the whole of the denture bearing area and the impression will be incomplete. Flow of cements is equally important. When a fluid is compressed between parallel plates, the load necessary to cause it to flow varies inversely with the cube of the thickness of the fluid film. This relationship explains why it is difficult, unless the conditions are correct, to produce a thin cement lute or to record an impression with only a thin layer of material.

The thermal contraction and expansion of a material is important from two main aspects. In the mouth, a range of temperatures occurs from ice-cream 0°C, to hot tea 65°C. The coefficient of expansion of all materials which are permanently in contact with tooth structure should be the same as that of the tooth dentine and enamel. If the coefficient of expansion of a filling is higher than that of the tooth structure, weak portions of the tooth may be fractured on drinking hot tea. On eating ice-cream the filling will shrink away from the tooth and leave a gap in which further decay can start. Secondly, in the laboratory, a material which is manipulated in a warm or hot condition will change its dimensions on cooling to mouth temperature. This cooling is accompanied by a contraction which must be allowed for when deciding upon the dimensions of the heated material. This effect is well illustrated when metals are melted and cast into a mould. On cooling, one contraction occurs on solidification of the metal and a further one on cooling down to room temperature. The mould into which the molten metal is poured must therefore be of larger dimensions than those required in the finished product.

A material of low density is more suitable than a heavy one for the construction of an upper denture, as the patient finds a light denture easier to keep in place. On occasions a little extra weight is an advantage in a lower denture. The weight of filling materials is not of any practical importance, since their bulk is not sufficient to make the patient conscious of their presence.

The dental pulp in the centre of the tooth is a delicate and sensitive structure and it responds sharply to a rapid rise or fall in temperature. Many of the filling materials are metals and transmit heat very readily. This is particularly noticeable in alloys containing silver, gold and copper. The metal filling replaces tooth structure which had a low thermal diffusivity and which acted as an effective insulator for the pulp. A big metal filling must have an insulating layer between it and the pulp if painful thermal stimulation of the latter is to be avoided. Similarly any galvanic currents which may be set up in the mouth between dissimilar metals may pass through the pulp and stimulate it unless an electrical insulating layer is present.

It is difficult to carry out many dental techniques within the restricted space of the oral cavity. The soft tissues such as lips, cheek and tongue restrict visibility and reduce the accessibility of the teeth; also some means of excluding the saliva must be used. If the best properties of a material are to be produced every time it is used, the technique involved must be relatively simple to carry out and applicable in the mouth.

More difficult techniques can be carried out in the dental laboratory, but a longer technique or one using expensive equipment raises the cost of the finished product and restricts its sphere of application.

The thermal expansion or contraction affects the dimensions of a filling or denture during its life, whereas any contraction or expansion during fabrication produces an inaccuracy in the original shape. Sometimes two contractions or expansions of different materials add together to create a large error in dimension. Other circumstances arise where an expansion of one material can compensate for the contraction of another. In passing from a mouldable condition to the finished set material, nearly all dental materials show a contraction or expansion and suitable compensation for this change in dimensions must be arranged.

Adhesion between filling materials and natural teeth is an advantage where part of a tooth is to be restored. By this means, leakage between the filling and the tooth could be eliminated and the possibility of further decay reduced. If orthodontic appliances could be attached directly to tooth enamel, this would simplify the technical problems involved. An adherent varnish applied to the natural tooth could reduce the incidence of dental decay, particularly in areas of the tooth which are difficult to clean, such as the pits and fissures on the occlusal surfaces of posterior teeth and the contact points.

Although most materials are selected because they are non-irritant to the living tissues, and have no effect upon them, a few have a desirable tissue effect. For example, the oil of cloves in some cements will 'quieten down' a mild toothache when placed within a tooth cavity. When a filling material prevents bacterial growth, it reduces the possibility of further decay in that tooth. All dental materials should resist bacterial growth in order to maintain normal cleanliness and health of the mouth.

Apart from one or two examples, the materials discussed in this book are relatively inert. In circumstances where metals or polymers are embedded within the skin, gums or bones, a lack of tissue reaction is of paramount importance.

It will be appreciated from the previous discussion that in many cases the values for the strength of dental materials cannot be directly applied to the construction of a dental appliance, particularly one which is to be made in the mouth. Most of the tests in Group 1 are of value in comparing the strength of new or modified materials with those which are already in use.

The chemical and simple physical properties of Group 2 can be directly applied to all dental structures.

The third group are really subdivisions of one test which is of the greatest importance in the evaluation of any material. This is clinical testing for the materials used in the mouth, and laboratory testing in dental technology for other materials. A material must be subjected to a period of practical use, before a sound opinion can be expressed on its suitability for dental use.

Section B

Cast and wrought metals

Chapter 5
Grain structure. Metallography

A metal can be defined according to various chemical and physical properties. For example, metals are usually heavy, can be deformed plastically, conduct heat and electricity, and have a metallic lustre. Metals also form positive ions when in solution. The metalloids and non-metallic elements form negative ions. The main metalloids of interest in dentistry are C and Si. These resemble metals in some respects and will combine with them to form alloys.

SOLIDIFICATION OF A METAL

If we take the temperature of a molten metal during its change from

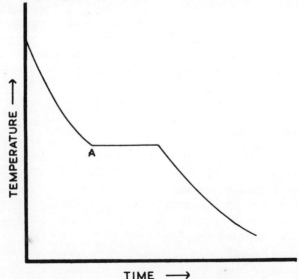

Fig. 19. Cooling curve of a pure metal

liquid to solid, and plot a time–temperature graph, a curve similar to that in Fig. 19 will be produced.

In a metal in the liquid state the atoms have sufficient energy to move about freely. As the temperature falls, the atomic movement becomes more sluggish until on reaching a certain temperature (*A*), the thermal energy is no longer sufficient to prevent groups of atoms from forming crystals of the metal. The change from liquid to solid is accompanied by the evolution of latent heat of freezing. This heat compensates for that lost to the surroundings and is always sufficient to keep the temperature constant while solidification proceeds. This portion of the cooling curve is therefore a horizontal line; it is called a *plateau*. Once solidification is complete, the temperature of the metal again falls.

Dendritic growth

Solidification of a molten metal starts at centres or nuclei of crystallization. Even in what might be called a pure metal, slight impurities exist and these act as centres of crystallization scattered through the metal. At these centres the first crystals or nuclei are formed: then further atoms attach themselves to the corners of these nuclei, growth taking place in three directions at right-angles (Fig. 20a). The six arms of the *primary dendrites* grow outwards and from each arm *secondary dendrites* grow at right-angles (Fig. 20b). This growth continues until contact is made with adjacent growths. Then the primary dendritic growth ceases and the remaining molten metal fills in the interdendritic spaces.

Grains and grain boundaries

The units of growth are termed *grains* and the boundaries between them are *grain boundaries* (Fig. 20c). The orientation of crystals and therefore of crystal planes will be the same throughout any one grain and will be that which occurred in the original nucleus. In adjacent grains, the orientation differs in a random manner since the initial nuclei form independently of one another.

The grain boundary may be regarded as a narrow region about two or three atomic distances wide. Since the orientation of crystal planes differs between adjacent grains, the grain boundary atoms are highly

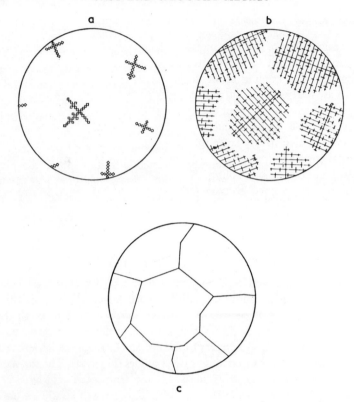

Fig. 20. Dendritic growth. This growth takes place in three dimensions, producing polyhedral equiaxed grains

disorganized and take up irregular positions between those of the atoms in the adjacent crystals.

Evidence of the dendritic mechanism or solidification may not be apparent in the solid metal. However, if a low melting point metal is poured on to a sheet of glass, some air may be trapped between the metal and glass, and into this space dendrites will grow. Another method is to take a small cast ingot of which the outer skin only has solidified, drill two holes in the solid crust, and pour off the remaining molten metal inside. After cooling, the ingot is sawn in two and the cavity is found to be lined with dendritic crystals. In some types of alloy, the primary dendrites are of a different composition from the rest of the crystal grain. The dendritic structure can be revealed on the surface of these alloys by selective chemical attack.

Grain structure of cast metal

The grain structure of a cast metal is dependent to a marked extent on the rate at which it cools from the liquid state.

Slow rates of cooling result in the formation of only a few nuclei which are fairly evenly distributed through the liquid. The amount of growth which occurs about each nucleus is roughly the same, and this gives rise to a coarse-grained structure (Fig. 21A). This would be observed in a relatively large mass of metal cast into a mould of low thermal conductivity.

With uniform rapid cooling, the large number of nuclei which form result in a fine-grained structure (Fig. 21B). This structure is considered

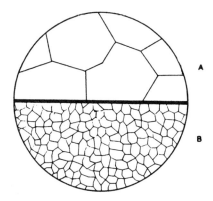

Fig. 21. Equiaxed grain structure. (A) Coarse. (B) Fine

to be the more satisfactory from the mechanical strength point of view. It occurs in castings of small bulk provided the casting is made from metal which is heated just above its melting point. If the metal is overheated, slower cooling takes place and a coarser grain is produced.

The arrangement of crystal grains within a solid mass of metal also depends upon the shape of the mould in which it cools, as well as on the rate of cooling. In a cylindrical mould, cooled from the outside, the crystal grains grow inwards along the radii. Whereas in a square mould the grains grow inwards at right-angles to the walls and meet along the diagonals. This line of junction is a weakness in the metal and therefore ingots are usually cast into rounded moulds and not into square ones.

Solidification shrinkage

The change from liquid to solid during the freezing of a metal is usually accompanied by a reduction in volume of 3 to 7 per cent. This contraction is in addition to that which occurs in the liquid metal while it cools prior to solidification, and also to that occurring in the solid metal after solidification is complete.

In a large bulk of metal cast into an open mould solidification starts at the sides and bottom of the mould and proceeds progressively inwards. As each successive layer of metal freezes, the level of the remaining liquid falls, forming a central *primary pipe* (Fig. 22a).

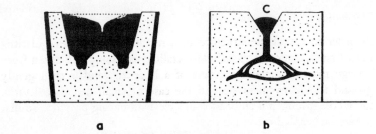

Fig. 22.   Primary and secondary pipe in castings

Solidification shrinkage also causes *secondary piping* in investment castings. In such a casting, the button of metal (C) freezes first, followed by the outer layers of the casting. These layers remain in contact with the walls of the investment mould. As the result of solidification shrinkage, insufficient molten metal remains to fill the mould and a central defect appears (Fig. 22b).

METALLOGRAPHY

The grains of a metal can sometimes be seen with the naked eye. When a brass door-handle has been in use for some time and has not been polished, the constant rubbing of hands over the surface smooths the brass, and sweat from the hand etches it. The grains can be seen as small crystals of varying yellow tones. In such brass specimens the grain-size is comparatively large and may be 5–6 mm across a grain. However, in the majority of metals and alloys, the grains can only be distinguished by the use of a microscope. For example, some steels have grains only 0·025 mm across.

Metallurgical microscope

Light cannot be transmitted through a metal specimen and so its surface is examined by reflected light.

The metallurgical microscope has an attachment just above the objective which throws a beam of light from a small bulb horizontally into the main tube of the instrument. This light beam is reflected down through the objective on to the specimen to give surface or incident lighting. After reflection from the specimen, the light passes back into the objective, and is collected in a normal eyepiece.

Preparation of the specimen

In order to reveal the structure of a metal, its surface irregularities must first be removed. Usually a metallurgical 'sample' is taken from a large mass of metal by means of a hacksaw, and is then gently ground to a convenient size. In the case of small dental structures, the whole specimen is embedded in a clear mounting polymer, so that it may be handled conveniently.

The specimen is abraded until the area which is to be examined is revealed and is flat, care being taken to avoid overheating the specimen. It is then ground on a series of silicon carbide papers of increasing fineness, well lubricated with running water, until only fine scratches remain. These fine scratches are then removed by mechanical or electrolytic polishing, or both. In mechanical polishing the surface of the specimen is held lightly on a horizontally rotating polishing disc, driven by an electric motor. The surface of the disc is covered with chamois leather or selvyt cloth, which is impregnated with fine abrasives and polishing agents, usually of diamond dust. By careful adjustment of the hand pressure which is applied and by using progressively finer abrasives, a highly polished surface free from scratches can be produced. Some difficulty is experienced with soft materials, as a layer of metal tends to smear over the surface. In such cases, the specimen is polished electrolytically.

After polishing, the specimen is washed with water and then with alcohol to produce a clean surface free from grease. If this surface is now examined under the microscope, no grain structure will be evident, but any porosity or pitting in the metal can be seen, together with any hard non-metallic impurities which may be present.

During polishing, the surface layer of the metal flows slightly and fills up the scratches from the fine SiC paper. The grain structure is thus covered by a thin film of heavily deformed crystals called the *Beilby layer*.

Etching

To reveal the grains, the Beilby layer is removed by chemical reagents during the process of *etching*. After this layer has been dissolved, the etching solution next attacks the grain boundaries. The atoms in these areas are less closely packed than those in the crystal grains on either side of them. They are therefore more reactive. This selective attack

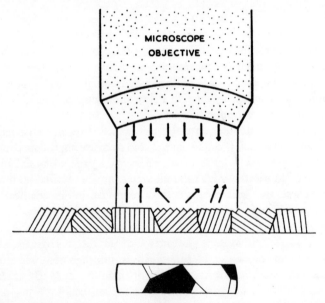

Fig. 23. Appearance of an etched metal surface under a metallurgical microscope

causes the boundaries to appear as shallow grooves. When the specimen is examined under the microscope these grooves scatter the light more than the surface of the grains, so that the grain boundaries show as black lines. Under suitable etching conditions, the black grain boundaries enclose crystal grains which vary in shades of the colour of the metal under examination. In a gold specimen some grains will be dark yellow while others will be brightly reflecting. This difference is due to the orientation of the crystal planes to the surface under examination. From the planes at right-angles to the surface, a large proportion of light will be reflected back, whereas from those at an angle, some of the light will be dispersed and the crystal grain will appear darker. In a pure metal, the dendritic structure is not seen under the microscope as all portions of a crystal grain are etched to the same extent. In some alloys or mixtures of metals, the primary and secondary dendrites may differ slightly in composition, and then their structure will be revealed by etching.

Some metals are etched in a few seconds and others may take several minutes to produce a clear picture. The etching reagents are usually aqueous or alcoholic solutions of acids or alkalis.

It is better to etch a specimen by progressive stages and to examine it at intervals, as too deep an etching does not give a clear picture of the structure.

Chapter 6
Deformation of metals. Softening heat treatment

When a metal is subjected to a stress, it deforms elastically at first, and then, when the stress becomes greater, part of its change in shape becomes permanent. At first, the stresses are opposed by primary interatomic bonds and the material behaves elastically, recovering its shape after the stress is removed. Application of stresses larger than the elastic limit results in the breaking of interatomic bonds and movement of atoms past each other. There is a permanent change in shape, and the material behaves plastically.

Slip

On permanent deformation, one layer of atoms moves over the surface of another and then takes up a relationship with new opposing atoms (Fig. 24). This movement is called *slip*, and the plane along which it takes place is called a *slip plane*. The movement is rather like a pile of coins being pushed sideways, each coin moving a little to the side.

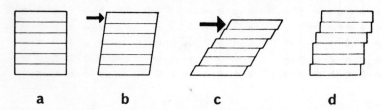

      a   b   c   d

Fig. 24. Deformation of metal by slip. (a) Metal unstressed showing possible slip planes. (b) Elastic deformation. (c) Deformation under greater stress. (d) Permanent deformation remaining after removal of stress

It might be assumed from this explanation of slip that crystalline structures such as metals were perfect in their crystal arrangements.

If this were true, then metals would display much greater strength than they do. 'Whiskers' of metal can be grown under suitable conditions which have no irregularities in their crystals, and these are very strong. Normally, however, crystals show lattice imperfections and the planes of atoms are not all complete. An incomplete plane is known as a *dislocation* (Fig. 24). Slip takes place by propagation of a dislocation along a slip plane. This requires much less energy than that necessary to move all the atoms of a complete plane. The presence of dislocations therefore enables slip to take place at a lower stress than if the crystal structure was perfect.

Deformation along slip planes can be seen as an irregularity on the surface of a piece of metal, as some portions of the grain are pushed up above the others. If a piece of metal is polished and etched, and then strained, a series of thin dark slip lines can be seen running across the surface of the individual grains. Slip planes are not continuous through grain boundaries because of the change of orientation which occurs in passing from one grain to the next. When the metal is polished after distortion these surface effects are removed.

The extent to which a metal may be deformed plastically depends on the type of atomic packing, on the size of the grains, and on the temperature of deformation. The type of space-lattice is particularly important as this determines the number of planes and directions in which slip can occur. Face-centred cubic metals can usually be deformed to a much greater extent than can close-packed hexagonal metals under similar conditions.

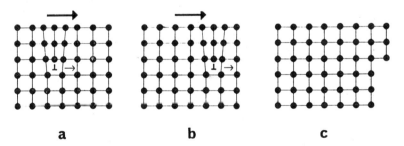

Fig. 25. (a) A dislocation or part of an extra plane of atoms is present. The dislocation is indicated by the sign: $\perp$. (b) Propagation of this dislocation due to a shear stress. (c) Resultant change in shape

Polycrystalline metals offer more resistance to deformation than do single crystals. This is only to be expected, since the deformation of any one grain in a polycrystalline mass is limited by the extent to which the surrounding grains will deform. In general, it is found that the strength and elasticity of metals increases with decreasing grain size. However, the extent of this increase is also dependent to some extent on the space-lattice of the metal concerned, and is more marked in hexagonal than in cubic metals.

A further factor which may be of importance in connection with grain size is the effect of the segregation of impurities at grain boundaries. In the case of a coarse-grained material which has a relatively small grain boundary per unit of volume, the concentrated impurities in these boundaries might markedly reduce the strength of the metal. With fine-grained material which has a large grain boundary area, the concentration of impurity per unit area of grain boundary is small, and hence the effect on the mechanical properties is less marked.

Twinning

Close-packed hexagonal metals also deform by twinning. Instead of movement along slip planes, a plane of atoms moves slightly relative to its neighbour and creates a similar crystal structure in a mirror-image orientation.

Cold work and strain hardening

Metals may be shaped by bending, swaging, rolling, drawing, etc. If shaping is carried out at a relatively low temperature, it is called *cold work*. During cold working the metal is deformed plastically, it becomes harder and stronger, and is said to show *work* or *strain hardening*. For further cold working, a greater stress must be applied to produce plastic deformation. In other words, elasticity is increased and plasticity reduced by cold working.

Strain hardening can largely be accounted for by the interaction of dislocations with one another and with obstacles such as grain boundaries and inclusions. During cold work, there is a large increase in the number of dislocations present. They move on intersecting planes and in various directions, and tend to tangle up rather like too many cars in a complicated network of city streets. This great resistance to motion of dislocations must be overcome or by-passed before further slip can occur.

In polycrystalline materials the grain boundaries or inclusions stop the progress of dislocations. When the propagation of one dislocation is halted, others build up behind it rather like a line of cars at traffic lights. Until a large force overcomes the blockage, further slip is prevented.

During cold working the grain structure is modified by the deformation process. For example, when a metal is rolled or drawn the grains are elongated in the direction of working, and a fibrous structure is said to develop. This fibrous structure causes a metal to have a directional difference in its mechanical properties. The metal will have a greater tensile strength along the grains than across them. Wire has such excellent elastic properties when subjected to a bending or stretching force because all its grains were elongated when pulled through the hole in the drawplate.

Although cold worked metals have increased mechanical strength and elasticity, they have poorer ductility and malleability than unstrained metals and may fracture if any further attempt is made to alter their shape. Cold working also lowers the corrosion resistance of a metal.

SOFTENING OR SOLUTION
HEAT TREATMENT

In a cold-worked metal the increased strength and hardness are associated with a distortion of the crystal structure on an atomic scale. Superimposed on this distortion are internal stresses which arise due to different parts of the metal having been deformed to different extents.

Stress-relief anneal (Recovery)

When cold working small metal structures in dentistry, more work may be carried out in one small area than along the rest of the structure. For example, a wire may be bent sharply at one point but to more gentle curves at others. If the wire is left in this condition it may fracture if further adjustment of the highly strained areas becomes necessary. By a stress-relief anneal, sufficient heat energy is applied for the dislocations to group into lower energy configurations. There is no change in grain structure. The mechanical properties are not greatly affected and may in some cases be improved. A *small* amount of further cold work may be carried out if necessary. Stress-relief annealing takes place at relatively low temperatures when compared with the melting point.

Recrystallization or annealing

If further heat is applied to the cold worked material, the increased thermal vibration of atoms is sufficient to allow them to move to less stressed positions. The number of dislocations falls and the previous grains are replaced by new, smaller, stress-free ones. The metal is said to have undergone *primary recrystallization* or to have become *annealed*. In this condition it possesses lower strength and hardness than the cold worked material, but has improved ductility and malleability and better corrosion resistance. Since a small grain structure results from primary recrystallization, cold work followed by suitable annealing provides a means of refining grain structure.

When working a metal or alloy, there is a limit to the amount of cold work possible as eventually the stress necessary to change its shape is equal to its ultimate strength and the material fractures. If further plastic deformation is necessary, the material must be annealed. This process of cold working and annealing can be carried out until the desired shape is achieved.

The recrystallization temperature for a given metal is not constant but depends on the amount of cold work which has been carried out. The greater the degree of cold work the lower the recrystallization temperature.

Now that the concept of recrystallization temperature has been introduced, it is possible to define the term cold work more accurately. Cold work is deformation carried out below the recrystallization temperature. Hot work, on the other hand, involves simultaneous deformation and recrystallization and is carried out at, or above, the recrystallization temperature. In the case of lead, room temperature deformation is accompanied by simultaneous recrystallization, and is therefore hot work.

Practical application

There is usually an optimum range of temperature for softening a metal. Above this range recrystallization takes place too rapidly and cannot be controlled with accuracy, and below it, the process takes too long.

Usually dental metals are softened by simply heating them in a bunsen or blowpipe flame. This method is rather inaccurate, and usually leads to over-annealing. Since the times and temperatures for softening vary with different alloys, a test should be carried out on all wrought metals to find the minimum softening which is necessary for cold work to be performed.

After a metal has been softened by heat it may be cooled rapidly by 'quenching' in water or oil, or it may be left to cool in air. With most non-ferrous metals, quenching will retain the recrystallized grain structure. On quenching steel, however, a harder material is produced, and steels are cooled very slowly in order to soften them.

Metals which are quenched should be plunged completely under the surface of the cooling medium so that the whole mass of metal is cooled at once. Irregular cooling will cause stresses to be set up within the metal with consequent distortion of its shape.

Both stress-relief and recrystallization are a function of time as well as temperature. That is, within limits, the same result can be obtained by heating at a lower temperature for a long time, as at a higher temperature for a shorter time.

Grain growth

During annealing care must be taken to avoid heating the metal to too high a temperature, as once primary recrystallization has started it will be succeeded by grain growth at a rate which increases rapidly with rising temperature. Grain growth is effected by migration of the grain boundary, whereby one large grain replaces many smaller ones. The resulting coarse-grained structure will have mechanical properties inferior to that of a material with a fine recrystallized grain.

In most metals or alloys, there is a critical amount of strain which leads to excessive grain growth—commonly referred to as *secondary recrystallization*. Such critical strains should be avoided in the cold working of metals or alloys used for dental structures as the danger of secondary recrystallization is great on any reheating.

Chapter 7
Alloys. Hardening heat treatment

An alloy is a combination of two or more metals, or of metals with a metalloid. Most of the metallic materials used in dentistry are alloys because, in general, a pure metal is not sufficiently strong to withstand the forces applied to it in the mouth. Sometimes a work hardened pure metal is used, as in this condition its strength is greatest.

The individual metals which make up an alloy are chosen because they impart to the mixture some desired property such as strength, corrosion resistance, or an alteration in the melting temperature. In making an alloy, it is usual to select a 'parent' or 'basic' metal which possesses the most suitable properties, and then to improve these properties by adding other metals. An alloy may be a mixture of a large number of different metals and metalloids, but the following discussion will be limited to the study of alloys containing only two metals. These are known as *binary alloys*.

Some idea of the physical properties of simple binary alloys can be derived from a knowledge of the constituent metals, and of the way in which the metals combine. When an alloy is made up of five or six metals, the combined effects of all the additions on the alloy can only be discovered by mechanical testing. This difficulty of assessing the properties of complicated alloys is illustrated by the fact that there are many different dental gold alloys on sale today, and each is claimed to have some properties superior to the others. These alloys differ quite appreciably in composition. If it were possible to predict the properties of a complicated alloy by simple reference to the effects of the constituents upon each other, only a few different alloys would exist.

THERMAL EQUILIBRIUM DIAGRAMS

An indication of the properties of an alloy can be gleaned from a study of the changes which take place in its structure when subjected to temperatures ranging from its melting point to room temperature. An even clearer picture is obtained if the thermal changes of a particular alloy are examined in relation to similar changes which take place within the entire range of alloys that can be formed between the two metals.

A *thermal equilibrium diagram* provides a graphical method of representing these changes. The diagram shows the phases which are stable at certain temperatures and the temperature boundaries within which they exist.

A number of methods are available for locating boundaries in equilibrium diagrams, but only the cooling curve method will be considered. In this method an alloy is cooled slowly from the liquid state and its temperature recorded at frequent regular intervals of time during the process of solidification, and after it is complete. Examination of the cooling curve obtained by plotting temperature versus time, indicates the temperatures at which changes occur. In the case of a pure metal, the cooling curve would show only one arrest, this being at the freezing point. With alloys, solidification occurs over a temperature range, so

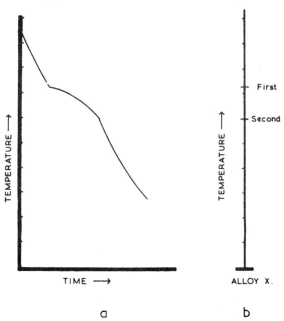

Fig. 26. Cooling curve of an alloy

that the start and completion of solidification will be apparent in the
cooling curve (Fig. 26a). We can plot these two marked changes in rate
of cooling against temperature, as in Fig. 26b.

To provide a picture of the thermal changes of all the alloys formed
by two metals, cooling curves are first prepared from alloys consisting
of the two metals in the following percentages 90–10, 80–20, 70–30,
etc., up to 10–90.

Then we draw a graph with percentages by weight of the two components A and B along the base-line and with temperature running vertically (Fig. 27). Since a reduction in the percentage of A means an

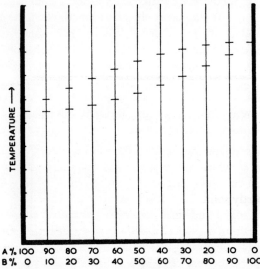

Fig. 27. Construction of a thermal equilibrium diagram

increase in B, the entire range of alloys can be accommodated between
100 per cent A and 100 per cent B. The melting points of pure metals
A and B are known and these are noted on the uprights of the graph.
Then, for each alloy, the temperatures at which a change in rate of
cooling occurs are entered vertically above its composition on the graph.
Now draw a line connecting all the first arrest points, and then the
second points. On removing the vertical lines, a graph such as that in
Fig. 28 will be left. For increased accuracy, further cooling curves may
be added for alloys which differ by only 5 per cent in composition.

The line CLD indicates the temperatures at which any alloy begins
to solidify. Above this line the alloys are liquid. This line of thermal

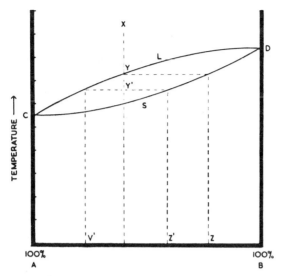

Fig. 28. Typical thermal equilibrium diagram of solid solution alloys

equilibrium is called the *liquidus*. The lower line *CSD* shows the temperatures at which alloys are completely solid, and it is appropriately called the *solidus*. Between these two lines the alloys are partly liquid and partly solid.

Hence, the initial and final melting temperatures of any alloy are obtained by raising a vertical line from its composition on the baseline of the graph, and noting where this cuts the solidus and the liquidus.

The complete thermal equilibrium diagram is often called a *constitutional diagram of an alloy system*. In Fig. 28 it is the *A–B* system or *A–B* constitutional diagram as these are the two metals involved. Each metal is a component of the system and the lines on the diagram show the temperatures at which a change of phase takes place.

TYPES OF BINARY SYSTEM

Because of the large number of binary systems that can be represented by equilibrium diagrams, many of which are merely modifications of others, it is desirable to consider them as types. The types of binary system that will be considered are as follows.

Solid solutions. Metals which are completely soluble in both liquid and solid states

This type of system is formed between metals which have similar valency and whose atomic size, crystal structure and electrochemical characteristics are similar. The diagram which was constructed in Fig. 28 from the cooling curves of alloys between A and B, is typical of that obtained when their alloys are all solid solutions. The two metals dissolve completely in each other in all proportions and the melting points of all the alloys lie between those of the two components. In certain systems, however, a minimum may be apparent in the liquidus and solidus curves.

It has already been noted that alloys freeze over a range of temperature, and to find out what happens during this period of cooling, we will take a solid solution alloy of 60 per cent A : 40 per cent B (Fig.28).

On slow cooling from X, the molten alloy remains unchanged until the temperature falls to Y on the liquidus. At this temperature the first portion of the alloy solidifies. The only alloy between A and B which can be solid at this temperature is that of composition Z, where this temperature cuts the solidus. So the first metal to freeze will be a dendrite of this composition. When the alloy has cooled a little further to Y^1, the portion solidifying will be of composition Z^1 and the remaining liquid of composition V^1. Therefore, the first solid portions of a solid solution alloy will be richer in B than those which freeze later on in the cooling period. However, under *very slow* cooling, the composition of the dendrites changes by a process of diffusion so that the microstructure of the solid alloy will be similar to that of a pure metal, and will show no evidence of the dendritic mechanism of solidification.

Coring

If the cooling of the alloy is rapid there will be insufficient time for the composition of the separated solid to change by diffusion. Then, the composition of each grain varies continuously from its central primary dendrite to the outside. When this structure is examined under the microscope, the difference in composition between the portions of the crystal grains appears as in Fig. 29.

This difference in composition between the first and last formed portions of a crystal grain is called *coring*. It occurs most readily when there is a large temperature distance between the liquidus and the

Fig. 29.   Cored structure

solidus. When an alloy solidifies over a small range of temperature little or no segregation takes place.

The small mass of precious metal solid solution alloy used in dental castings cools quickly, and often shows a cored structure. Coring reduces the corrosion resistance since some portions of the alloy may have too little of the corrosion-resisting component, and the dissimilar alloys present may form a galvanic couple.

Homogenizing anneal

To remove the cored structure from a cast alloy, and produce grains which are of the same composition throughout, sufficient heat must be applied so that the atoms can diffuse through the metal, and eliminate the differences in composition. Homogenizing is carried out by heating the alloy at a temperature not far below the solidus for a period of time. It takes place more readily in a grain structure which has been cold worked.

A homogenized solid solution alloy shows a microscopic structure identical with that of a pure metal.

Types of solid solution alloy

In the solid state, the crystal structure of these alloys is made up of atoms of both metals.

Solid solutions may be of the *substitutional* or *interstitial* types. In the former case atoms of the added element substitute for those of the parent metal in its space-lattice, whereas in the latter case atoms of the added element fit into the spaces between those of the parent atoms. The substitutional solid solution is the more common. In this type of solid solution it is not essential for the space-lattices of the two metals to be identical, unless a complete range of solid solutions is to be formed, but the 'atomic size' of the different atoms must be similar.

Alloys of Au, with Ag, Pt, Pd, Ni, Cu, and of Pd with Ag, form a series of substitutional solid solutions.

Advantages of solid solutions

If the atomic size of the added metal is slightly smaller or larger than that of the parent metal, the crystal structure will be distorted at the points where the new atoms are located. This distortion interferes with the movement of dislocations, and renders the alloy more resistant to permanent deformation. This effect is known as *solution hardening*. The grain structure will remain that of a pure metal, and the alloy can be cold worked if necessary, although it requires a greater force to change its shape. Like pure metals, it has a high corrosion resistance. An increase in the number of alloying atoms causes greater distortion and gives greater strength to the alloy. The maximum amount of alloying metal which can be added depends upon the solubility of the alloying metals in each other. When there is complete solid solubility, the greatest strength is usually obtained in an alloy containing an equal number of both atoms, or 50 per cent atomic of each metal.

Ordering or superlattice

If, in a substitutional solid solution, the atoms of the added metal take up positions at random in the parent lattice then the solid solution is said to be *disordered*. In certain cases, however, solid solutions are disordered at higher temperatures but undergo an atomic rearrangement on slow cooling. Atoms of one kind segregate to one set of atomic positions leaving the other atoms to occupy the remaining sites (see Fig. 34). In this way an *ordered solid solution or superlattice* develops. The composition range over which ordering occurs approximates to simple formulae such as *AB* or *AB₃*.

Eutectic alloys. Metals which are soluble in the liquid state but insoluble in the solid state

In a series of alloys of this type, the addition of increasing amounts of one metal to the other markedly reduces the melting point, until at a certain composition the lowest melting alloy is found. This particular alloy is called the eutectic alloy, from the Greek word *eutēktos*, meaning easily melted.

The constitutional diagram for two metals which form a typical eutectic system is given in Fig. 30.

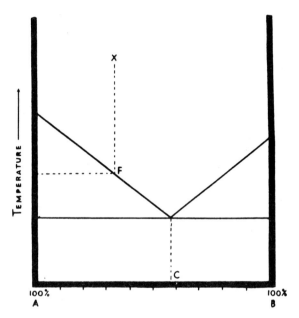

Fig. 30. Thermal equilibrium diagram for a eutectic type alloy

When an alloy between *A* and *B* freezes, it first of all deposits crystals of the metal which is in excess of that necessary to give the eutectic composition. When it has thrown out sufficient of this metal and has cooled to the eutectic temperature, the remaining liquid freezes at a constant temperature.

For example, an alloy *X* begins to solidify at *F* by depositing dendrites of metal *A*. It continues to form these until the liquid is of composition C. Then the eutectic liquid solidifies by the simultaneous rejection of both A and B. The solid eutectic structure is an intimate mechanical mixture of the two component metals. Its microscopic appearance may show a laminated pattern of straight or curved lines, or finely dispersed particles of the two metals.

Alloys which differ from the eutectic composition show a micro-structure of primary metal dendrites embedded in a matrix of eutectic.

To be perfectly correct, the term 'eutectic alloy' should be applied only to the one alloy of eutectic composition, but it is applied loosely to describe alloys between metals which combine to give a *eutectiferous system*.

Advantages of eutectic alloys

Continuity of slip planes may not exist across a eutectic mixture and it may behave as a 'composite'. The dispersed phase interferes with slip producing good mechanical properties. Because they are com-posed of two separate and dissimilar metals, their resistance to cor-rosion is poor. The main advantage of a eutectic alloy is that it possesses a low melting point. In dentistry where one is restricted to the rela-tively simple methods of melting alloys, a low melting point can be of great advantage. Solders and low-fusing alloys are usually eutectic mixtures.

By careful choice of suitable low-fusing constituents, a eutectic alloy can be made which melts below 100°C. These low-fusing alloys are discussed in Chapter 14.

Intermetallic compounds

In certain metallic systems the component metals may combine to form an intermetallic compound. These compounds frequently occur when the electrochemical characteristics of the two metals are mark-edly different. Intermetallic compounds are hard and brittle, and often have high melting points. If present in an alloy in massive form they have a weakening effect, but in a finely divided form they can mark-edly increase the mechanical strength. Intermetallic compounds, like ordered solid solutions, approximate in composition to simple for-mulae, but unlike the latter they exist over much narrower ranges of composition.

**Metals which are soluble in the liquid state, insoluble in the
solid state and which form a compound by a peritectic reaction**
This type of system is illustrated in Fig. 31. Alloys of compositions
lying between 100 per cent *A* and *Z* undergo a peritectic reaction
during solidification. Alloys of composition to the right of *Z* solidify
like the eutectic alloys previously discussed.

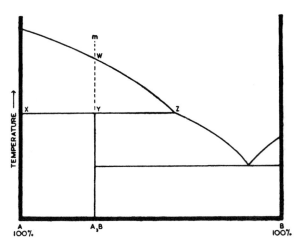

Fig. 31. Thermal equilibrium diagram showing the formation of an intermetallic compound by a peritectic reaction

The solidification under slow cooling conditions of an alloy in
which the peritectic reaction goes to completion will be considered,
i.e. an alloy of composition *m*. On cooling from the liquid, separation
of solid *A* occurs when the liquidus is reached at *W*. As the temperature falls, more solid *A* will separate and the remaining liquid composition follows the liquidus line *WZ*. Eventually the peritectic
temperature is attained at *Y* when solid *A* is in equilibrium with
liquid of composition *Z*. At this temperature the solid and liquid
react to produce a new solid, in this case the intermetallic compound
A_3B. When the reaction has gone to completion cooling continues to
room temperature. In alloys lying to the left or right of the composition
m there will be an excess of solid *A* or liquid *Z* respectively, once the
peritectic reaction has gone to completion.

Peritectic reactions frequently take a considerable time to go to completion, since the layer of reaction product which forms between the reacting liquid and solid tends to stifle it.

Other equilibrium diagrams

In practice, it is frequently found that metals form equilibrium diagrams which are extremely complex in that a number of changes are involved. For example, in the Cu–Zn system (the brasses) a number of peritectic reactions occur, in addition to other changes.

In some systems reactions may occur in the solid alloy at temperatures well below that at which solidification is complete. One such reaction, which is of particular interest in connection with steel, is known as a *eutectoid* reaction. This involves the breakdown of a solid solution at a definite temperature to produce an intimate mechanical mixture of two solids which may be very like a eutectic in appearance.

HARDENING HEAT TREATMENT

Order hardening

Many dental gold alloys are of the substitutional solid solution type. In these alloys, hardening can occur on slow cooling due to ordering. The ordered structure, or superlattice, produced by this heat treatment may have a space-lattice similar to the disordered solid solution from which it forms, or the atomic rearrangement may result in a change in the shape of the lattice. For example, when alloys of composition approximating to CuAu undergo ordering, the atomic rearrangement results in the unit cell changing from a cubic to a rectangular box or tetragonal shape (Fig. 34). This causes a large elastic strain field to be set up round each ordered region as the result of contraction of one axis of the unit cell. Dislocations have difficulty in surmounting these strain fields in order to move.

Although ordering may develop on slow cooling it is sometimes more satisfactory to quench to room temperature from above the temperature at which ordering commences, and so suppress the change initially. This disordered alloy can then be progressively ordered by heating at a predetermined temperature for a period of time. In this way a more careful control of the increased mechanical strength associated with ordering can be obtained.

Precipitation hardening

Some metals are completely soluble in the liquid state but only
partially soluble in the solid state, the degree of solubility falling
with temperature. This type of system is a eutectic one but, during
solidification, the primary separation involves a solid solution instead of a single metal, and the eutectic consists of a mixture of solid
solutions and not of single metals.

If an alloy a (Fig. 32) is cooled slowly from temperature $t°$, rejection
of β solid solution from the a solid solution occurs on crossing the solid

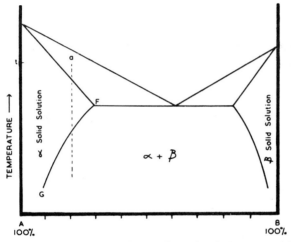

Fig. 32. Thermal equilibrium diagram of metals which are partially soluble
in each other in the solid state

solubility boundary FG. As the temperature falls further, the composition of the a follows the solubility boundary with further rejection
of β. However, if the alloy is cooled rapidly from $t°$, then there is
insufficient time for rejection of β to occur, so that a supersaturated
solid solution is obtained at room temperature. If this solid solution
is subsequently heated to some temperature between room temperature
and the solubility line for a period of time, the gradual rejection of β
in a very finely divided form occurs. This dispersion of β within the
grains may be so fine that it is not visible under the optical microscope. But it interferes with the slip process by creating strain fields
which resist the movement of dislocations. Thus, the alloy is harder and
stronger.

If the alloy is 'quenched' from just below its solidus temperature, no ordering or precipitation hardening occurs and the alloy is a simple solid solution. After any necessary cold work has been carried out it can be hardened by reheating and cooling it slowly through the range of temperature at which either or both of these hardening effects occur.

This procedure is called *hardening heat treatment* and is of particular importance in dental gold alloys.

In the metallurgical field the terms *precipitation* and *age hardening* are synonymous, although there is an increasing tendency to use the former term.

As a basis of deciding whether increased strength is due to precipitation hardening or order hardening, it is suggested that the former term is used when the precipitated phase has a markedly different composition from the solid solution out of which it is rejected. Whereas order hardening indicates that the hardening is associated with the formation of an ordered solid solution whose composition is either identical with, or only slightly different from, the disordered phase from which it forms. A system of the type shown in Fig. 32 would show precipitation hardening, whereas order hardening would be associated with the system shown in Fig. 33 (page 75).

Chapter 8
Gold. Yellow and white gold alloys

Pure gold is very malleable and ductile and can readily be cold worked. In the cast condition the metal is too soft to maintain its shape under the forces of mastication. However, its strength can be greatly improved by cold work, and it is in this condition that pure gold is used in a filling.

PURE GOLD FILLINGS

Since Au does not readily oxidize in the atmosphere at room temperature, it is possible to obtain a clean metal-to-metal contact between two thin pieces of Au. If a force is applied pressing two pieces firmly together, metallic bonds are formed at their point of contact and the Au is welded together without the application of heat. This property of *cold welding* is utilized when building up a gold filling.

Cohesive gold is available in two basic forms. First as very thin gold sheet or 'foil' and secondly, in a variety of structures which can be compressed or completed. Gold foil, approximately 0·001 mm thick, is purchased in the form of cylinders or pellets. These are rolls of one or more layers of foil, slightly compressed and prepared in a fully annealed state, care being taken so that all the surfaces are perfectly clean. On condensation, each addition of foil bonds with the material already in the cavity. For larger cavities, a rope of gold foil may be used. Alternative forms are mat (sponge or crystal) or powdered gold. Mat gold is a fine interlacing meshwork of Au usually in the form of a small cylinder. It is produced by a variety of means including the sintering of gold powder, rapid electrolytic deposition or the evaporation of mercury from a gold amalgam. A very porous readily collapsed structure is produced but the weight of Au per cylinder is, of course, much less than that in gold foil. Powdered gold is made from a very fine powder which after being moulded into a pellet, is enclosed in a wrapping of gold foil.

The cohesive property of pure Au disappears if the metal is exposed to gases which adsorb on its surface. Similarly, the presence of dirt or grease will prevent bonding. In some cases, the cohesive property of Au is not desired in the construction of the filling and *non-cohesive gold foil* is used. It is usual, however, to make use of the cold welding properties and most gold 'foil' fillings are made of cohesive gold.

Cohesion

In order to achieve good welding between the pieces of Au, any adsorbed gases which are present on the foil due to storage, etc., must be removed by heating. To prevent adsorption of gases, the flame used to heat the Au should not come into contact with it. The ideal method of heating is by small electric furnace, but this is not always convenient. Usually the Au is placed on a clean mica tray above a gas or alcohol flame, and is heated to 200–300°C. This ensures a clean surface, without annealing the Au unduly. If the foil is annealed fully, it will cohere more readily, but a softer filling is produced. The tooth to be filled is isolated from the saliva and thoroughly dried. It should preferably be screened from the patient's moist breath, as condensed moisture will prevent cohesion. The Au is carried to the cavity in tweezers and is 'plugged' or condensed into place.

Gold pluggers are hand instruments with flat or lightly serrated 'points' about 1 mm in diameter. With these the Au is pushed into place. Then it is condensed either by hand, with an automatic mallet, or by the application of a mechanical vibrator. The automatic mallet delivers a fairly high force at relatively infrequent intervals, whilst a pneumatic or electrically driven condenser delivers frequent, light blows. Ultrasonic vibration of the condenser tip produces a less porous filling, particularly when using mat gold. The energy applied how-ever, overheats the filling and may damage the pulp unless care is taken. The force applied closes up most of the air-spaces present, welds the metal together and work hardens it. The tooth and its supporting structures must withstand this rather harsh treatment, and adsorb the energy applied. Fortunately, both the dentine and the periodontal membrane are resilient.

A pure Au filling similar in hardness and strength to a cast alloy, can only be obtained by appropriate cold work, but often the living tissues limit the amount of force which can be applied. For instance, much harder fillings than are possible in the mouth can be made by condensing gold foil into a hole in a steel plate, as this will withstand a much greater force, and the Au will be subjected to more work hardening.

When small increments of foil are condensed, a harder filling results as more work hardening is achieved.

The amount of work hardening varies with the size of the plugger point and therefore with the area to which the force is applied. With a plugger point of small area, hardening is achieved with a relatively small force. Unfortunately a very small point will perforate the Au instead of condensing it. This tends to distort the filling and to pull it away from the cavity walls. A large point requires a greater force than the patient will tolerate. Therefore, plugger point sizes are limited for practical reasons between 0·4 and 1·0 mm² in area.

The surface hardness of a filling varies from place to place due to differences in the degree of condensation and work hardening. The BHN should be between 45 and 60 if sufficient work hardening has taken place. If the filling is not sufficiently condensed, a value as low as 18–20 is produced.

The advantages of a gold foil filling are that it is completely resistant to corrosion, it is as hard as the softer cast inlay golds and does not have the disadvantage of a soluble cement lute. In areas where little or no force is applied to the filling in use, or where the cavity is completely surrounded by tooth substance, gold foil is the most permanent filling material.

The different forms of Au lead to various techniques for filling the cavity. Sometimes a layer of non-cohesive gold is first placed in position followed by the use of cohesive material to complete the filling. Generally, the time taken to fill the cavity is greatest when using mat gold due to its lower metal content per cylinder. On the other hand, the highly compressive nature of mat gold enables one to fill all the cavity detail, particularly that designed for retention of the filling. Mat gold tends to produce a somewhat porous surface unless compacted very vigorously and burnished well, and a layer of gold foil may be placed over the surface to complete the filling, thus ensuring a more solid superficial layer. Powdered gold, whilst it enables one to fill the cavity rapidly, produces a restoration which is softer and less dense than with gold foil or mat gold. Its use should therefore be limited to non stress-bearing areas.

GOLD ALLOYS

Gold alloys are available in dentistry in the wrought condition, as sheet or plate metal, and in the form of wire. They are also supplied in small ingots, or portions of thick plate ready to be melted and cast. The 'nobility' of a gold alloy is indicated by its *carat* or *fineness* number.

Carat or fineness

The carat and fineness numbers denote the proportion of Au which is present within the alloy.

In the carat grading, pure Au is 24 carat; it is 24/24ths Au. The carat number of any alloy shows how many twenty-fourths of the metal by weight are Au. For example, 18 carat is 18/24ths or 75 per cent Au, whereas 9 carat is 9/24ths or 37·5 per cent Au. Quite often the percentage of Au present within an alloy cannot be related accurately to a carat number, since each one represents an increase in Au content of over 4 per cent.

The system giving fineness employs a scale of 1000 parts and is therefore more precise. Pure Au is 1000 fine. The fineness figure for an alloy is ten times the percentage of Au within it. As an example, a 75 per cent gold alloy is 750 fine (and is also 18 carat).

Neither of the systems takes any note of the metals with which the Au is alloyed, they refer simply to the proportion of Au which is present within the alloy.

YELLOW GOLD ALLOYS

Gold is alloyed with Cu, Ag, Pt, Pd, Ni, Zn, and Sn. A study of some of the binary alloys between each of these metals and Au gives an indication of the correct methods of handling gold alloys so that their best properties are brought out.

Yellow gold dental alloys are basically mixtures of Au with Cu and Ag, to which other metals are added in small amounts. Sometimes, however, Pt may be present in similar quantity to that of the Ag or Cu.

Gold-copper

Gold and Cu dissolve in each other in all proportions to form solid solution alloys. Unlike the typical solid solution thermal equilibrium diagram, the one for Au–Cu shows a reduction in the melting point of the alloys below that of either component metal (Fig. 33). This is similar to the effect of a eutectic alloy but, nevertheless, a true solid solution alloy is always formed. In this diagram the solidus and

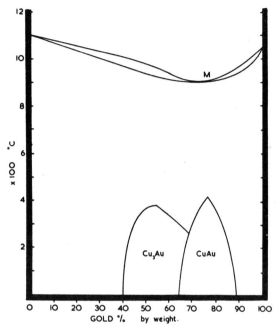

Fig. 33. Thermal equilibrium diagram of Au–Cu alloys. (The liquidus and solidus actually coincide at M but *do not cross*)

liquidus are very close together, particularly within the range of alloys which are used in dentistry, that is 75 per cent Au and upwards. There is, therefore, little coring even on rapid solidification. This short distance between the liquidus and solidus also indicates that when the alloy is to be cast its melting point will be clearly defined.

The addition of Cu and Au improves its strength and hardness. Maximum hardness is achieved with 20 per cent of Cu, but this is too high for dental use. Even a small addition, however, causes a large improvement in the strength of the alloy.

An important function of Cu in dental gold alloys is its *order hardening effect*. Gold and Cu both have face-centred cubic lattices, and all alloys between them consist of substitutional solid solutions. In the *disordered* condition, the lattice sites are occupied at random by Cu or Au atoms. At temperatures between 200–450°C, the atoms in certain Au–Cu alloys diffuse within the solid metal to preferred sites within the space lattice. In alloys containing between 40–65 weight per cent of Au, an *ordered* superlattice based on Cu_3Au is formed. From 65 to 87 per cent of Au, an ordered tetragonal superlattice of CuAu is formed (Fig. 34).

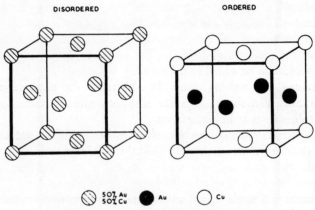

Fig. 34. Ordering or superlattice of CuAu

Since gold alloys must contain at least 75 per cent Au to resist corrosion, the ordered structure CuAu is the one of dental importance.

The tetragonal CuAu superlattice being of different dimensions from the normal lattice limits the movement of dislocations and reduces slip. This improves the hardness, strength and elasticity of the alloy, while reducing its ductility.

Gold–silver

These metals dissolve in all proportions to form solid solutions whose melting points are between those of the two component metals. A small addition of Ag improves the strength and hardness slightly due to solution hardening. Silver lowers the melting point. When Ag is melted in a blowpipe flame, it adsorbs gases, particularly oxygen. A high silver content alloy which has been overheated will show porosity, due to the release of these gases as the alloy cools.

Gold–platinum

Platinum also combines with Au to form a series of solid solutions, but there is a wide interval of temperature between the liquidus and solidus. This may be as much as 300°C, so that coring may readily arise during solidification. It has been found that the cored structure in a Pt-containing cast gold alloy is not always completely removed by the homogenizing anneal usually recommended by the manufacturers, that is 700–750°C for 5–10 minutes. A longer period of time is necessary to produce a homogeneous grain structure. On melting an ingot of platinized casting alloy some difficulty will be experienced in fusing the alloy completely due to the wide melting range. Platinum also increases the melting temperature, and therefore the amount of this metal which can be added to a gold alloy is limited.

In raising the melting point, Pt also raises the recrystallization temperature. Platinized alloys are therefore more suitable for use when soldering is to be carried out.

Under standard conditions of cooling, Pt brings about a refinement in the grain structure of a casting, and thereby improves its hardness, strength and elasticity. Platinum also assists in producing order hardening effects with other constituents of gold alloys.

Platinum is a noble metal, and it raises the corrosion resistance of an alloy, despite its tendency to produce a cored structure. It can therefore replace the Au content to some extent.

Gold–palladium

Due to the high cost of Pt, its place in dental alloys has been taken to a certain extent by the cheaper Pd. Gold and Pd form solid solution alloys with a narrow freezing range. The melting point is raised more sharply by Pd than by Pt despite the former's lower melting point. This reduces the amount of annealing which takes place on soldering, as a rise in the melting point causes a similar rise in the recrystallization temperature. In casting alloys, Pd has a similar effect to Pt, but its effect in refining grain size is not quite as marked. Palladium adsorbs gases on melting and care must be taken not to overheat alloys containing a high percentage of this metal.

Casting alloys containing a large amount of Pd together with Ag are called *white golds*.

Gold–nickel

Up to 2 per cent of Ni may be present in wrought alloys. It is not usually present in casting alloys. Nickel is added to harden and strengthen.

Gold–zinc

Zinc is added to casting alloys in quantities up to 2 per cent to protect the more important constituents. When melting a gold alloy, either during manufacture or in use, the base metals such as the Cu will oxidize. After melting, the composition of the alloy will be different from that originally present. Zinc oxidizes more readily than the other metals, and will reduce any of their oxides which are formed. The zinc oxide is removed by the flux, or is taken from the molten metal as a 'slag'. The zinc is called a *scavenger* since it cleans up the molten alloy by removing other oxides. If oxides remain in an alloy, they collect at the grain boundaries, and make the alloy brittle.

Gold and Zn form a eutectic mixture, and therefore the addition of Zn lowers the melting point to a marked degree. Since a gold solder must melt at a lower temperature than the alloy which is being soldered, a solder of correct carat can be made by replacing a portion of the Ag in an alloy by Zn. Tin has a similar effect on the melting point but does not act so effectively as a scavenger.

Other metals

A fine grain size is important as many dental structures are of relatively small dimensions. With a coarse grain structure, a thin section may contain only one or two grains across its width and thus be very weak. Some metals of the platinum group such as Ir, In, Os and Ru refine the grain size when present in only very small quantities.

WROUGHT AND CAST YELLOW GOLD ALLOYS

The dental application of gold alloys is extremely exacting for many reasons. In the mouth, metals are continuously exposed to wide variations in acidity and alkalinity, and they must be sufficiently 'noble' to resist this corrosive attack. This reduces the amount of alloying which is possible and limits the proportions of strengthening metals which can be added. Appliances or fillings are usually of thin and irregular sections, yet they have to withstand fairly large stresses during use. Also, the shape of many dental appliances is complex, and requires an alloy which can readily be worked within the limitations of dental laboratory equipment. In engineering, the properties of an alloy are improved by cold working. In dentistry this is not always possible, particularly with small pieces of varying section. Moreover, soldering with its attendant annealing effect may reduce the strength of any work hardened structure.

Because of these difficult conditions, the type of gold alloy in use today tends to be of the heat hardening type rather than of the work hardening variety.

WROUGHT GOLD ALLOYS

Applicable specifications: Brit 3520; Amer 7; Austral 1625.

Wrought gold wire is used for clasps on partial dentures and to a small extent for orthodontic appliances. After the wire has been drawn during manufacture to the correct diameter, it has a fibrous crystal structure running lengthwise. Usually this is annealed by the manufacturer to give a very fine grain structure which will allow some cold work to be done. If the amount of bending to be done is considerable, an intermediate anneal may be necessary. Many of these alloys can be heat hardened mainly by the effect of ordering to improve their mechanical properties. Some wires are available in three-quarter hard condition when they still have a fibrous structure but are amenable to some cold work.

Two main types of wrought gold wire may be found, usually described as high and low precious metal content, that is, total content of Au, Pt, Pd, and other metals of the Pt group. The actual Au content of the high precious metal group may be as low as 35 per cent, but with a total precious metal content of 65–75 per cent. These alloys may contain a little Ni. The low precious metal content wires may contain as little as 15 per cent of Au but have a total precious metal content of 40–70 per cent, together with 2–6 per cent Ni. Heat treatment of the low precious metal wires is more critical than that of the higher precious metal type. Over-hardening causes embrittlement.

Typical mechanical properties of high precious metal content wires:

	Annealed	Heat hardened
PL N/mm²	900	1050
UTS N/mm²	980	1350
Mod. of elast.	118 × 10³ N/mm²	
	(unaffected by condition)	
Elongation	20 per cent	5 per cent
VHN	200	320
Fusion temperature	1000°C	

The lower precious metal content wires have a slightly lower PL and UTS and less elongation after heat hardening. Their fusion temperature is usually about 100°C lower.

YELLOW GOLD CASTING ALLOYS

Applicable specifications: ISO R 1562; Brit 4425; Amer 5; Austral 1620. These may be divided into two types, first those used for inlays, and secondly, those for partial denture bases.

The mechanical strength of cast gold alloys depends upon three factors:

1. The solution hardening effect imparted to them by the inclusion of Cu, Ag, Pt, Pd and Ni in their composition.
2. The formation of a fine grain structure on cooling by the inclusion of high melting point metals of the Pt group and by the use of a correct casting technique.
3. Hardening due to ordering or precipitation.

Heat treatment of yellow gold casting alloys

On melting the alloy, any metallographic structure which it possessed as an ingot is lost, and a new crystal structure is created as the metal 'freezes' inside the mould.

It is important to quench the casting before it cools to the range of temperature within which heat hardening takes place. Usually the mould is left until the gold visible in the sprues of the casting is no longer at red heat. This indicates that the internal metal temperature is about 600°C. Then the mould is plunged into cold water in order to chill the metal quickly, and also to cause disintegration of the mould. Rapid cooling keeps the cast alloy in the soft state.

An alloy which is allowed to cool slowly to room temperature will undergo heat hardening. Before any alteration in the shape of such a casting is attempted, it must be softened by cooling rapidly from above 600°C.

Dental alloys containing Pt and Pd generally have a cored structure and they should undergo a homogenizing anneal. This removes most of the coring, and tends to produce a solid solution structure similar to that of a pure metal.

While in the soft condition the casting may be adjusted to fit the model and the patient's mouth. This should not be necessary if an accurate technique has been followed, but on occasions a slight adjustment of clasp arms is required. On bending a clasp to fit, stresses may be introduced into the material. Similarly, uneven heating or cooling of the casting during soldering may set up stresses, and may also introduce a degree of heat hardening. These effects are removed by a further softening heat treatment. After all alterations and additions of metal to the casting are complete, and after it has been polished, it is hardened to make it suitable for oral use.

Hardening heat treatment

In yellow gold dental casting alloys, hardening is due both to ordering and to precipitation. The changes which will occur are difficult to predict in an alloy of six or seven constituents. The best hardening effect is discovered by physical testing after various hardening heat treatments have been applied.

The casting can be hardened by reheating it to above 450°C and cooling slowly. Moreover, the degree of hardness can be controlled by the speed of cooling. It can also be hardened by maintaining it at a temperature below 450°C for a period of time.

Summary of heat treatments

1. Quench the casting after it has solidified.
2. Clean the casting. Homogenize anneal at 700°C for 10 minutes and quench.
3. Polish the casting and check its fit in the mouth.
4. If any bending was necessary in fitting clasps or if soldering has been carried out, re-anneal (stress-relief).

5. Harden by heating to above 450°C and cool slowly in 15–30 minutes to 200°C or maintain at 350°C for 30 mins. Quench.

6. Repolish and add teeth to the denture.

The precise details of the heat treatment vary with the different alloys, and the manufacturer's directions should be followed. In general, however, they are similar to these suggested times and temperatures.

If, at this stage, any further alteration of the metal base is required the teeth must be removed, and the appliance heated to 700–750°C for 10 minutes and quenched. After adjustment the casting can be re-hardened by heat treatment as before.

Practical application

Softening heat treatment or homogenizing may both be carried out in an open flame, by heating the casting to a bright cherry-red colour and then quenching it. Uneven heating of large pieces can occur by this method, and the most satisfactory treatment is to heat the casting in a pyrometrically controlled furnace. To prevent oxidation, the casting should be covered with a flux and must be supported by sand or other refractory material so that it will not sag under its own weight at the annealing temperature.

Hardening heat treatment should preferably be carried out in a furnace with a pyrometer in order to produce consistent results. The casting should again be supported in sand, but need not be covered with flux as only mild oxidation takes place.

Too much heat hardening will make the casting very brittle, while too low a temperature or heat treatment for too short a time, will leave the casting too soft, and clasps and other thin sections will be distorted in use.

INLAY GOLDS

Gold alloys for casting inlays are subdivided into three groups or types according to Brinell (or Vickers) hardness:

Soft	Type I	BHN 40–75	VHN 50–90
Medium	Type II	BHN 70–100	VHN 90–120
Hard	Type III	BHN 90–140	VHN 120–160

The partial denture casting golds are included in this classification as Extra Hard, Type IV, BHN above 130, VHN above 160.

Yellow gold alloys for inlays should have good corrosion resistance, since they are cleaned in the mouth and are not as accessible for cleaning as the metal of a removable denture. They should have a moderate fusion temperature around 900–950°C and should freeze as homogeneous solid solutions. Since there is always a thin layer of cement between the inlay and the tooth substance, it is preferable that these alloys be sufficiently soft to allow burnishing. By this means the alloy can be made to cover the thin cement lute and thus shield it from attack and solution by the saliva.

The strength of a cast inlay obviously varies with the bulk which is employed and also upon the amount of support it has from tooth substance. The stronger alloys are hard and cannot be burnished so that the casting technique must produce an accurately fitting inlay.

Soft inlay golds

These alloys usually contain 90–94 per cent of precious metals. They are not amenable to heat hardening and show the following typical properties:

PL	98 N/mm^2
UTS	255 N/mm^2
Mod. of elast.	78 × 10^3 N/mm^2
Elongation	35 per cent
BHN	40–75
Melting range	950–1100°C

Some of the alloys of this type have melting points up to 1200°C. An oxygen-gas torch is therefore necessary to melt them rapidly.

Alloys with a lower precious metal content of 60–70 per cent are also available. These are much stronger and harder but less resistant to corrosion than the alloys which meet the present specified composition limits.

The soft inlay golds are suitable for restorations which are well supported by tooth structure and which do not have to resist large masticatory forces. The high figure of elongation indicates the ease with which this type of gold alloy can be burnished. It also shows how much change of shape by flow can be expected if a large force is applied to the filling. These alloys are suitable for inlays in the non-occluding surfaces of teeth.

Medium inlay golds

These alloys are harder, they resist abrasion and are not distorted by the forces of mastication when they are used in moderately thick sections.

Approximate composition:

Au	78·0 per cent
Ag	12·0 per cent
Cu	7·5 per cent
Pt/Pd	2·0 per cent
Zn	0·5 per cent

An inlay of medium gold is left in the 'as cast' condition as these alloys are not amenable to hardening heat treatment.

Typical properties:

PL	155 N/mm^2
UTS	340 N/mm^2
Mod. of elast.	78×10^3 N/mm^2
Elongation	24 per cent
BHN	70–100
Melting range	920–980°C

As the accuracy of inlay casting techniques has improved, the necessity for a very soft inlay gold has largely disappeared. No longer is it necessary to cover up discrepancies in the fit of an inlay by burnishing its edges. The medium inlay golds therefore find almost universal use for restorations which are of moderate bulk.

Again due to the high cost of gold, alloys with a precious metal content as low as 30 per cent are available. These show good mechanical properties though their elongation is usually a little less than that of the high precious metal alloys.

Hard inlay golds

When strength is required in very thin sections a stronger alloy is used. In some techniques only a thin layer of enamel is removed from the inner or lingual surface of a tooth, and this is replaced by a thin casting. When this type of preparation is used as the support or abutment for one end of a fixed bridge, the thin casting must withstand a considerable amount of stress.

Hard inlay golds contain a greater percentage of Cu, and Pt or Pd, and should be heat hardened before they are cemented into place.

Approximate composition:

Au	75 per cent
Ag	10 per cent
Cu	10 per cent
Pt/Pd	4 per cent
Zn	1 per cent

Typical properties:

	As cast	Heat hardened
PL N/mm²	195	295
UTS N/mm²	360	540
Mod. of elast. N/mm²	78×10^3	83×10^3
Elongation	20 per cent	10 per cent
BHN	90–140	120–170
Melting range	900–1000°C	

Inlays cast in this type of alloy must be made to the highest standards of accuracy, so that the cement lute is as thin as possible. Burnishing of the edges can be carried out before the alloy has been heat hardened, but not after.

Type IV, partial denture yellow gold casting alloys

Cast partial dentures usually include clasps or other devices for retaining the denture which must be flexible and show elastic properties throughout the life of the appliance without permanent distortion. To achieve a sufficiently high proportional limit, more Pt/Pd is present in this type of alloy. This tends to raise the melting point and since these alloys are melted in moderate weights of up to 60 g (2 oz) at a time, it is more convenient if their fusion temperature is within the range of the gas-air blowpipe flame. To achieve this, more Cu and Ag are added to the alloy. This tends to reduce the corrosion resistance. However, the appliances are removed from the mouth for cleaning, and therefore any slight discoloration can be more easily removed than in the case of an inlay which is fixed in a tooth.

The properties of this type of alloy indicate a small capacity for cold work in the soft state, as evidenced by their figure for elongation of 15 per cent. In the hard condition any attempt at altering the shape of the casting will result in fracture, since their elongation may fall to 7 per cent or less.

Approximate composition:

Au	70 per cent
Ag	11 per cent
Cu	12 per cent
Pt/Pd	6 per cent
Zn	1 per cent

Typical properties:

	As cast	Heat hardened
PL N/mm^2	350	590
UTS N/mm^2	490	790
Mod. of elast. N/mm^2	98×10^3	103×10^3
Elongation	15–25 per cent	7 per cent
BHN	130–190	230–290
Melting range	870–950°C	

Alloys with a lower precious metal content are available, usually containing more Pd and often a little Ni. These show mechanical properties often better than those of yellow gold alloys but they are more readily corroded in the mouth. Their cost is lower, and where an appliance is removed and cleaned regularly, the tendency towards corrosion can be accepted. The decision to use such alloys is an economic one and it is advisable to confirm, before using such an alloy, that its mechanical properties are at least as good as those of the Type IV yellow casting alloys.

Gold alloys are also available which are specially designed for use in the making of metal/ceramic structures. These and other alloys suitable for this purpose are discussed in Chapter 10.

WHITE GOLDS

The white golds are essentially alloys of Pd and Ag with only a small percentage of Au.

Typical composition:

Ag	45 per cent
Pd	24 per cent
Au	15 per cent
Cu	15 per cent
Zn	1 per cent

Typical properties in the softened condition:

PL	390 N/mm²
UTS	490 N/mm²
Mod. of elast.	98×10^3 N/mm²
Elongation	12 per cent
BHN	150–200
Melting range	920–1025°C

White gold alloys are lighter than the yellow alloys, having a density approximately two-thirds that of Au. They are sometimes preferred because of their less conspicuous appearance in the mouth. The effect of Pd upon the melting point of silver alloys is not as marked as it is in gold alloys. Nevertheless, the melting point of the white alloys tends to be rather high, as Pd melts at 1549°C. None of the white golds show as precise a melting point as the yellow golds, but fuse over a range of temperature and therefore require more care in melting. Both Pd and Ag adsorb oxygen when they are molten. Care must be taken not to overheat the alloy, or the resultant casting will be porous, due to the liberation of gas after the metal has passed into the mould. A 'noisy' flame with too much air produces sounder castings from some alloys. Borax is generally more suitable than a reducing flux. It should be noted that a denser casting is obtained by centrifugal force, than when using steam or air pressure. During centrifugal casting there is more opportunity for gases to escape compared with the other methods where the gas pressure tends to keep the adsorbed gases within the alloy.

On comparing the properties of the white golds with those for cast yellow denture golds on page 86, it will be noted that the proportional limit of the white golds is well below that of the hardened yellow alloys, and that in the softened condition, their elongation is only slightly greater than that of a hardened yellow gold. This combination of properties indicates that the white golds will fracture in use, and this point is borne out in practice. Thus clasps often fracture after a short period of wear in the mouth. The frequency of fractures may be due partly to the fact that these alloys readily work harden. After an initial bending, the elongation is reduced to a very small figure, so that any further flexure beyond the elasticity of the metal will result in fracture. It has further been suggested that the flexural fatigue strength of white golds is not as high as that for yellow golds.

Heat treatment

White golds are amenable to the same hardening heat treatment as yellow golds, but though this raises the proportional limit, the elongation may be reduced to as little as 2 per cent, and the alloy is exceedingly brittle. It is therefore usual to quench white gold castings quickly from above 750°C and use them in the mouth in the softened condition. With some alloys, a modified hardening heat treatment at 300–350°C for 15 minutes gives increased strength without causing too great a reduction in the value for elongation. After any soldering, or 'fitting' of clasps by bending, the casting must be resoftened at 700–750°C for 5–10 minutes. At temperatures above 850°C, the white golds show very rapid grain growth, and therefore overheating during annealing must be avoided.

Wrought white gold

White gold wire and plate, containing a little more Pd than the casting alloys, is also available. Since palladium alloys respond readily to cold work, it would seem advisable to make the flexible components of a white gold denture from wrought metal and to attach these to a casting of the more rigid and thicker sections.

The white gold alloys tend to discolour in the mouth as the percentage of Au and Pd present is not sufficient to prevent corrosion.

In partial denture construction, white golds can be used for the more simple type of denture. Dentures with numerous thin sections such as continuous clasps, stress breakers, etc., should be constructed in a stronger material.

To conclude, it can be said that white gold alloys are hardly satisfactory for skeleton denture castings, but that they find a limited use for the more simple denture designs where a high degree of strength and elasticity is not essential.

Remelting precious metal alloys

With care in melting, there is little deterioration in the properties of the modern precious metal alloys. At least one-third of a new yellow gold alloy should be used for each 'melt' and for white gold alloys, it is advisable to use 50 per cent of new alloy. Zinc is the main constituent to be lost on remelting. When all the Zn has been oxidized, the other constituent metals are no longer protected by its scavenging action. An addition of new alloy provides the necessary amount of Zn.

Before remelting a button of gold, it should be cleaned by sand-blasting to remove any adherent investment material. It is also preferable to break a large button into small pieces so that fusion takes place more rapidly.

Pickling

Precious metal castings are usually cleaned by placing them in 10 per cent H_2SO_4 at 70–80°C. This is a slightly slower method than dropping the hot casting into HCl but it is less dangerous to the person. Fused $KHSO_4$ may also be used. To remove any acid present on the casting, it may be reheated and quenched in 70 per cent alcohol.

Some silica may remain embedded in the gold and may carry with it plaster from the investment. To remove the silica, the gold may be immersed in HF, taking the usual precautions with this extremely corrosive liquid.

A casting may also be cleaned by electrolytic polishing. It has been suggested that this process could be continued to adjust the dimensions of a slightly oversized inlay, or to make room for the cement lute, particularly over the pulpal floor of the cavity.

Chapter 9
Base metal casting alloys

Whilst the gold alloys show mechanical and working properties very suitable for dental applications, the cost of such alloys has always been high. Consequently attempts are constantly being made to produce base metal alloys which can be used for the casting of partial and other denture bases, for crowns and for inlays.

COBALT-CHROMIUM ALLOYS

Applicable specifications: Brit 3366, 3531; Amer 14; Austral T28.

An alloy of Co and Cr was first introduced to the dental profession in 1929 under the trade name 'Vitallium'. This alloy arose from investigations of Haynes in 1907 who was engaged in finding a durable alloy for the points of car sparking-plugs. Cobalt–chromium alloys show a high resistance to corrosion even at high temperatures, and were used as a material for the turbine blades in jet engines. These alloys are also used for making cutting tools in engineering, and in the engineering world are known as *stellites*.

Their resistance to corrosion is due to the large percentage of Cr present. Chromium quickly forms an inert or 'passive' Cr_2O_3 layer over its surface, and this protects the remainder of the metal from attack.

Compositions vary rather widely but the following indicates the range:

Co	46–65 per cent
Cr	20–35 per cent
Ni	0–10 per cent
Mb	4–6 per cent
C	0·2–0·35 per cent

Other metals such as W, Mn, Fe, Al, Be, Ti, Ta and Si are also present in some alloys.

Effect of constituents

Replacement of part of the Co by Ni causes a loss in strength but an increase in ductility and a decrease in melting temperature. When used for implants, the Ni content should not be above 2·5 per cent but the elongation of the alloy should still be greater than 8 per cent by modification of the other constituents. There is a slight danger of tissue sensitivity to the Ni in the alloy even when it is not embedded but in contact with the mucosa.

Molybdenum reduces the grain size slightly and strengthens the alloy. Tungsten has a similar but lesser effect.

Manganese and Si may be present to act as scavengers and remove oxides and so improve the soundness of the casting. Iron and Al may act in a similar manner. Beryllium is sometimes added but it should be noted this metal is cytotoxic, that is, it poisons living tissue cells. Although Be reduces the grain size and melting point, the resultant alloy should not be used for surgical implants. It has been suggested that there is also possible danger to staff when working with alloys containing Be. Adequate ventilation of the area in which the alloy is melted and at the grinding and polishing areas should be provided.

Carbon has the most important effect. Carbon is always present to a limited extent though its amount may be increased by pick-up during the melting of the alloy. Carbon is only slightly soluble in the solid solution formed between Cr and Co and is usually seen metallographically as a finely dispersed carbide within the solid solution matrix. Since the carbides are associated with the last liquid to freeze, they appear between the dendrites of the cored solid solution. The amount of interdendritic carbide affects the hardness of the alloy. Too much carbide makes the alloy very brittle, particularly if this phase is continuous and not dispersed.

It has been suggested that improvements in the proportional limit and the percentage elongation of Co–Cr alloys can be achieved by the inclusion of Ta or Ti, together with a reduction in carbon. Additions of up to 12 per cent of Ta are claimed to increase the figure for proportional limit and to increase elongation to about 10 per cent. Tantalum forms a new phase, CoTa. This phase forms a relatively large strain field in its area and dislocations have to overcome this 'hurdle' in order to move. Whilst the new phase resists deformation and strengthens the alloy, it does not reduce ductility. Similar claims have been made for the addition of small percentages of Ti. Difficulties arise in making sound castings of the alloys containing Ta and Ti. Whilst under controlled conditions in a research laboratory, specimens can be cast to produce better properties than those in other alloys without Ta or Ti, it is often found in practice that such properties are not always reproducible in normal dental technological practice.

As with gold castings, those of Co–Cr alloys tend to show a rather large grain structure so that a cross-section of a clasp arm, for example, may show only two or three grains. Grain size is reduced by casting at as low a temperature as possible. It is also refined by the addition of trace amounts of Ga or Ir.

Typical properties:

PL	530 N/mm^2
UTS	690 N/mm^2
Mod. of elast.	$200 \times 10^3 \text{ N/mm}^2$
Elongation	3–8 per cent
BHN	370
Melting point	1250–1500°C

Melting point

As the Co–Cr alloys melt at temperatures between 1250 and 1500°C, and also have a higher specific heat than the Au alloys, a more intense source of heat than the gas-air blowpipe is required to melt the alloy quickly and so reduce the time during which oxidation can take place. High-frequency induction is the ideal method of melting these alloys so that their composition is not greatly affected. This method requires expensive equipment and as an alternative an oxy–acetylene flame is used.

The properties of the alloy are affected by the quality of the flame used. An oxidizing flame provides the hottest conditions but will cause too rapid conversion of the alloy into oxide which then appears as inclusions in the casting. This flame has a sharp bluish inner cone surrounded by a small blue enveloping flame. A harsh note is produced by the burning of the gases. A little more acetylene or a reduction in the oxygen creates a neutral flame. This has a short white inner cone with rounded apex which is enveloped by a larger pale blue flame. It is accompanied by a mild hissing sound. The carburizing flame contains too much acetylene. It burns quietly and has a white 'feathering' flame round the blunt inner cone. The carburizing flame will add carbon to the alloy, thus reducing its ductility. This makes clasps and other flexible portions of the casting too brittle.

Overheating can be caused by holding the blowpipe nozzle too near the alloy, and a flame distance of 3-4 inches has been suggested to improve the quality of the resultant casting.

Usually a multi-jet burner is used to cover an area of alloy. This has the slight disadvantage that the individual cones of flame are not identical, those towards the centre being more oxidizing. When melting alloys in a crucible, the flame is also affected by the enclosing effect of the crucible walls, and usually a very slightly carburizing flame provides the best melting conditions.

Casting

A fine grain structure in the completed casting is obtained when the alloy is cast as near to its melting temperature as possible. If the alloy is overheated, a coarse grain size will result and in small dental structures such as clasps the proportional limit will be too low.

A high casting force is required to fill the mould rapidly before solidification occurs. Centrifugal force must be used and the machine must be capable of producing a high initial acceleration.

As already noted, a high carbon content makes the alloy brittle. Alloys supplied for oxy-acetylene melting therefore contain less carbon than those for induction melting, since some carbon pick-up from the flame always occurs.

If the casting is quenched immediately, the carbide remains as a fine dispersion between the dendrites. The resultant structure is moderately strong, but its value for elongation indicates that it can be bent only to a limited extent if necessary. Slower cooling allows further precipitation of carbides to take place in the solid state. These carbides separate out as layers or *lamellae* at the grain boundaries. Since they are precipitated from a solid, they are known as *lamellar eutectoid*. An increase in this component at the grain boundaries improves the strength but reduces the value for elongation. Slow cooling of the casting over several hours, or subsequent ageing at 850°C, are therefore not advised as these treatments render the casting too brittle. Such heat treatments might be applied to thicker structures without clasps. When clasps are present, bench cooling of the casting within an hour appears to be the best compromise.

Remelting

Provided that melting conditions have been carefully controlled, the 'button' of alloy from one casting may be used for another one. Excess carbon or inclusions in this used alloy are not eliminated by remelting, however, and if doubt exists, new alloy should be used.

Only after several remelting procedures is the alloy composition affected, mainly by a loss of Cr. As with gold alloys, some new alloy should be included in each melt.

Finishing the casting

The greatest expense in the fabrication of a Co–Cr partial denture lies in the time which is taken to trim the casting and to polish it. There are two main reasons why the finishing process is difficult.

First, the alloys are extremely resistant to abrasion; indeed, this is one of their great assets when they are used in engineering. In dentistry their abrasion resistance is an asset once the denture has been polished, as the polished surface will be maintained for a long period of wear. The Co–Cr alloys can only be ground by suitable abrasive stones rotating at high speed. In Chapter 29 reference is made to the optimum surface speeds for efficient grinding to take place, and in trimming Co–Cr alloys this optimum must be attained. When using small dental stones of 12 to 3 mm diameter, spindle speeds of 20,000 to 70,000 rpm are necessary. By using larger abrasive wheels, the spindle speed necessary can be reduced.

The second reason for difficulties in finishing is due to the coarse nature of some investment powders. In some techniques, a thin layer of powdered flint, or Zircon ($ZrSiO_4$), suitably bonded, is sprayed on to the wax surface in order to improve the cast metal surface.

After casting, it is usual to sandblast the metal to remove any surface roughness or adherent refractory material and to clean away the oxide film. After a very careful waxing up and investment technique, electrolytic polishing (Chapter 16) may then be carried out. At the first immersion in the bath the thicker sections only should be treated and the clasps covered with a varnish. By this method, no coarse grinding of the broader surfaces of the casting is done, except where sprues are attached. Trimming of the edges and abrading the surfaces with a fine flexible abrasive wheel is all that is necessary before final polishing.

With care during the preliminary stages of construction a denture can be polished in 30–40 minutes, compared with 3–4 hours by a more careless technique.

For final polishing a very high peripheral speed of the polishing buff is essential.

Fracture of Co–Cr dentures

Defects in the casting account for most of the failures of dentures in service. Dirt, or fracture of small pieces of the investment mould are obvious causes of internal defects. Oxidizing conditions of melting increase the number of inclusions. An inert atmosphere such as Ar creates more favourable conditions. Voids may be gaseous or due to contraction. Correct melting conditions and the provision of thick sprues feeding the casting in the direction of centrifugal force are essential. If the design of sprues is such that the alloy is expected to flow 'uphill' against the casting force, an increase in microporosities can be expected.

The Co–Cr solid solution matrix of these alloys is quite ductile. Fracture of a component of a denture can therefore be attributed either to presence of inclusions, to a large precipitation of eutectoid, to a large grain size or to fatigue failure.

The first aim, therefore, is to produce a sound casting and radiography of castings is necessary to ensure this has been achieved. Secondly, either by care in melting or by incorporating other elements, the amount and the bulk of eutectoid precipitate can be reduced. If a large amount of such an incoherent precipitate is present, fracture proceeds readily through the boundary of this continuous brittle phase. Fatigue fracture and fracture after work hardening in a correctly cast alloy both appear to be transcrystalline rather than at the grain boundaries themselves.

ALLOYS FOR PARTIAL DENTURES

An alloy which is suitable for the base of a denture must have a high modulus of elasticity, so that it maintains its shape rigidly under occlusal stresses. It must also have a high proportional limit so that it will not become permanently deformed during wear or whilst it is being cleaned. On the other hand, the clasps which help to hold the denture in place must be flexible so that they do not require the application of too great a force to push them over the bulging tooth contours.

In other words, the alloy for a clasp should possess a lower modulus of elasticity. Yet a clasp alloy must have a high proportional limit too, so that it will display an elastic deformation over a relatively wide range of flexure. Therefore, the only way that one alloy can fulfil these varying requirements is by using it in sufficient bulk for the rigid portions, and in thinner sections where flexibility is required. But the thickness of the metal must not be too critical. For example, an alloy with a very high modulus can be used in relatively small bulk for the base, but retention devices will have to be made very thin indeed to ensure that they are flexible within the range of movement required for a clasp. During the construction of the pattern for a casting, some freehand or non-measurable carving is carried out. It is not easy to maintain accurately the cross-section of a thin piece of metal, as a little error in trimming the pattern or the casting may cause the part to be either too rigid or too weak.

Comparison between yellow cast denture golds and cobalt chromium alloys

When one compares the typical properties of the Type IV yellow gold alloys after heat hardening and the Co–Cr alloys as cast, the following facts emerge:

> Cobalt–chromium alloys have a density less than half that of the gold alloys.
> The modulus of elasticity of Co–Cr alloys is just over twice that of the gold alloys.
> Their proportional limit is the same or slightly less.
> Their percentage elongation is slightly less in many cases.
> Their hardness is almost twice that of the yellow gold alloys.

Thus, for the base of a partial or complete denture, the Co–Cr alloys are very suitable. Not only can they be used in thin sections with adequate stiffness of structure, but they are much lighter in weight. This is an advantage for dentures in the upper jaw, where the force of gravity must be resisted by the retention of the denture. Table 4 gives dimensions for some components of partial dentures which, in clinical use, have shown themselves to be satisfactory.

Table 4. Dimensions of some components of partial dentures

	THICKNESS	WIDTH		
		Co–Cr	Yellow gold	White gold
Palatal bars	mm	mm	mm	mm
	0·8	12·5	20·0	24·0
	0·9	10·0	14·0	18·0
Less than 3 cm long	1·0	8·0	10·0	12·5
	1·1	6·5	9·0	10·0
	0·7	9·0	12·5	16·5
	0·8	5·0	9·0	10·0
More than 3 cm long	0·9	4·5	6·5	8·0
	1·0	*	4·5	5·0

* Not practicable

The following dimensions are for Co–Cr components only:

Lingual bar. Half pear-shaped

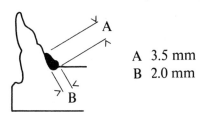

A 3.5 mm
B 2.0 mm

Sublingual bar. Half pear-shaped

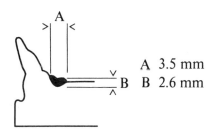

A 3.5 mm
B 2.6 mm

Occlusal rest. Minimum thickness 0.5 mm

The high modulus of elasticity of Co–Cr alloys, however, causes difficulties in the construction of clasps. A clasp of the same cross-section would be much stiffer in Co–Cr than in gold alloy. A greater force would therefore be required to flex the clasp outwards in order to move it over the bulge of the tooth. During this flexion, the stress developed in the Co–Cr alloy would be approximately twice that in the yellow gold alloy since its modulus of elasticity is almost double. But the stress at which the proportional limit of Co–Cr occurs is slightly less than that for gold and therefore there would be a greater chance of permanent deformation of the clasp. In the design of engineering structures, one normally works with a safety factor of at least two. That is, the stress applied at maximum is only half the proportional limit. A Co–Cr clasp may be working to the limit of its elastic properties.

A reduction in thickness decreases the force necessary to push the clasp over the bulge of the tooth but leaves the clasp arm exposed to the dangers of bending during cleaning and handling of the denture. By a reduction of undercut to approximately half that engaged by a gold clasp and also using a slightly thinner cross-section, a clasp of moderate retention and adequate functional life can be designed. The use of very small undercuts, however, requires precise positioning of the clasp arm and this is not always easy to achieve. Consequently, one frequently finds Co–Cr clasps which are either too retentive initially and which lose this retention after a period of wear due to permanent deformation, or alternatively, clasps engaging rather too small an undercut are made and these have barely adequate retentive properties. To control the clasp section accurately, preformed patterns of wax or a polymer are essential for Co–Cr work. The yellow casting golds in the heat hardened condition show the nearest approach to the correct properties for clasps according to our present ideas on the design of these structures.

The best of both worlds, therefore, is to use Co–Cr alloy for the base and connectors and class IV yellow gold alloy for clasps and other retentive devices. Whilst it is possible to solder these structures together, corrosion at the joint is not uncommon and where possible, the gold clasp should be attached to the denture via the polymeric denture base material.

The Co–Cr alloys have a higher hardness than gold alloys and a greater resistance to abrasion; they take and retain a high polish very well indeed. Although the abrasion resistance of the Co–Cr alloys is very high, there is no evidence that they abrade the enamel of the tooth to any significant degree. Any apparent erosion of enamel under clasps is usually due to decalcification in the somewhat stagnant conditions under a clasp arm. As already noted, loss of retention can be attributed mainly to permanent deformation of the clasp arm.

Sometimes difficulties arise with gold alloy dentures when dissimilar metal fillings are present in the teeth. Galvanic currents may be produced and cause discomfort or pain to the patient. Co–Cr alloys show less galvanic activity.

Extreme accuracy of construction of Co–Cr dentures is essential as little adjustment by bending can be done. The alloys show only a small figure for elongation in the 'as cast' state. They also work harden very readily. Thus, after initial bending, their elongation falls to a very low value and the alloy becomes brittle and breaks on further bending. Whereas by suitable softening heat treatment, yellow gold alloy castings can be adjusted where necessary and then their properties restored again by heat hardening.

When a Co–Cr denture is carefully and accurately made, the difficulties of finishing the material can be reduced. But compared with the finishing of gold alloys, more equipment is required. Although the initial cost of the alloy may be as low as one-thirtieth that of yellow gold, the outlay on equipment and length of technique makes the final cost of appliance construction some half to two-thirds of that for a yellow gold denture. The costs of production decrease as the number of dentures increases.

Some Co–Cr alloys are used in metal/ceramic work. They are discussed in Chapter 10.

Wrought wires of Co–Cr alloy are discussed on page 121.

Some patients prefer the appearance of a gold-coloured denture instead of the slightly bluish colour of the Co–Cr alloys. Cobalt–chromium castings can be gilded after an initial layer of Ni has been laid down, though the Au plating does not have a very long clinical life.

NICKEL-CHROMIUM CASTING ALLOYS

Alloys of the following approximate composition:

Ni	75–80 per cent
Cr	15–20 per cent
Si	3·5 per cent
Bo, C, Mn, Fe	2·0 per cent

have the following typical properties:

PL	230 N/mm^2
UTS	600 N/mm^2
Mod. of elast.	220 × 10^3 N/mm^2
Elongation	5–25 per cent
VHN	260
Melting range	1150–1250°C

It will be noted that these alloys have a much lower proportional limit than those based on Co–Cr. Their use for removable partial prostheses is therefore doubtful.

ALUMINIUM BRONZES

Alloys of Cu and Al containing up to 10 per cent of Al are called bronzes although they contain no Sn. Their corrosion resistance is good and it is improved by the presence of Ni. These alloys were developed primarily for marine use where their corrosion-resistant properties are of considerable importance. These properties are due to the formation of a film of Al_2O_3 on the surface which soon 'heals' after scratching. Interest in these alloys was first shown some 35 years ago but they have not yet achieved a wide use. Perhaps one of their main attractions is their golden colour.

Typical composition:

Cu	80 per cent
Al	9·5 per cent
Ni	4·5 per cent
Fe	5·0 per cent
Mn	1·0 per cent

Typical properties:

UTS	720 N/mm^2
Mod. of elast.	125 × 10^3 N/mm^2
Elongation	18–30 per cent
BHN	Soft 120–170
	Hard 230–300
Melting range	1055–1080°C

Whilst a gas-air torch is just adequate to melt the allow, oxy–acetylene or induction melting is faster. Linear casting shrinkage is approximately 2·5 per cent and therefore some difficulty arises in obtaining precise castings. The alloy can be hardened by heat treatment at 500–650°C for 1–2 hours. It can be soldered with a high carat gold solder. During clinical use, the alloys quickly lose their polish and in some circumstances, the oral corrosion is unacceptable. Successful electroplating with a Sn–Ni alloy has been reported.

BASE METAL ALLOYS FOR INLAYS AND CROWNS

A copper alloy containing Zn, Ni, In and Co shows the following properties:

PL	185 N/mm²
UTS	462 N/mm²
Mod. of elast.	92 × 10³ N/mm²
Elongation	15 per cent
BHN	95–100

This alloy shows a rather high casting shrinkage but it can be cast with accuracy into a gypsum-bonded mould which is expanded both hygroscopically and thermally using cristobalite investment. In tissue compatibility tests, it was shown to have satisfactory histocompatibility. In clinical use, it can be readily burnished to the cavity margins, giving a good marginal finish to the restoration. It can be used for inlays and for short pontic fixed bridge restoration. It has a similar application to white golds in the construction of partial dentures. That is, a somewhat thicker section than normal has to be used.

Alloys of 75–85 per cent Sn with Ag or Sb have also been used for inlays. The alloys melt at 225–360° and are relatively easy to cast with accuracy. They are unfortunately extremely weak and brittle and because of their relatively poor mechanical properties, have not been successful. In general, dental amalgams have better properties.

Chapter 10
Alloys for metal/ceramic structures

Dental porcelain, described in Chapter 30, has excellent aesthetic and compressive properties but is very easily fractured in tension. In addition, precision of fit of a porcelain restoration is difficult to achieve. Hence the development of the metal/ceramic restoration which consists of a core or thimble of a suitable alloy veneered with porcelain (Fig. 35). The core is strong and fits well, whilst the porcelain veneer resembles tooth substance.

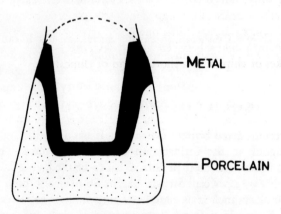

Fig. 35. Section of metal/ceramic jacket crown

For use as a core, an alloy must possess certain properties. It must be cast readily and precisely by the relatively simple dental techniques. The temperature at which the alloy anneals must be above the fusing temperature of the porcelain so that the casting maintains its shape and does not sag or creep during the relatively long heating cycle necessary to fuse the porcelain veneer. The alloy should bond with the porcelain veneer other than by simple mechanical retention, that is, ionic bonds or van der Waals' bonds should be formed. So that the core can be made of thin section, the alloy should have mechanical properties similar to those of class III yellow gold alloys in the heat hardened state and like the yellow gold alloys, should show some heat hardening effect at or below the temperature at which the porcelain is fused. For preference, however, the modulus of elasticity should be greater than that of gold alloys and similar to that of the Co–Cr alloys. In addition, the coefficient of thermal expansion of the alloy should be the same or slightly greater than that of the porcelain veneer. When the porcelain has a slightly lower coefficient of expansion than the metal core, it is subjected to a small compressive stress on cooling. The application of a subsequent tensile stress reduces the compressive stresses without creating tensile stresses against which porcelain shows but little strength.

Three types of alloy are in use today. The first type to be developed was a high content Au alloy. The second types of alloy which are whiter in colour are based on Pt or Pd and the third, more recently developed alloys, are based on Ni–Cr. Some Co–Cr alloys are also used. The alloys are usually designed for use with a particular porcelain, though in some cases more than one porcelain has compatible properties. If incompatibility between alloy and porcelain is present, the veneer flakes or chips after a short period of clinical use.

GOLD COLOURED ALLOYS

A high precious metal content is necessary since the porcelains fuse at temperatures up to 1000°C. Platinum and Pd raise the fusion temperature. Tin, Ni or Cu may be added to produce a bond with the porcelain. Nickel and Cu, however, produce a green discolouration at the junction line and Sn is preferred. Indium is usually present to produce a fine grain size and also to assist in bonding. Iron may be present to take advantage of a heat hardening effect due to $FePt/FePt_3$ phase changes. A typical composition might be:

Au	84–89 per cent
Pt/Pd	5–14 per cent
Zn	1 per cent
In	0·5 per cent
Fe	0·5 per cent
Sn	0·5 per cent

Other alloys contain 12–15 per cent Ag.

Typical properties:

	Annealed	Heat hardened
PL N/mm^2	300	400
UTS N/mm^2	490	520
Mod. of elast.	80–85 × 10^3 N/mm^2	
Elongation	5 per cent	2 per cent
BHN	140–160	170–180
Bond strength	30–75 N/mm^2	
Melting range	1200°–1500°C	

The melting point of these alloys usually demands the use of a phosphate-bonded investment. In some circumstances, however, gypsum-bonded refractories are suitable. It has been suggested, however, that the use of gypsum-bonded refractories can lead to a weakening of some alloys due to the formation of Pd_4S on the breakdown of gypsum at higher temperatures. The alloys usually have a coefficient of thermal expansion of about 10–14 × 10^{-6}/°C and the porcelains for use with such alloys usually have a difference of only 1–2 × 10^{-6}/°C in thermal expansion. The alloys are not easy to cast since their melting temperature is fairly high. A gas/oxygen flame is used when induction melting is not available. On melting alloys containing Fe by gas/oxygen flame, there is a marked reduction in Fe content, greater than that which occurs on induction melting. At least 33 per cent of new alloy should be used for each melt. Sag or distortion of castings may occur at the temperature of porcelain fusion. Marginal adaptation at the edge of a crown is usually affected more if a chamfer is used rather than a shoulder preparation.

In the as-cast state, the structure is usually dendritic, showing marked evidence of coring. On veneering the alloy with porcelain, most of the alloys undergo homogenization. Since, however, they are not strain hardened, there is no change in the grain structure itself.

It will be noted that the properties of this type of alloy are not as good as those of the type III golds in the hardened condition. The absence of Cu from the constituents means that precipitation and order hardening due to a Cu-Au phase, cannot take place. Some of these alloys soften with the heat treatment received during porcelain fusing but can be hardened afterwards. Others harden at the temperature used for applying the porcelain veneer. If the alloys are not amenable to precipitation hardening due to $FePt/FePt_3$ transformations, then the properties of this type of alloy are not ideal for intraoral use and they must be employed in moderately thick sections. For example, rapid wear of the alloy may occur where it is subject to high masticatory forces. In addition, distortion of the base under occlusal stress will inevitably lead to fracture of the porcelain veneer. In the construction of a bridge, therefore, those components which are not to be veneered with porcelain should be constructed from a type III gold alloy and soldered to the gold/ceramic components. This can be carried out in a furnace, or with care by using a gas/air blowtorch. Slow warming up and cooling of the invested components is essential.

WHITE COLOURED ALLOYS

These vary widely in composition. Some have a moderate Au content of up to 50 per cent. Others are mainly Pd and Ag with small amounts of Ru, In and Sn. Others are Pt–Ir alloys. The properties vary somewhat. Some show heat hardening effects at the porcelain firing temperatures due to the formation of intermetallic compounds containing Sn or In.

In general, these alloys fuse at a much higher temperature than the gold-coloured alloys, thus giving a greater margin of safety on fusing the porcelain. Their high melting temperature necessitates the use of phosphate-bonded investment materials but the alloys can be melted with a gas/oxygen flame. Difficulties arise in making accurate castings in these higher fusing alloys and this limits the breadth of their application in general dental laboratories.

NICKEL-CHROMIUM ALLOYS

Because of the high cost of the Au and Pt/Pd based alloys, various Ni–Cr alloys are available. Some alloys are based simply on Ni 80 per cent, Cr 20 per cent. Others have a more complex formulation indicated by the following:

Ni	40–80 per cent
Cr	10–18 per cent
Co	1–11 per cent
Fe	2–4 per cent
Al	0–2 per cent

Mo	2 per cent
Pd	0–25 per cent
Si	0·5–1·0 per cent
Be	1·2–1·6 per cent

plus traces of Ag, Cu, Mn, Ti.

Typical properties:

PL	550–600 N/mm²
UTS	800–900 N/mm²
Mod. of elast.	180–200 × 10³ N/mm²
Elongation	3–15 per cent
BHN	280–350
Bond strength	25–100 N/mm²

The base metal alloys, therefore, are stronger, harder and have a higher modulus of elasticity than the gold alloys but have a similar value for elongation. Some alloys harden on heating between 600–800°C with a maximum effect at about 700°C. After this treatment, their elongation reduces quite markedly. For some alloys, an elongation as high as 20 per cent is claimed, reducing to 10 per cent on heat hardening. Other alloys soften a little during the fusion cycle.

Some of these alloys are difficult to cast with accuracy, particularly in thin sections. In general, however, they do allow the use of thinner castings than is possible with the other alloys from a structural point of view. Due to limitation on the amount of tooth substance which can be removed from a vital tooth, there are therefore advantages in the use of these stiffer base-metal alloys. However, the design of the metal substructure is important in ensuring sufficient strength and rigidity. For example, extra thickness round the neck of a tooth is possible, as is thickening on the lingual or palatal surfaces.

One of the main advantages of the base metal alloys is that they show less 'sag' at the porcelain fusion temperature. Unless a relatively large bulk of the gold based alloys is present, then a long structure such as a bridge may deform under its own weight at the temperature at which the porcelain is fused. This does not happen to the same extent when one uses the base metal alloys.

Most of these alloys require the use of the more refractory phosphate-bonded type though some can be cast into gypsum-bonded investment moulds. Whilst accurate castings can be made, suitable for inlays and crowns, the technique is not as simple as that for gold alloys. An investment of high strength and high thermal expansion is required.

Some investment materials are mixed with a silica suspension to increase their strength and also the setting and thermal expansions of the mould. A total setting and thermal linear expansion of the order of 1·5–1·7 per cent is necessary for accurate castings to be produced. In addition, with some alloys, thermal expansion of the wax pattern is also necessary in an attempt towards achieving compensation for thermal shrinkage of the alloy. A very fine grained refractory is necessary. It is essential to remove air from the investment mix by vacuum and to vibrate the material into position. The viscosity of the mix should also be somewhat lower than that usually employed when making refractory moulds for cast Co–Cr dentures. When using fine-grained phosphate-bonded investments, back pressure effects are reduced by scraping the layer of more compact investment from the base of the ring as well as by restricting the thickness of investment between the pattern and the end of the ring to 3–4 mm. Overheating of the alloy must be avoided.

After casting, the work is trimmed, preferably with the use of porcelain-bonded abrasives and is then prepared to obtain a bond with the porcelain veneer.

THE METAL/CERAMIC BOND

The strength of the joint between the metal core and the porcelain veneer appears to have three component factors. These are mechanical retention, adhesion and retention by compression of the porcelain by the alloy surrounding it.

After the casting has been trimmed to shape, preferably by the use of porcelain bonded abrasives, the surface is sandblasted. This increases the surface area available for bonding, provides some mechanical retention, as well as producing a clean metal surface. Sandblasting is preferred to pickling in acid as some acid or salts may remain on the surface of the alloy. The use of a sandblasting grit of size 80 appears to produce the most suitable roughness of surface. A very rough surface, for example that produced by a file, may leave grooves which are incompletely filled by the porcelain, so reducing the area of contact and leaving voids at the interface. At the sharp edges of ridges left from filing the metal surface, stress accumulation may occur leading to fracture of the porcelain during service.

Good wetting of the metal base by the porcelain is essential and the contact angle at the firing temperatures should be low. The difficulty is one of producing a frit which flows readily at the firing temperature so that good bonding is achieved, yet one which retains the carved shape required in the finished article.

Adhesion plays probably the most important part in the strength of the metal/ceramic bond. It is produced via the oxides on the surface of the metal core and those present as pigments within the porcelain veneer. In the high gold content alloys, diffusion of Sn and In occurs across the interface. With base metal alloys, bonding is by Ni, Cr and Mn oxides. These oxides have uneven, electrical charge distribution and van der Waals' forces act between these permanent dipoles. However, covalent and ionic bonds also contribute to the strength of the bond, particularly in the case of the gold based alloys.

Some manufacturers advocate the use of a *bonding agent* which is fired on to the casting before applying the porcelain veneer. With gold alloys, this is probably a colloidal suspension of gold, together with other alloying elements. This layer bonds to the casting and also provides mechanical attachment and oxide bonding to the porcelain. The bonding agents also assist in producing an oxide film of even colour all over the surface of the casting. This creates a uniform colour background for the porcelain.

All cast alloys have adsorbed gases present and unless these are removed, they will be released when the porcelain is being fired on to the surface of the metal under vacuum. After sandblasting, therefore, the casting is degassed at 900–1000°C under a partial vacuum for 10–15 minutes. A high degree of vacuum is ideal but the degree of vacuum obtained in normal dental furnaces appears to be adequate. If an attempt is made to fuse porcelain at a reduced atmospheric pressure on to a metal core which is not degassed, bubbles of gas appear at the interface and prevent wetting by the porcelain, giving a poor bond. Degassing and oxidation of the surface layer take place at the same time and the surface is then ready for the porcelain. When once an oxide film has been produced, the surface should not be contaminated in any way. It should not be touched either by the fingers or with instruments. Only the surfaces which are not to be veneered should be handled.

The bond strength increases if degassing and porcelain firing are done in an inert atmosphere. Argon and hydrogen have been recommended.

In general, multiple firing as the crown is gradually built up gives better bonding than when a single firing technique is used.

It has been suggested that the strength of the bond between alloys containing Cr and a porcelain veneer is affected markedly by the presence of Cr_2O_3. Even if an inert atmosphere is used when firing the porcelain, the formation of this oxide increases stress at the alloy/ceramic interface and contributes to bond failure. The inclusion of Cr_2O_3 in a porcelain frit reduces its coefficient of thermal expansion to a level at which it is incompatible with the alloy. In addition, the green colouration produced can be wrongly attributed to the use of too thin a veneer of porcelain and the assumption that one can see the metal beneath. Some base metal alloy/ceramic systems, however, appear to have overcome these difficulties of bonding and bond strengths have been reported which are higher than those of gold alloy/ceramic systems. Variations in the values given for bond strength are related to the method used to determine this property. Only time will tell whether the system of bonding being used will withstand the stresses imposed on these relatively delicate structures during use.

Developments in the nickel–chromium type of alloy appear to be taking place towards the development of a suitable casting alloy for inlays and crowns with or without porcelain veneers which might eventually replace the yellow gold casting alloys whose price has now become almost prohibitive.

Modified Co–Cr alloys are also available which can be used for metal/ceramic constructions. However, the accuracy of casting appears to be higher and the bond appears to be better with the Ni–Cr alloys.

Chapter 11
Steels

Steel is an alloy of Fe with C which usually contains less than 2·0 per cent of the latter element. Alloys containing more than this amount of C are known as *cast irons* and do not show the inherent strength of steel.

The changes which occur in the manipulation of steels and in their metallographic structure have been the subject of a very large amount of study, and no attempt will be made to cover them in detail.

The equilibrium diagram of alloys between Fe and C is a little complex. Figure 36 is a simplified version of part of the diagram. It

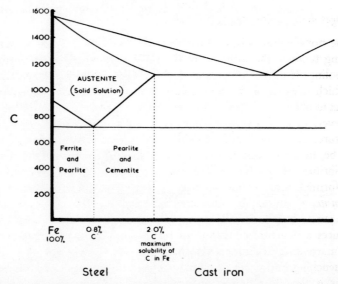

Fig. 36. Simplified thermal equilibrium diagram for alloys between Fe and low percentages of C

shows that C is soluble in the high temperature (face-centred cubic) form of Fe up to a maximum of 2 per cent, forming an interstitial solid solution known as *austenite*. On cooling, the solubility of C reduces with temperature, until at 723°C, the austenite contains 0.8 per cent C. At this temperature the solid solution austenite breaks down to form a mixture of two components, one containing virtually no C and the other being rich in C. The first component is the low temperature (body-centred cubic) form of Fe, termed *ferrite*, and the other an intermetallic compound Fe_3C, known as *cementite*.

This structure is like a eutectic, but since it is produced in the solid state, it ii known as a eutectoid.

A steel containing 0.8 per cent of C is the eutectoid steel, and appears metallographically as an intimate mechanical mixture of ferrite and cementite. During the preparation of this material for micro-examination, the ferrite is removed more rapidly than the harder Fe_3C, giving the specimen a ridged surface. At low magnifications, the diffraction and diffusion of light from this undulating surface produces a play of colours similar to that seen with mother-of-pearl. For this reason the eutectoid structure is called *pearlite*.

Changes during quick cooling (Quenching)

In the non-ferrous alloys which were discussed in Chapter 8, quick cooling retained the structure of the alloy as it existed at the instant of cooling. If a mass of carbon steel is cooled from the temperature at which it exists in the solid solution or austenitic state, we might expect to obtain a solid solution type of grain structure. It is impossible, however, to cool a plain carbon steel so as to retain the austenitic structure. Even during rapid cooling, some austenite transforms. There may be, however, insufficient time available for the formation of the equilibrium phases ferrite and cementite. Instead, the austenite is transformed into a body-centred tetragonal structure known as *martensite*, which may be considered as ferrite distorted by the presence of excess C in solution. Thus, rapid cooling of a plain carbon steel produces a structure consisting of retained austenite and martensite. This martensitic structure is very hard but may be brittle.

Quenching into water or oil may be used to produce rapid cooling. Water is the most drastic quenching medium, but the quenching stresses superimposed on the transformation stresses may cause cracking or distortion. Oil is less severe in this respect, producing a less brittle product.

Tempering

In the quenched condition, the modulus of elasticity of a steel is very high and its hardness and strength are maximal. However, thin sections such as the cutting edge of a bur or chisel would be brittle and would chip readily when pressed against a material such as tooth enamel. The adjustment of the hardness of the steel to suit the purpose for which it is to be used is called tempering. This consists of reheating the hardened steel up to a relatively low temperature, holding for a short period of time, and then cooling it rapidly from this temperature. The changes brought about depend on the tempering temperature. At temperatures up to 200°C relief of the internal stresses associated with quenching occurs.

PLAIN CARBON STEELS

These are used for making dental instruments and parts of dental equipment which must be strong without being of large bulk. Carbon steel instruments can be ground to a sharp edge and, because of the high modulus of elasticity and high proportional limit of the steel, will maintain this edge over a long period of use.

Plain carbon steels find only a limited use for dental hand instruments today because they corrode too easily. Some carbon steel instruments are chromium-plated except at the cutting edge or point. When cutting instruments are to be sterilized by boiling them in water, some corrosion resistance is desirable. However, for surgical knives and other cutting instruments where extreme keenness of the edge is essential, carbon steels are still used as their edge-strength is greater than that of the corrosion-resistant alloys. Corrosion of steel instruments during sterilization is reduced if film-forming amines are added to the water used in an autoclave. Neutralizing amines such as cyclohexylamine in a concentration of only 0·1 per cent not only form a monomolecular protective layer on the surface of steels, but also neutralize the acidity of the atmosphere inside the autoclave by combining with the CO_2 present.

These steels are tempered at a low heat, and if an instrument or knife is ground on a dry grindstone without cooling water, the heat evolved will raise the temperature of the thin cutting edge above its correct tempering heat. This makes the edge soft and it will not cut. To reharden such an instrument, heat it to red heat (750°C) and quench. Then clean the surface and temper at 230°C or until the steel assumes a pale straw colour.

ALLOY STEELS

Applicable specifications: ISO R 1795, 2157; Brit 2965, 4178; Amer 23; Austral 1086.

Today, small amounts of Cr and other metals are usually added to the steel of most dental cutting instruments. Chromium increases tensile strength, proportional limit and hardness, whilst rendering the alloy a little more resistant to corrosion. In a chromium alloy steel for a cutting instrument, the amount of C present would be such as to make a hypereutectoid steel, i.e. one containing more than 0·8 per cent C. For instruments which must be less brittle a hypoeutectoid or eutectoid steel would be used. The amount of Cr present in such steels is usually only 0·5 to 1 per cent, and its effect in reducing corrosive attack is not very great.

Other alloy steels contain Ni, W, Co, Mn or Si in small amounts in order to make them suitable for particular purposes. The number of alloy steels is so great that it presents a subject in itself. Usually the addition of an alloying element to steel alters the temperature at which changes within the steel take place. Therefore, it is extremely difficult for the dentist or technician to heat treat an alloy steel correctly unless he knows its composition and is aware of its correct heat treatment. The best way of avoiding trouble with steel instruments and equipment is never to overheat them. When grinding or sharpening a cutting instrument, the abrasive wheel should be wet and the instrument applied to it for only short periods of time. This is particularly important in surgery instruments, as these are of only thin section and heat up rapidly on grinding.

Chapter 12
Wrought base metal alloys. Stainless steels

STAINLESS STEELS

Applicable specifications: Brit 2965, 2983, 3507, 3531, 4106, 4681, 4750, 5211; Austral T24, T32, T42, 1086, 1264.

If sufficient Cr is added to steel it resists corrosive attack. When adding Cr only, at least 13 per cent is necessary to render a steel stainless for general use.

The important discovery of the value of adding Cr to steel was made accidentally by Brearley of Sheffield in 1913. The stainless steels resulting from this work were first developed for the manufacture of table cutlery, but they have since been applied to a great variety of purposes where resistance to corrosion is required.

Composition

Two types of stainless steel are in general use: first those in which the austenitic solid solution breaks down on cooling, in a manner similar to carbon and alloy steels, and secondly those in which the solid solution remains at room temperature. The first, or martensitic, type can be hardened by heat treatment, while the austenitic variety only harden by cold work. The difference between the two types of stainless steel lies in the amount of Cr, Ni and C which each contains.

Nickel lowers markedly the temperature at which the austenite decomposes, besides imparting strength and corrosion resistance to the alloy. Chromium slows down the speed at which austenite breaks down on quenching and also causes a eutectoid to be formed at a smaller carbon percentage than occurs in plain carbon steels. When a sufficient amount of both Ni and Cr is present, their effects combine to slow the breakdown of austenite. In steels containing more than

18 per cent of Cr, 8 per cent of Ni and less than 0·1 per cent of C, rapid cooling completely suppresses any breakdown, so that a fully austenitic alloy is obtained at room temperature. A similar effect is obtained with 12 per cent of each metal.

The solid solution or austenitic type of steel is unsuitable for making cutting instruments as its physical properties can only be improved by cold work. Even in the work hardened state it is not suitable for making a sharp cutting edge. For this reason stainless steels of the hardenable type containing less Cr and little or no Ni are used for dental cutting instruments while the more highly corrosion-resistant steels are used for mixing and other non-cutting instruments.

Hardenable stainless steels are available in two main types. These are plain chromium steels and high chromium–low nickel steels.

Plain chromium steels

These have a varying C content which controls their hardness. The greater the amount of C the harder and stronger the steel.

A chromium steel which finds an application in the manufacture of dental instruments is *modified cutlery steel*. This contains approximately 0·65 per cent C and 16·5 per cent Cr, and combines corrosion resistance with a good cutting edge. It is heat treated by oil quenching from 1000°C, followed by tempering. This may be carried out at a temperature only a little above 200°C. During sterilization, therefore, dental instruments such as probes must never be heated over 200°C. Good control of the temperature of autoclaves or dry heat sterilizers is essential.

Martensitic stainless steels

Other hardenable stainless steels contain Ni. A typical composition would be Cr 16·5 per cent, Ni 2·5 per cent, Carbon 0·16 per cent. Its corrosion resistance is superior to the lower chromium stainless steels. After quenching from 950–1000°C, the steel is tempered at 400–650°C.

This type of steel is used for some hypodermic needles because of its corrosion resistance and high edge strength. This alloy, however, work hardens readily and fractures easily when bent. Bent needles should never be straightened or used again as they might fracture on reinsertion in the patient's tissues.

During recent years, semi-austenitic stainless steels have been developed which have excellent corrosion resistance, can be worked readily, yet which can be precipitation hardened.

Typical composition:

Cr	17·0 per cent
Ni	7·0 per cent
Al	1·0 per cent
C	0·1 per cent

After a solution heat treatment at 1000°C these steels are austenitic in structure and work readily. This austenitic structure can be broken down to a martensitic one by a precipitation hardening heat treatment at 450–600°C.

AUSTENITIC STAINLESS STEELS

For all dental instruments which do not require a cutting edge, and for dental equipment such as bowls and sterilizers, resistance to corrosion is more important than mechanical strength and hardness. Steels for this purpose contain sufficient Cr and Ni to prevent the decomposition of austenite on rapid cooling.

The austenitic stainless steels show a simple pure metal grain structure, and slip occurs readily. The alloys are extremely malleable and ductile. On cold working, their mechanical properties improve very rapidly indeed. They are readily workable and resist corrosion extremely well due to the formation of a tenacious passivating layer of Cr_2O_3.

18–8 stainless steel

Austenitic stainless steels are known by various trade-names and reference numbers, but this type of alloy is generally known as 18–8 stainless steel. These numbers refer to the amounts of Cr and Ni present in their composition. The amount of C present is usually less than 0·1 per cent.

These steels show the following typical properties:

	Soft	Work hardened by rolling, swaging, etc.	Hard drawn wire
PL N/mm²	275	1080	1850
UTS N/mm²	590	1180	1950
Mod. of elast. N/mm² ($\times 10^3$)	195	195	225
Elongation	50 per cent	6 per cent	1 per cent
BHN	170	250	350

The great reduction in the figure for elongation shows the extent to which these steels are affected by cold work. Though the improvement in the strength of the metal which accompanies this change is an advantage in the finished appliance, the rate at which work hardening takes place sometimes causes difficulties in shaping the metal.

The manipulation of 18–8 stainless steel

For dental use these steels are supplied in the form of sheet, wire or ribbon. Sheet metal is purchased in a fairly soft condition while wire and ribbon may be obtained either hard, moderately soft or fully softened. Except for wire in the fully softened condition, the material is usually highly polished so that final polishing of an appliance should not be a lengthy procedure.

The only satisfactory method of forming sheet stainless steel to make a denture is to change its shape swiftly in one movement. Slow changes in shape by beating or swaging are unsatisfactory since work hardening makes further changes in shape difficult to achieve. A hydraulic press and metal dies may be used, but hydraulic forming is preferable. High oil pressures are used to shape the sheet stainless steel to a die of artificial stone or a polymer such as polyester or epoxide. When forming curves of short radius, i.e. deep palates, an intermediate anneal may be necessary.

Annealing 18–8 stainless steel

In circumstances where a great deal of cold work has to be done, it may be necessary to recrystallize the stainless steel and so enable further slip to take place.

Austenitic stainless steel is a solid solution of iron, nickel, chromium and carbon. If this structure is heated between 400 and 900°C, Cr_4C precipitates out and forms at the grain boundaries. This causes a loss of Cr from the solid solution adjacent to the grain boundaries, rendering these regions more susceptible to corrosion. In a corrosive environment the grain boundaries are rapidly attacked, and on stressing the material, it may then disintegrate.

This effect on the austenitic stainless steels when they are heated between 400 and 900°C is known as *weld-decay*. When large pieces of stainless steel are joined together in engineering construction, the welded joint is heated above 900°C. The metal at the join is therefore not subject to weld-decay. But on either side of the weld the temperature to which the metal is heated is much lower and a strip of metal here will be susceptible to weld-decay. Hence the origin of the term.

The amount of weld-decay which takes place can be reduced in two ways. First, a reduction in the carbon content of the steel will create less favourable conditions for carbide precipitation. Unfortunately, a low carbon stainless steel is not economical to manufacture. Secondly, metals such as Ti or Nb can be added to the steel. These metals will form carbides in preference to the chromium in the weld-decay temperature range, and their carbides are not precipitated in the grain boundaries. The Cr remains in solution so that the corrosion resistance of the steel is unimpaired. Such steels are known as *stabilized stainless steels*.

To soften cold worked stainless steel and produce recrystallization, it is heated to 950–1050°C for a few minutes. Thorough degreasing and cleaning is essential before heating to prevent contamination of the surface and subsequent corrosion. The recommended method is to boil the steel in a 10 per cent NaOH solution followed by thorough washing in hot water. When steel has been worked to its limit of malleability, there is a danger of spontaneous cracking due to the relief of stress, if the metal is placed in a hot furnace. It is therefore preferable to place the steel in a cold furnace. After heating, the steel is quenched in water. Annealing causes the surface of the steel to oxidize unless the furnace is filled with an inert gas. The metal is pickled in a solution such as:

10 per cent by volume commercial HNO_3

$3\frac{1}{2}$ per cent by volume commercial (60 per cent) HF

$86\frac{1}{2}$ per cent H_2O

The high polish which was originally present on the surface of the sheet metal is therefore lost during annealing, and more time is required to finish the denture ready for the mouth. Also some loss of corrosion resistance is evident unless great care is taken to ensure the correct annealing temperature. Annealing should therefore only be resorted to when difficulties occur during the swaging of a stainless steel denture base. It is inadvisable to attempt to anneal stainless steels in a blowpipe flame. A pyrometrically controlled furnace should be used.

Stainless steel wire

The manipulation of wire and ribbon for making orthodontic appliances involves various degrees of cold work and a material in a suitably annealed state should be chosen. Wires are sold in soft, half-hard, hard and spring temper grades. Hard stainless steel wires can be worked to a limited extent, but numerous alterations in the shape of a piece of wire must be avoided. If the steel is overworked, it will break when any further adjustment of the appliance is carried out. The amount of cold work is frequently not the same throughout the length of a wire forming part of an appliance. Where a sharp loop or bend has been formed, large stresses will remain. If this portion is adjusted later it may fracture. A stress-relief anneal at 370–450°C for 1–2 minutes reduces the possibility of fracture on further cold work. With some wires, this heat treatment also improves their elastic properties. The lower temperature is preferable as it avoids the possibility of weld-decay.

The tensile strength and proportional limit of hard stainless steel wires generally increases as their diameter decreases, due to the greater work hardening effect on drawing the thinner wires. The modulus of elasticity, however, rises very little.

The modulus of elasticity of stainless steel is twice that of gold orthodontic wires. An orthodontic spring is designed to apply a small constant force to a tooth in order to move it, and therefore to apply a similar force, a stainless steel spring is made of thinner wire than a gold one. Ideally, a spring should apply the same force throughout a wide range of movement so that repeated adjustment of the spring due to tooth movement is not necessary. Because of its higher modulus of elasticity, and the use of a thinner gauge wire, the stainless steel wire only applies its force over a small range of movement and so requires frequent adjustment.

WROUGHT NICKEL–CHROMIUM WIRES

On soldering thin stainless steel wires some loss of elasticity takes place due to recrystallization above 700°C. In a small mass of metal such as a thin wire, softening will take place very rapidly after a few seconds at temperatures between 700 and 800°C. Many silver solders melt at or near 700°C, and gold solders fuse at temperatures up to 870°C. If the soldering time is at all prolonged, sufficient softening of a stainless steel wire will take place to make it unsuitable for use as an orthodontic arch wire or spring. Turbine silver solders fuse at slightly lower temperatures, usually between 570 and 700°C. These reduce the degree of annealing which takes place, but it is difficult to control accurately the heating of a thin wire, and overheating can readily take place when soldering a thin wire to a thicker one.

A wire made of an alloy of Ni and Cr possesses good mechanical properties in the work hardened state. The alloy used is *nichrome*, composed of 80 per cent Cr with 20 per cent of Ni. This alloy has a high electrical resistance, and is used in the form of wire or tape for the elements of electric heaters. Nickel and Cr form a series of solid solutions, but the alloy is rather expensive to manufacture. For this reason 15–25 per cent of Fe is often added when making electric elements. Nickel–chromium alloys are also used for base metal thermocouples.

For dental purposes, the simple Ni–Cr alloy is preferred. Its corrosion resistance in the mouth is excellent. This is due to the passivity of the Cr coupled with the low galvanic activity of Ni.

Typical properties:

	Hard drawn
PL	1190 N/mm^2
UTS	1240 N/mm^2
Mod. of elast.	215 × 10^3 N/mm^2
Elongation	1 per cent
BHN	200–220

Nichrome wire work hardens in a manner similar to stainless steel, and no hardening heat treatment is possible. Annealing of nichrome wires may be carried out at 850–1050°C, but usually wires are purchased in a moderately hard condition, so that a small amount of cold work can be performed without the necessity for annealing. Like stainless steel, this wire will fracture if it is work hardened to too great an extent.

After a stress-relief anneal at 450–480°C for 2–3 minutes, these alloys show an improvement in proportional limit, tensile strength and modulus of elasticity, with a marked decrease in ductility.

The recrystallization temperature of nichrome is above the melting point of both silver and gold solders, and therefore little change in mechanical properties occurs on normal soldering. Even if soldering takes ten minutes—an excessive time—the mechanical properties fall by only a third.

OTHER WROUGHT WIRES

Wires of Co–Cr alloy are also used both for clasps and for orthodontic appliance construction. They may be soldered together in a manner similar to stainless steel and Ni–Cr wires, and like Ni–Cr wires, are not so easily softened during soldering. One alloy contains approximately 16 per cent Fe with a low C content of 0·15 per cent. The alloy can be annealed by a solution treatment at 1150°C followed by quenching. Strength and hardness are increased by heating the wire at 450–480°C.

Typical properties:

	Hard drawn
PL	980 N/mm²
UTS	1700 N/mm²
Mod. of elast.	165 × 10³ N/mm²
Elongation	1 per cent
VHN	250–400
Fatigue limit	32 per cent of tensile

An alloy of Ti–Ni containing equiatomic amounts of each metal exists as an intermetallic compound with unusual properties. It has a modulus of elasticity of 69 × 10³ N/mm², being less than one-third of that of hard stainless steel. It has a relatively high proportional limit and therefore exhibits the properties required for an orthodontic spring in that it applies a relatively small force over a large range of movement. The alloy also has the unusual property of returning to its original shape after being bent if it is heated at relatively low temperatures.

Chapter 13
Tungsten carbide

Applicable specifications: ISO R 1795, ISO 2157; Brit 4178; Amer 23.

For many years, dental burs have been made from carbon and alloy steels. Although a blade of this metal will cut tooth dentine satisfactorily, it shows little capacity for cutting the harder tooth enamel, and it rapidly becomes blunted in the attempt. Similarly, during cavity preparation it is often necessary to trim an edge of enamel with a sharp hand instrument or chisel. Most hand instruments are made from alloy steels containing Cr, but these do not maintain a good cutting edge against a hard material such as tooth enamel.

Tungsten carbide (WC) is an exceedingly hard and high-fusing compound. For use in cutting instruments, 'sintered' carbide is used This consists of fine carbide particles embedded in a matrix of pure Co. Small amounts of Ti or Ta carbides may be present also. As may be expected from such a composite structure, the less the percentage of Co and the finer the tungsten carbide grains, the harder will be the material. Sintered WC is made by the process known as powder metallurgy. If finely divided metals are compressed and heated, they will join together at a temperature lower than their normal fusion point. The mechanism of fusion in the case of WC appears to be the formation of a solid solution of WC in Co, affecting the outer surface of the WC grains. To make dental instruments, WC and Co powders are moulded to the approximate shape of cutting head required and are then sintered at a high temperature. The cutting portion is then soldered or welded to a stainless steel shaft before it is ground to the required shape.

Mechanical properties

The hardness of WC is beyond the range of the Brinell machine, and a reading can only be obtained with a hardness tester using a diamond indenter. The Vickers hardness is usually between 1300 and 1700 VHN. This hardness is maintained even at elevated temperatures, so that the efficiency of a bur is not reduced by the heat evolved while it is cutting tooth structure. The modulus of elasticity is extremely high, being 540–640×10^3 N/mm^2 and the material deforms elastically up to its point of fracture. Thus a sharp cutting edge is maintained longer than with a steel instrument. Unfortunately, the amount of elastic deformation of WC which can take place before fracture occurs is not as great as that of steel, that is, the resilience or amount of energy absorbed is not as high. Thin sections are therefore contra-indicated. The angle between the faces forming the cutting edge of a WC instrument is usually twice that between the same faces in a steel instrument (Fig. 37). Fracture of the edge will take place on the

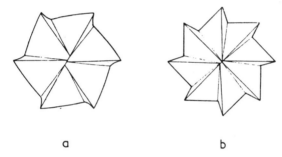

a   b

Fig. 37. End-on view of dental burs. (a) Tungsten carbide. (b) Steel

application of a sudden impact stress, such as dropping the instrument. Again if a bending stress is applied to a thin fissure bur which has penetrated tooth substance, the carbide will break. To prevent large stresses on the single blades of a bur, it should be applied to and removed from the tooth while rotating at full speed so that all the edges contact in quick succession. Only a light pressure should be employed, consistent with control of the cutting action. The bur must run true within the handpiece, or its blades will be broken by the large stresses set up on one or two teeth in eccentric rotation.

For smooth finishing of cavity margins, 12-bladed and 40-bladed tungsten carbide finishing burs are available.

When using WC chisels or scalers, no bending stress must be applied to the carbide tip, or it will break.

Sterilization

Sterilizing of instruments must be carried out with care, as some chemical sterilizing agents attack the Co matrix, and also dissolve any soldered joint between the head and the shaft. If the Co matrix is dissolved, the carbide particles disintegrate causing loss of material at the cutting edges and a reduction in cutting efficiency. Iodine, H_2O_2, solutions evolving Cl, or those containing quaternary ammonium salts should be avoided. In general, chemical sterilization is not advised. Autoclaving at 134°C is the preferable method. An alternative is dry heat at 160°C. The use of dry heat at 180°C causes slight surface effects. Boiling in plain water causes marked deterioration of both the surfaces and edges of the blades.

Tungsten carbide is also applied as an abrasive coating on the surface of rotating cutting instruments, in a similar way to the use of diamond dust.

Chapter 14
Die and counterdie alloys. Fusible alloys

Whilst most denture bases are now cast, a number of swaged stainless steel based dentures are still provided. A swaged denture base can be made very thin (down to 0·5 mm), whilst there is a limit to the practicability of casting a thin Co–Cr plate. In consequence, the swaged denture is less obvious to the patient and is lighter in weight. The swaged plate has a smooth, highly polished surface which is not abrasive to the soft tissues. Additions can be made to the swaged base by welding or soldering, whilst bonding of polymers directly to stainless steel has been reported. Even with the use of a silane coupling agent, however, the bond strength reduces markedly with time in the mouth.

In the fabrication of a denture base, the stainless steel is cold worked by swaging it between metal dies and counterdies. A fairly large force is necessary to swage a sheet of metal of the size suitable for a denture. The dies used must withstand this load without distortion, and there should be little alteration in the form of the counterdies.

The usual method of casting a metal die is to prepare an open mould in sand. Molten die metal is poured into this mould and allowed to cool to room temperature. Then counterdie metal is poured over the working surface of the die.

Zinc, with a melting point of 419°C, and a BHN of 54 is the common metal used for dies. It is readily melted but oxidizes if overheated. In sections of 2–3 inches it shows sufficient strength to withstand swaging forces. The thermal contraction of Zn on cooling causes an error in the dimensions of the die unless it is compensated by the use of an expanded cast for the mould.

To provide a die of higher strength for use in a hydraulic press, alloys of Zn with Cu, Al and Mg are used. These are much harder than Zn alone but do not melt so readily in a simple gas furnace.

Other alloys give a more accurate die than zinc:

Babbitt metal

Sn	60–70 per cent
Sb	18–22 per cent
Cu	10–12 per cent
Melting range	260–280°C

This alloy oxidizes rather easily on melting, and tends to segregate on cooling. Babbitt metal is no stronger than Zn, but shows less contraction on freezing due to the presence of Sb. This constituent expands on solidifying.

Type metal

Pb	50–70 per cent
Sb	18–25 per cent
Sn	10–25 per cent

This alloys expands on solidification and thus produces the sharply defined type with which this page is printed. Type metal is used to make moulds for flexible facial prostheses.

Zinc becomes contaminated after a period of use, but can be cleaned by stirring into the molten metal some NH_4Cl (sal ammoniac). Iron forms alloys with Zn and the iron ladle should be protected by a coating of lime or whitening. A separate ladle should be kept for Zn to prevent contamination with other metals.

Counterdies may be made of the above alloys or of Pb and its alloys. Lead with Sn is used, while Sb is added to harden Pb for stainless steel swaging.

The hydraulic forming technique employs dies of artificial stone or of one of the epoxy resins.

FUSIBLE ALLOYS

Smaller dies and counterdies are used for shaping small pieces of sheet gold during the construction of metal crowns. The gold sheet used for this purpose is thinner than that for dentures and the force necessary for swaging is much less. It is more convenient for this type of work to use an alloy which melts readily in the bunsen flame, as with such an alloy a less refractory material than sand can be used for the mould. Usually a clay-like moulding material is used.

The term fusible alloy is applied to any alloy whose melting point is below that of pure Sn, that is 232°C.

Dental fusible alloys are essentially alloys of Bi, Sn and Pb, with additions of Cd or In. The low melting point of these alloys arises because the components form ternary or quaternary eutectic alloys with each other.

Chapter 15
Soldering and welding

In the construction of an appliance from wrought materials such as sheet metal or wire, it is frequently necessary to join component parts together.

Definitions of the terms

In dentistry there are two basic methods of joining metals together; these are soldering and welding. In the case of soldering, an alloy is melted between the metals to be joined. When the solder alloy solidifies, it joins the pieces of metal together. No intermediate alloy is used when joining two pieces of metal by welding, but the surfaces of the two pieces of metal are joined directly to each other.

SOLDERING

Solders are divided into two types, soft and hard. Soft solders are eutectic alloys of lead and tin. They are used mainly for joining lead, brass or copper together. In dentistry, soft solders find only a limited use. Hard solders are used in joining parts of appliances for the mouth. These may either be precious metal or silver solders.

Mechanism of joining in soldering

In a good soldered joint, the solder wets and comes into intimate contact with the metallic surfaces of the pieces to be joined. Metallic bonds may then form between the surface atoms of the solder and those of the metals being joined. Provided that the atoms of molten solder and of the solid metals come into close contact, a good adhesive bond is produced. The presence of an oxide film, dirt, etc., naturally produces much weaker adhesive forces. To make a good joint, the metal surfaces must be clean and free from any oxide film at the moment when the solder is molten. Mechanical interlocking of the solder into surface irregularities at the interface can also cause an attachment of the solder to the components. There is evidence that no diffusion of atoms across the joint takes place in a joint which is soldered quickly.

Certainly when using soft solders on higher fusing metals and alloys, the joint is only a mechanical one. But when the melting points of solder and pieces to be joined are not separated by a large temperature difference, some *slight* surface alloying may occur. If much alloying occurs across the interface, or if inclusions or an oxide film are present, the strength of the soldered joint is markedly reduced. The chemicals used to prevent the formation of an oxide film or to remove it as soon as it is formed are called *fluxes*.

Fluxes

For soft soldering, a concentrated solution of $ZnCl_2$ (killed spirits) is used, or a soldering resin.

A flux suitable for use with hard solders to join precious metals, brass and copper alloys would be:

Powdered borax (dehydrated) ($Na_2B_4O_7$)	55 per cent
Boric acid (H_3BO_3)	35 per cent
Silica (SiO_2)	10 per cent

A flux for hard soldering stainless steel, Nichrome or cobalt–chromium alloys must contain a fluoride. Mixtures of borax or boric acid with potassium fluoride (KF), or acid potassium fluoride (KHF_2), are all suitable to break down the tenacious oxide film.

In practice, the metal parts are cleaned, and then a thin film of flux is applied to protect the surface during heating. If the application of flux is left until the metals are hot, some patches of oxide may remain despite the flux and a weak joint will be produced. To ensure an even covering of flux, and to reduce efflorescence, it is usually applied either as a watery paste, as a concentrated solution, or in powder form.

On overheating, borax forms beads of metallic borates. These are difficult to remove from the surface of the metal after the completion of soldering. Therefore, care must be taken to prevent overheating of the flux during soldering.

Antifluxes

To restrict the flow of solder on clean metal surfaces, a layer of graphite, whitening or rouge can be applied over the metal away from the joint. The simplest method is to draw a line with an ordinary lead pencil about 2 mm away from the joint and then cover the metal beyond this line with a thin graphite film by 'scribbling' with the pencil.

Methods of soldering

Two methods are in general use in dentistry. These are *freehand* and *investment* soldering.

Freehand soldering is done by taking suitable lengths of wire or of strip metal and coating them with solder at the point where the joint is to be made. Then these coated sections are held together in a flame until the solder fuses. After cooling, the wires are bent to the precise shape required.

This method of soldering is very quick. It produces the minimum effect upon the crystal structure of the metals since they are heated rapidly to the soldering temperature and quickly cooled. There is little possibility of accurate positioning, however, and further bending of the wires has to be done. The use of soldering jigs improves the accuracy of positioning. If the joint is overheated, the wire will fracture on being bent due to the coarse grain structure which is produced. The solder will not bend very readily, as it is brittle, and no attempt should be made to bend the joint itself.

To solder a clasp in position on a denture, or to join the pontic of a bridge to its retainers, an accurate relation of the component parts must be maintained. No adjustment is possible after soldering and therefore the freehand method is unsuitable. Investment soldering must be used.

The metal components are first joined together by a hard sticky wax. If a large gap (over 1 mm) is left between the parts, soldering will be difficult as the solder will not bridge the gap. A moderate gap (0·4–0·8 mm) allows soldering to be effected but contraction of the solder on solidification will tend to approximate the components. On the other hand, if the components are placed in firm contact on assembly, they expand on heating and push each other apart, causing a change in relation. For gold soldering a gap of 0·15–0·20 mm is preferable. This gap can be achieved by placing a small piece of tinfoil of gauges 1, 2 or 3 between the parts before sticking them together. A gap of this dimension allows the solder to flow freely and also reduces the possibility of porosity within the solder.

The assembled structure is invested in a small mass of investment material. A cristobalite investment is preferable. After setting, sticky wax and foil are removed and preheating and soldering carried out as quickly as possible. Less distortion is found if the invested piece is heated uniformly to the soldering temperature in a furnace. With a blowpipe, localized heating usually takes place, producing some distortion.

Wrought gold parts of a denture or appliance may be embedded within a casting ring, and will join with the molten cast metal as it enters the mould. It is important to prevent the formation of an oxide or sulphide film on the metal surface and thus produce a sound joint. An investment material containing a considerable amount of a reducing agent such as graphite may be used to counteract oxidation, and the refractory should preferably be cristobalite. This achieves its maximum expansion between 400 and 450°C and this temperature will not affect the grain structure of the embedded metals. Under ideal conditions, the joint made by this method is as good as one which is soldered.

Methods of heating

Solder may be melted either by a flame, by a laser beam, by placing the components and the solder and flux in a furnace, or by utilizing the heating effect of the passage of an electric current.

The flame produced by the ignition of coal-gas with air at atmospheric pressure is not sufficiently hot for rapid hard soldering, except when only small masses of metal are being joined. Such a flame can only be used for joining two wires together. The addition of air under pressure to a coal-gas flame raises the flame temperature.

The control of the proportion of air and gas in a blowpipe flame is most important. If too little air is added to the gas, a generally reducing flame is obtained but this will be lacking in heat due to incomplete gas combustion. With too much air the blast of cold gases from the blowpipe will cool the metal and will also blow the solder away from the joint.

Temperatures of the various flames:

Bunsen burner	1250°C
Coal-gas, air (blowpipe)	1800°C
Coal-gas, oxygen	2200°C
Oxy-hydrogen	2420°C
Oxy-acetylene	3500°C

These are temperatures of the flames themselves and not the temperatures to which metals can be heated. Usually the maximum melting temperature which can be achieved is just over half of these figures.

Table 5. Colour temperatures

	°C	°F
Lowest visible red	475	890
Dull red	550–625	1020–1150
Cherry red	700	1300
Red heat	750	1380
Light red	850	1560
Orange	900	1650
Full yellow	950–1000	1740–1830
Light yellow	1050	1920
White heat	1150 or above	2100 or above

When an object is heated, it passes through a range of colours which vary from a dull red to white heat. These colours can be interpreted as temperatures, if the heated object is examined in comparative darkness. The colour, particularly at lower temperatures, is seen much more clearly when the material is in an enclosed furnace than when it is examined under artificial or natural lighting conditions.

A laser beam can be concentrated on a small area and quickly fuses hard solders.

Whilst heating in a furnace gives good temperature control, the method is preferably applied to cast alloys whose structure is not affected by the time and temperature used.

When an electric current passes, it causes a rise in temperature. The heating effect of a relatively large current can be utilized to melt solder and thus join metals together. The method is usually applied to the soldering of thin orthodontic wires. The apparatus consists of a transformer which has a large current output at 2–5 volts. This output current is fed to two electrodes. One 'earth' electrode is in the form of a clamp which holds the components near the joint. The other is an insulated hand electrode connected to the transformer by a flexible lead. This electrode may be in the form of a carbon rod which itself heats up. The parts are clamped in position and the flux and solder applied. The hand electrode is then applied to the solder and the joint until the solder fuses. This is usually accomplished in a second or two and the movable electrode is immediately withdrawn.

Speed of soldering

Prolonged heating of the components to be joined will cause recrystallization and grain growth, particularly in strain hardened structures. For example, a wrought stainless steel wire which is used in the fully hard condition will rapidly lose its elasticity if it is heated for more than a few seconds during soldering.

Form of the solder

Solder is obtained in the form of thin strip, wire, or as a powder. It should never be used in thick sections since the amount of heat necessary to melt a large mass of solder will affect the metals being soldered. A mixture of finely divided solder and flux is available as a 'soldering paste'. Solder in tube-form which contains flux within its lumen may also be purchased.

Melting point of solders

The melting point of the solder should be definite, and should not spread over a wide range of temperature. When there is a wide range of fusion, the solder flows very sluggishly at first, since some of it is still in the plastic or semi-molten state. A joint made with solder in this condition is much weaker than one made with solder which is completely molten. Overheating the solder also gives a weaker joint. In this case the solder will be porous due to the oxidation of the lower melting point metals. There is a greater danger of overheating a solder which melts slowly than one which shows a definite and precise change to the fluid state. A solder alloy should therefore have a small range of temperature between its liquidus and solidus.

Molten solder will flow from the cooler to the hotter parts of the work. Thus some control can be exercised over the solder by moving the blowpipe flame along the joint; the solder will follow the flame along.

Strength of the soldered joint

The strength of most solders is not as great as that of the metals which they join. This is due to the fact that the composition of a solder is decided mainly in accordance with the melting point and corrosion resistance requirements rather than for strength. Also, the solder in a joint is a cast metal. If it is connecting wrought wires or sheet metal, the strength of the solder will be much less than that of the work hardened metals which it joins.

It has been shown, however, that the strength of a thin soldered joint may be greater than that of the solder itself. This is due to the fact that distortion of the thin solder film is restricted by the surrounding stronger components. The relatively weak solder within the joint resists stress to a greater degree than if it were freestanding. Thus, if a soldered joint is tested in tension, the stress in the joint may not be simply a tensile stress in the axis of the applied load. Stresses in the two other axes at right angles to the tensile stress may also be present. This effect is known as *triaxiality*.

When using hard solder it is not necessary to build solder round the sides of a joint to improve its strength. In fact, the increased temperature and time taken to melt the larger mass of solder may affect the properties of the metal being joined and so reduce the strength of the joint. The amount of solder should be the smallest that will fill the area of the joint.

General principles of soldering

Scrupulous cleanliness of the parts to be soldered. Remove all oxide, dirt and grease. Remove all sticky wax in investment soldering.

Small gap between the parts to be joined.

Apply just sufficient flux to cover the metals thinly—no excess.

Heat up quickly and solder in a few seconds.

If the solder does not flow, cool the metals, reclean and start again.

Use the minimum of solder.

PRECIOUS METAL SOLDERS

Applicable specifications: Brit 3384; Austral 1623.

A solder for joining wrought or cast gold alloys is composed basically of Au, Ag and Cu, with small additions of Zn and Sn. Zinc and Sn

lower the melting point of gold alloys. The amount of Au present
must be sufficient to impart a satisfactory corrosion resistance to the
alloy.

When a gold solder is being purchased, it is usual to refer to it by a
carat number. For example, one may purchase 18 carat solder. This
carat number does not indicate that the solder contains eighteen
twenty-fourths of Au, but that its melting point, colour, and corrosion
resistance are such that it is suitable for soldering 18 carat alloys.

This system of designating solders is not sound, however, as the
modern yellow gold alloys containing Pt and Pd have melting points
which differ from those of the more simple alloys of the same carat.
In order to make sure that the colour and melting temperature of the
solder is correct, it is advisable to use the solder which is recommended
by the manufacturer for the particular alloy being soldered.

An 18 carat solder would have the following typical composition:

Au	65 per cent
Ag	16 per cent
Cu	13 per cent
Zn	4 per cent
Sn	2 per cent

Typical properties:

	Quenched	Heat hardened
PL N/mm²	175	270
UTS N/mm²	350	430
Elongation	10 per cent	1 per cent
BHN	110	190
Melting point	750–800°C	

Heat treatment of precious metal solder joints

Solders are amenable to the usual heat treatments, but the figure for
elongation after heat hardening indicates that the joint would be very
brittle after such treatment.

When soldering yellow gold castings the investment method is
almost invariably used and therefore the casting itself is annealed.
After soldering, any stresses set up by uneven heating are removed
by reheating to 700°C, followed by quenching. Then the casting is
heat treated by cooling at a rather faster rate than normal, so that less
hardening is achieved.

White gold solders

The melting point of white golds is higher than that of the yellow gold casting alloys and a yellow gold solder can be used to join the white alloys. Special solders are available and these should preferably be used to avoid the possibility of galvanic action and to obtain an invisible joint. The solders are basically similar to the white gold alloys, but have an increased proportion of the lower melting point metals.

A slightly higher temperature is required when soldering with white solders in order to obtain good flow of the solder. But, the white gold casting alloys show rather rapid recrystallization and grain growth at temperatures within 50–100°C of their melting points. Therefore, it is particularly important that these alloys are soldered as rapidly as possible. Wrought white golds contain a higher percentage of Pd, and are not as easily softened during soldering as the cast alloys. It will be found that the difference in melting points between cast white gold alloys and their solders is about 150°C, so that grain growth is avoided to some extent.

No hardening heat treatment is applied to these alloys, and both the solder and the casting are left in the fully softened condition.

Soldering technique alloys

Applicable Specification: Austral 1622.

For practice work in the teaching of dental technology, silver solders are used in place of gold solders, for reasons of economy. Their melting point is lower than that of gold solders and is also well below that of the technique metals. Therefore, soldering is much more simple. A flux of plain borax is quite satisfactory for this type of work.

Soldering stainless steel

For soldering stainless steel, the melting point of the solder employed should be below 700°C. Above this temperature Cr_4C is precipitated rapidly within the grain boundaries of the steel, resulting in a lower corrosion resistance and a tendency for the metal to disintegrate from intergranular corrosion. Annealing of the steel also takes place above 700°C and the wrought metal will lose its excellent cold worked properties.

Gold solders can be used to join stainless steels, but to produce an alloy with a sufficiently low fusion temperature the proportion of Au must be reduced to less than 45 per cent, or about 10 carat. The corrosion resistance of such an alloy is very poor and there are no advantages in its use.

The high silver content solders can be used for joining stainless steel, but their fusion temperature is rather high. A solder containing less Ag and which fuses at a lower temperature is known as a *turbine solder*.

Typical compositions:

	Silver solder	Turbine solder
Ag	63 per cent	45 per cent
Cu	27 per cent	25 per cent
Zn	10 per cent	15 per cent
Cd	—	15 per cent
Melting range	700–730°C	580–660°C

The mechanical properties of both these solders are superior to those of yellow gold solders. The elongation of silver solders is usually between 10 and 15 per cent, so that the appliance can be adjusted near the soldered joint without fear of fracture.

None of the silver solders are corrosion resistant in the mouth, and therefore it is not usual to join stainless steel by soldering when constructing a permanent appliance. The only exception is where the joint will be completely covered by a non-metallic denture base and thus protected from the oral fluids. Silver solders are used extensively in making stainless steel orthodontic appliances which are only used for a few months, and which can be inspected and repolished from time to time.

At one time it was considered that the union between stainless steel and silver solders was simply one of attachment, and that due to the passive layer on the surface of the steel, no adhesion took place. It appears, however, that a small amount of adhesion does take place. The strength of a silver solder joint between stainless steels is greater than that of the solder alone due to the triaxiality effect when the solder is stressed. During clinical use, a soldered joint of stainless steel or Ni–Cr wire tends to undergo *crevicular corrosion* at the edge of the solder. Attempts have been made to reduce corrosion by electrodeposition of Au or Ni on the wire before soldering. Only a small benefit is achieved with stainless steel, but joints on Ni–Cr wires are better.

Practical points in soldering stainless steel

When once a coloured oxide film has formed on the surface of stainless steel the flux will not remove it and soldering cannot take place. The flux must therefore be applied to the wire or sheet while it is cold or very slightly warm. When soldering a thin wire to a thicker one by the freehand method, the thin wire should be covered with flux only. The thicker wire is coated with solder, and as the solder melts, the thin wire is placed in position and the solder flows across the joint. This reduces the amount of softening which takes place.

Investment soldering is a little more difficult to carry out rapidly, and every attempt should be made to shorten the soldering time. The mass of investment used must be as small as is practicable. If, during soldering, a brown or blue film of oxide forms, soldering will not be achieved.

Soldering by passing an electric current appears to cause the least change in the structure of the stainless steel.

Soldering Co–Cr and Ni–Cr alloys

These alloys can be soldered with yellow and white gold solders or with turbine solders.

When soldering gold clasps to a Co–Cr casting, a coating of yellow gold solder is first fused on to the casting at the joint. Then the gold clasp is soldered to this initial layer.

Cobalt chromium and Ni–Cr wires can be tack welded in place before soldering with any of the above solders. Investment material can be used to hold the parts in their correct relation, but the joint itself should be completely free from any surrounding investment material. Then heating of the joint is rapid.

The main difficulty in making attachments to Co–Cr castings is the formation of an oxide film on heating. This can be avoided by melting the solder in a reducing atmosphere. The method is to tack weld the parts together and support them on sand or alternatively, to invest them. They are then heated together with the solder in a furnace filled with a reducing gas such as hydrogen, bearing in mind the explosion danger when using this gas. The temperature of the furnace is raised quickly until the solder melts. Melting the solder by a laser beam or by the passage of electric current is again a very suitable method.

Speed is essential in all these soldering techniques to prevent annealing or grain growth, particularly in strain-hardened wires which may be near their critical limit for secondary recrystallization to occur. In a similar manner, gold or other wrought wires embedded in the invest-ment mould will, due to the high mould temperature, undergo grain growth and may fracture after a period of use. Even when soldering is carried out quickly, however, there is a marked reduction in the elastic properties of Co–Cr wires attached by soldering. If possible, they should be attached by the polymer denture base rather than by soldering.

WELDING

If two pieces of clean, pure gold are pressed or hammered together, they join permanently without the use of heat or a flux. Other metals will join if they are pressed together at an elevated temperature.

Sweating

Hot welding of metals finds little use in dentistry, though the simple Au–Cu–Ag alloys may be joined together by *sweating* or *autogenous welding*. Two pieces of gold sheet are held in contact and then heated until their surfaces just fuse together. Control of the heating tem-perature is rather critical to prevent complete melting of the metal, particularly when different thicknesses of metal are being joined. Local hot welding may also be achieved by using a laser beam of higher energy than that used for soldering.

Spot welding

Reference has already been made to the heating effect of an electric current. If the electric current is passed through only a very small section of the material, the local generation of heat may be sufficient to melt it at this one point.

In spot welding the two pieces of metal which are to be joined are pressed firmly in contact at one point by means of two electrodes, one on either side of the joint. Then an electric current of high amperage is passed through the electrodes and through the metal pieces. This current produces sufficient heat in the small area through which it passes to cause partial fusion of the metal surfaces. These join when pressed together at the instant of fusion. The electrodes are made of a thick section of Cu–Cr or Cu–Be alloy so that little heat is produced by the passage of current through them. Also their ends are pointed so that the current is concentrated in a narrow path through the metals. One spot weld is not sufficient to make a strong joint and numerous welds are made.

The resistance of the metal to be joined and its heat conductivity play an important part in spot welding. Those metals which conduct heat and electricity easily do not weld satisfactorily as less heat is produced, and this tends to be dissipated through too large an area of the metal. Stainless steel and Ni–Cr are satisfactory alloys for spot welding.

If the metals are not in contact at the spot to be welded, the current must take a longer line of passage through them and the heat will be lost over too wide an area, giving a poor weld. Loads ranging between 10–140 N at the electrodes are preferable for welding in dentistry. The point to be welded must be the only one which contacts the electrodes. If a stray piece of wire connects them, the current will be divided between the two contacts.

When two pieces of stainless steel of different thicknesses are being joined together, it is an advantage to shape the electrodes so that the thinner gauge of metal contacts a broader electrode surface than the thicker gauge. By this means the heat is concentrated on a small section of the thick metal but on a broader area of the thin metal. There is less tendency to overheat the latter than when identical electrodes are used.

The current necessary to spot weld varies with the thicknesses of metal being joined. Currents up to 5000 amperes are employed. This current is usually produced by a suitable step-down transformer which reduces the mains voltage to 2–6 volts. The period of time during which the current should pass is preferably 5–10 milliseconds. Such small intervals of time cannot be controlled accurately by mechanical devices and welding tends to be irregular. Electronic timing synchronized to the wave-form of the primary mains supply produces more consistent results. Energy storage welders store up energy in a capacitor and discharge it into the primary circuit of the transformer. Welding is again well controlled, but the total power available tends to be limited. The important controlling factor is the energy expended, which is a time/amperage relation.

If too little current is passed, only a very weak weld is made which can be broken quite easily. Such a *tack weld* is useful for checking the positioning of the metal parts before joining them permanently by stronger welds or by soldering.

Too large a current will fuse the metals between the electrodes completely, and the pressure applied will squash this molten metal to a very thin section. Such a weld will break easily when bent.

From a constructional point of view, the disadvantage of spot welding is that the metals to be joined must be placed flat over each other in an overlapping joint. It is not easy to butt-join metals as one does in soldering. This difficulty in making suitably designed joints is one of the chief factors in the restriction of the use of stainless steel for partial denture construction. In the design of orthodontic appliances, however, overlapping joints can easily be made, and it is in this field that spot welding finds its widest application. For orthodontic use, the electrodes of the spot welding machine should be suitably grooved, so that good contact with round wires is obtained. Otherwise, the current will arc between the electrode and the wire, causing a loss of welding power with burning of the surface of the stainless steel.

The disadvantage of spot welding lies in the effect of the heat produced upon the properties of the metal. At each welded joint, the heat of spot welding will cause some recrystallization of the grain structure. This reduces the strength at the very place where strength is required. The annealing effect is more pronounced with thin springy wires for orthodontic use. When such a wire is welded to a thicker one, the thin wire will frequently break at the weld on further bending. Many methods have been suggested to overcome this difficulty, and details will be found in books on orthodontics.

At the centre of each spot weld on stainless steel, the metal is heated to a temperature above 900°C. No weld-decay occurs in this area. However, surrounding each weld a ring of metal has been heated to within the range of temperature at which weld-decay may take place. During spot welding, which is accurately controlled in time, only a little weld-decay takes place.

Chapter 16

Electrodeposition. Electrolytic polishing.
Corrosion

ELECTRODEPOSITION

If a positive electrode of metallic copper is placed in a solution of $CuSO_4$, and connected through a battery to a negative electrode, a current can be passed within the solution from the positive to the negative electrode. The positive electrode is called the *anode*, and the negative one the *cathode*. The current passes within the electrolyte from the anode to the cathode. To carry this current, the positively charged Cu^{2+} ions move to the cathode, where they take up two electrons. These neutralize the positive charges of the copper ions and they become metallic Cu. The cathode thus receives a coating of Cu which may adhere to its surface. The SO_4^{2-} ion goes to the copper anode, gives up its two electrons and forms SO_4. This attacks the Cu and forms $CuSO_4$. In this way Cu is transferred from the anode to the cathode, and the electrolyte remains at a constant strength. The positive electrode is called a *soluble anode*.

Sometimes an anode is used which is not attacked, and the metal salts in the electrolyte are gradually exhausted.

Speed of deposition

The amount of metal deposited on the cathode depends upon its chemical equivalent and on the amount of current passing through the electrolyte. But the amount of metal carried across from anode to cathode by a certain current may be deposited over a small cathode, or one of large area. With a small cathode, the metal will be deposited rapidly, giving a plating which is rough or even porous and spongy in texture. To achieve a smooth fine plating, the metal must be deposited slowly.

Thus the important factor which must be carefully controlled in electroplating is the amount of current passing per unit area of the cathode. This is called the *current density* or c.d., and is expressed as amperes or milliamperes per unit area. The current density to produce a fine plating varies with the composition and strength of the electrolyte and with the metal being plated.

If in a plating bath the current density is adjusted to the correct level for the size of the cathode, it will be found that the potential difference across the anode and cathode is always the same, provided that the electrodes are kept the same distance apart, and that the strength of the electrolyte is constant. Therefore, in a plating apparatus, a voltmeter across the bath will give an indication as to whether the current density is correct for the area of the article being plated.

Anode–cathode distance

When an object with an irregular surface is plated, those portions of the cathode nearest to the anode will receive a thicker deposit of metal than those further away. The capacity of the electrolyte to deposit an even film over an irregular cathode is called its throwing power. This varies between different solutions.

To obtain an even thickness of plating over the whole surface of an irregularly shaped cathode, two methods are available. For small cathodes, such as impressions of single teeth, the anode and cathode are arranged, so that the distance between the nearest and most distant part of the cathode is small in relation to the total distance between anode and cathode. When the anode and cathode are far apart, the voltage must be increased to maintain the same current density, as the resistance of the electrolyte is greater. A second method is to shape the anode to conform to the cathode so that the distance between them is constant. For large pieces, a cylindrical anode enclosing the cathode will give a more uniform plating than a flat sheet. As large an anode as possible should be used both for long life and evenness of plating.

Polarization

After a short period of plating time, the rate of deposition tends to fall. The rate of diffusion of ions within the electrolyte is slower than the rate of deposition. Consequently, there is an accumulation of products of electrolysis at the anode, and depletion of electrolyte at the cathode. This causes an opposing emf and the plating current falls. This effect is known as *polarization*, and the electrolyte should be stirred to maintain the rate of plating.

METAL PLATING

This is used to form a metallic surface on small impressions in the construction of dies. The metal used may be silver, copper or nickel.

Making the impression conductive

The materials used for small impressions are compound, hydrocolloids, and elastomeric impression materials. None of these are conductors of electricity, and some means of making them conductive must be found before they can be electroplated. The surface of the impression is made conductive by coating it with powdered metal, with graphite or with a silver mirror.

Bronze or silver powder or flakes will adhere to the surface of the impression and so form a conducting layer. Adhesion to impressions is better if the powders are mixed with a mild solvent. Ethylene dichloride on compound impressions, or chloroform on polysulphide impression materials appear to be satisfactory. On plating, the metal particles are joined together to form a continuous coating.

An emulsion of colloidal graphite in water or in a resin can be painted over the surface of the impression and on drying forms a thin conducting film. The emulsion with water is only suitable where plating takes place rapidly, as the graphite film tends to soften when the impression is placed in the electrolyte. The resin emulsion forms a tougher film.

Several methods have been suggested for depositing a layer of Ag on to the impression surface, and the reader is referred to the literature for details. A silver mirror is the most highly conductive initial layer, but unfortunately such a film is not always easy to produce.

It is often preferable to produce an initial deposit or 'strike' before plating. When plating with Cu the prepared impression is filled with electrolyte and finely divided Fe is dusted in. Iron replaces Cu from the electrolyte and a thin film of Cu is deposited. When using Ag, a strike can be made by inserting the impression in a more concentrated electrolyte at a higher c.d. for a few seconds. The current should be switched on before immersing the impression.

The plating bath

When a conducting surface layer has been formed on the impression it is immersed as the cathode in an electrolyte and current is passed to it from the anode. For copper plating, a bath containing $CuSO_4$, H_2SO_4 and phenol is used. A silver plating bath contains the double cyanide $KAg(CN)_2$ together with a slight excess of free KCN. For nickel-plating a bath containing $NiSO_4$, $NiCl_2$ and H_3BO_3 at a pH of 4·0 is used.

After a period of use, electrolytes become too concentrated due to loss of water by evaporation. This decreases the throwing power of the solution and plating becomes uneven. The plating bath should be covered at all times to prevent evaporation, and all electrolyte removed in impressions should be collected in a dish of water. When the level of solution in the bath falls, it should be topped up with this dilute solution.

If the acid concentration of the copper solution falls, plating takes place more slowly. The acid in the electrolyte reacts with any impurities in the Cu anode to form a sludge in the bottom of the bath. From time to time, the electrolyte should be filtered to remove this deposit and at the same time the acid concentration should be checked.

A silver-plating solution with a high metal content is the most effective for all types of elastomer. However, this solution is *highly poisonous* and great care must be taken when it is used in the dental laboratory. The solution should be kept in a fume cupboard since accidental contamination with acids releases an extremely toxic gas of HCN.

Plating procedure

All metal parts, such as the connecting wire, must be insulated from the solution or the current will pass via these instead of through the conductive film.

When several impressions are to be placed in the same bath, care should be taken to see that they are all at the same stage of plating. If a newly coated impression is placed in a bath containing other impressions which are already covered with a film of metal, it will receive very little current as its resistance is comparatively high. As a result, little or no plating of the new impression will take place. Ideally, each impression should have its own plating bath and circuit so that plating conditions can be controlled.

The fine initial deposit of Cu must be light salmon pink in colour; any tendency towards a brown deposit indicates too high a c.d. The initial Ag deposit should be almost white. When the impression surface is completely covered, the current density can be increased in order to thicken the film. Initial plating should take about 1 hour, and thickening a further 3 to 8 hours.

Plating of Cu and Ag is fortunately quite readily carried out at about room temperature (17–20°C). A higher temperature of 45°C is essential for nickel-plating.

ELECTRODEPOSITION OF OTHER METALS

Because of the expense of using gold alloys for dentures, attempts have been made to render base metal alloys non-tarnishable by coating them with a film of either Au, Rh or a Sn-Ni alloy.

For gold plating, an electrolyte consisting of a 6 per cent solution of $KAu(CN)_2$ is used. An anode of pure Au is used, of at least the same size as the article to be plated, with an anode–cathode distance of 50–70 mm. Copper and its alloys take the best deposit, but other metals can be given a coating. The surface of any metal which is to be plated should be scrupulously clean and smooth, and entirely free from grease. The plating bath is kept at a temperature of 50°C and the current is passed from a 2 or 4 volt supply. If a cold solution is used, together with a low current density, the deposit is pale in colour. A darker tone is produced on increasing the current density and raising the temperature.

Rhodium has also been used for protecting base metals as it resembles Pt in colour and is impervious to chemical attack in the mouth. Unfortunately, during a short period of wear in the mouth, both Au and Rh deposits wear away and the base metal is uncovered. A plating of an alloy of Sn 65% and Ni 35% onto aluminium bronzes, employing a fluoride–chloride bath, has been reported as satisfactory in clinical use.

Gold or Ni plating is also used in an attempt to improve the joint when soldering stainless steel or Ni-Cr wire. The wire is given a 'flash' of metal which alloys with the silver solder.

Electroforming of dentures

Metals such as Ni can be electroformed to produce a simple denture base such as that for a complete upper denture. Whilst the adaptation of an electroformed plate is good, the mechanical properties are much lower than those of wrought or cast structures.

ELECTROLYTIC POLISHING

During electroplating, a current is passed within the electrolyte from the anode to the cathode, and this current causes a soluble anode to ionize. If the anode is removed from the electrolyte after a period of plating, its surface will be found to be clean and rounded in contour.

This leads us to a method of cleaning metallic surfaces, and, under suitable conditions, of smoothing out surface irregularities. If a rough metal surface is connected as the anode in a bath of a strongly acid electrolyte, a current passing between it and a cathode will cause the anode to ionize, and thus lose a surface film of metal. With a suitable electrolyte and the correct current density, the first products of electrolysis will collect in the hollows of the rough metal surface and so prevent further attack of these areas. The prominences of the metal surface will continue to be dissolved and in this way the contours of the surface are smoothed.

Electrolytic polishing is applied to stainless steel and to Co–Cr alloys. The electrolyte usually consists of a mixture of H_2SO_4 and H_3PO_4, together with glycerine and H_2O.

A current density of 0·5–1·0 amp per square mm is passed for a few minutes at room temperature, with a voltage of 4–10 volts. The cathode gases freely due to the release of hydrogen, and rise in temperature of the solution is noted.

The use of too low a c.d. causes the metal surface to be etched, and this effect is utilized in preparing specimens for metallographic examination. Too high a c.d. removes the effect of polarization and the entire metal surface is attacked.

The term 'polishing' is hardly correct in defining this process as there is no formation of a Beilby layer. Perhaps a better name would be electrobrightening.

This process is invaluable for producing a bright surface on complicated orthodontic appliances and on the fitting surface of Co–Cr dentures. It is also used for reducing the section of wrought stainless steel wires. The method is also used for increasing the thickness of the cement lute under gold inlays. The margins and the polished surfaces of the inlays are protected by wax. The remaining surfaces are reduced electrolytically so that the restoration fits closely only at the margins.

CORROSION

The conditions in the mouth are very suitable for the occurrence of corrosion. The oral cavity is warm and damp, and during the ingestion of food, conditions of considerable acidity or mild alkalinity, as well as ranges of temperature between 0 and 65°C are experienced. The decomposition of food debris left between the teeth can produce a local condition which is ideal for an attack upon metals to take place.

Electrolytic corrosion

The acids contained in the juices of fresh fruits and vegetables will have a direct, though rather transient, effect upon the surface of metallic restorations.

Hydrogen sulphide may be present in solution within the saliva and will react with Cu and Ag to form black sulphides. Amalgam fillings, blacken after a short period of time in the mouth of a patient who does not keep the metal surface clean with a tooth brush. The amount of metal lost by direct action is very small indeed in the mouths of patients who keep their teeth clean.

When two dissimilar metals are partly immersed in an electrolyte and are connected together, a current will pass between them. The strength of the current and the direction in which it passes depends upon the electrode potentials of the individual metals. The electrode potential of a metal indicates its tendency to produce ions in an electrolyte. The more reactive metals such as Zn, Mg and Al readily give up positive ions to the electrolyte, and so become negatively charged. Gold, Ag and Pt, however, show a tendency to receive positive ions from the electrolyte and so become positively charged.

Within the electrolyte, the current flows from the metal with a more negative potential to the one with a more positive potential. The first metal dissolves, whereas the second, more positive metal remains intact.

In the mouth, electric couples can be formed when any of the following are present, the saliva acting as the electrolyte:

Different metals and alloys.
Cored or eutectic structures.
Metals in a cold worked condition.

Differences in oxygen tension between portions of the surface of the same metal.

Different metals

It is fairly obvious from the above discussion that if an amalgam filling is placed next to a gold filling and is in contact with it, electrolytic action can take place when both are bathed in saliva. Varnishing of one or both dissimilar metallic restorations which are to be in contact reduces the possibility of corrosion. Electrolytic corrosion also occurs between amalgam alloys of different composition which are placed in contact. A metal denture which touches a filling made of another metal or alloy can set up galvanic action. A filling in one jaw or the occlusal rests of a denture have intermittent contact with fillings in the opposite jaw during mastication and a couple is then formed.

Corrosion of solders in a metal denture is commonly seen as the solder differs in composition from the remainder of the denture. Wherever possible, soldered joints should be embedded in polymethyl methacrylate and not exposed to the saliva. This is particularly so when silver solder is used at the joint between dissimilar alloys.

Various potential differences may be recorded between the dissimilar metals used in the mouth. A small p.d. of about 10 mV may be recorded between two apparently identical amalgams made from the same alloy. Cobalt–chromium alloys and stainless steels produce a low millivoltage when in contact with most of the other metals and alloys used in the mouth. Yellow gold alloys in contact with amalgams show a relatively high p.d. of 500 mV. White golds and amalgams give a slightly higher value. The highest millivoltages are produced when Al, Fe or base metal components are in contact with a high positive potential metal such as Ag.

Cored or eutectic structures

A cast restoration from a solid solution alloy may have a cored structure, and a eutectiferous type alloy such as a solder will show surface variations in composition. These different components are joined together in the body of the metal and form a couple on the surface with the saliva as the electrolyte.

Cold-worked metals

Metals which have been bent, rolled or drawn have stress present in their atomic arrangement and a couple consisting of stressed metal-unstressed metal can be set up. The stressed area is more reactive than the unstressed and corrodes. For this reason, some authorities do not advocate burnishing metals, as this produces an uneven stressed condition on their surface.

Difference in oxygen tension

Corrosion may also be brought about by a difference in oxygen tension between parts of the same metal. If two strips of iron connected with a galvanometer are placed in a solution of NaCl, no current will pass. On bubbling air over one strip, a current flows externally from the aerated strip to the unaerated one. Within the electrolyte, ions pass from the unaerated strip and it dissolves.

An area of a metallic restoration covered by plaque is anodic to adjacent areas which are exposed to the air. The area under the plaque will show signs of corrosion. If the surface of a filling is left rough and unpolished, the areas at the bottom of the surface concavities will be without oxygen, being covered with porous food debris and mucin. These areas will dissolve and increase the roughness of the surface, producing pitting of the filling. All surfaces of a restoration must therefore be highly polished. This applies particularly to those surfaces in contact with adjacent teeth as the patient finds difficulty in keeping these areas clean. Similarly, if an amalgam filling is not in close contact with the sides of its cavity, the filling material at the bottom of the crevice between filling and tooth will dissolve.

EFFECTS OF THE CURRENT PRODUCED.
GALVANIC PAIN

Whenever electrolytic corrosion takes place, an electric current passes between the two dissimilar metals which are in contact. The electric circuit is usually completed by the saliva, though it may involve gum tissue, or tongue, or tooth structure and its supporting bone. It has been shown that when an electric current passes through gum tissue or the tongue, an inflammation leading to ulceration can occur. This may be due to a sensitivity to the metallic ions produced by electrolytic action. Such a reaction is fortunately rare, and usually takes a long time to develop. When it does occur it can only be cured by replacement of all the fillings, using the same material. The possibility of such a reaction to dissimilar metals should always be borne in mind, and all fillings in a mouth should ideally be of the same material. Non-metallic fillings can of course be inserted.

When dissimilar metals, one or both of which is a filling, are brought into contact in the mouth, the patient may experience a sharp pain in a tooth. This is usually caused by intermittent contact of dissimilar metallic fillings in opposing teeth during mastication, or the connection of dissimilar fillings with metal instruments which are being used in the mouth by a dentist. It may also occur by the contact of a silver fork against a filling when a patient is placing food in the mouth. In these cases the tongue often acts as a conductor to complete the circuit, as its resistance is less than that of the other oral tissues. Galvanic pain is due to the sudden passage of an electric current through the tooth to the dental pulp with consequent painful stimulation of this sensitive structure.

Fortunately currents of sufficient magnitude to cause damage to the gum or to promote pain are infrequently produced. A good cavity lining or varnish insulates the pulp from the electric current. In addition, polarization quickly reduces the current to a low value.

Metals in permanent contact, therefore, bring about corrosion of the more electronegative metal, and only rarely produce other symptoms. Metals in intermittent contact may, on occasion, produce galvanic pain.

PASSIVITY

Some relatively reactive metals such as Al, Cr, Pb, Zn and Ni, show little tendency to undergo rapid oxidation or to take part in electrolytic action. On exposure to air, these metals form a very tenacious surface film of oxide or carbonate and this prevents further attack on the metal beneath. This film is called a *passive layer*. Chromium forms a clear passive layer and is useful for decorative purposes, whereas Al becomes dull after a short exposure to the atmosphere.

When assessing metallic materials for corrosion, the potential difference which must be applied to overcome the effects of the passive layer is an indication of the reaction of the material to intraoral corrosion.

ANODIZING

The low specific gravity of Al makes it suitable for use in dentures and orthodontic oral screens. For use in the mouth, the passive layer can be artificially improved so that it is much harder and thicker than that produced by simple exposure to the atmosphere. This process is known as *anodizing* and is carried out as follows:

The surface of the Al is polished and cleaned and then is immersed as the anode in an electrolyte mainly of H_2SO_4 in water. A Pb or C cathode is used, and a current passed of 16 mA per square mm. The bath should be at room temperature. The cations of the acid pass to the anode and react with its surface, forming a clear, hard film of Al_2O_3 together with salts of the acids present. This layer is afterwards sealed by boiling in water, when it swells and becomes non-porous. By incorporating acid dyes in the electrolyte the film can be tinted. The anodized Al is easy to clean, but must not be polished, nor should it be subjected to acids or alkalis during cleaning, especially if the film has been dyed.

Section C
Dental precision casting

Chapter 17
Waxes and similar thermoplastic materials

At some stage in the construction of a denture, inlay, crown or bridge, a pattern of the completed article, or a portion of it, is made in wax or in a synthetic polymer. From this pattern an open (two-part) or closed (one-part) mould is made, the pattern is removed and its place taken by a polymer or an alloy. The accuracy and detail of the finished product can be no greater than that of the pattern from which it arises, and a dimensionally accurate and stable pattern is always required.

Waxes are characterized most readily in terms of their physical nature rather than their chemical composition. They may be described as thermoplastic materials of low mean molecular weight and low mechanical strength. Waxes are mixtures of various organic compounds and it is their polycomponent nature which gives them their useful properties.

There are three main types of wax; hydrocarbon, natural ester and synthetic; the hydrocarbon group may be subdivided further into paraffin and microcrystalline waxes.

Paraffin waxes soften at 37–55°C and melt at 48–70°C. They crystallize either in flat plates or needles depending upon the temperature and the conditions under which they are cooled.

Microcrystalline waxes have a higher molecular weight and a fine crystal structure. They consist of branched or cyclic chains. These waxes melt at 65–90°C and when added to paraffin waxes raise the melting point markedly, but lower the softening point, giving easier manipulation.

Natural ester waxes vary widely in their properties, depending upon their source of origin. They are excreted by animals and plants and include beeswax, carnauba and candelilla waxes.

Synthetic waxes may be entirely man-made, e.g. polyethylene type, or prepared by modifying petroleum or other natural waxes such as montan. Since natural waxes vary in properties with their place of origin, there is an increasing use of synthetic materials with constant wax-like properties.

PROPERTIES OF WAXES

Waxes show only weak intermolecular bonding which is very temperature and time dependent. Bonding is by secondary forces only. Changes in crystal form occur on heating. For example, with paraffin waxes these change from an orthorhombic to a hexagonal lattice. At low temperatures waxes are brittle with a low strength. At higher temperatures and particularly during the solid/solid change of crystal state, they are mouldable under light stresses.

A typical cooling curve of a wax shows two or more arrests indicating a reduction in the rate of cooling due to the energy released as molecules become arranged within the wax. These arrests may indicate the crystallization of the various constituents of the wax. Alternatively they may result from a change in the crystal structure of the wax with temperature. After the molecular arrangement is established the shape of the wax is not easy to change and the end of the last arrest indicates the end of mouldability or the *transition point* of the wax. For most dental waxes the transition point should be about 40–42°C, that is, a few degrees above mouth temperature.

Stress relief

When wax is at a temperature above its transition point, it can be readily moulded as the molecules have sufficient heat energy to arrange themselves in a comfortable or unstressed relation with each other. On the other hand, if an attempt is made to alter the shape of a piece of wax after it has cooled below its transition temperature, stresses will be produced by the disturbance of the molecular arrangement.

These stresses will be released if the temperature is raised once more after cooling. If the stressed wax is left at room temperature for any length of time, however, relief of stress will occur by the gradual movement of molecules and subsequent distortion of the wax. At 0–5°C, the energy of the molecules is small so that little stress relief can take place on storage for several hours. Stress-relief distortion of wax is therefore a function of both time and temperature.

All waxes must therefore be manipulated while fully softened in order to reduce the amount of stress and possible distortion at a later date.

Flow

To determine the suitability of waxes for dental use, their flow is measured at various temperatures. Flow is determined in the laboratory by measuring the percentage reduction in length of a cylindrical specimen, when subjected to a load for a period of time at a certain temperature. A wax should have good flow above mouth temperature though it should retain sufficient 'body' to be workable. That is, it should neither become fluid nor should the constituents begin to separate. Ideally, below mouth temperature, waxes should show no flow, so that the accuracy of the pattern is maintained.

Thermal expansion and contraction

In order to avoid stresses from the disturbance of molecular arrangement within the wax, the ideal state in which it should be moulded is that of a liquid. Then there is complete freedom of molecular movement. Unfortunately all waxes have a high coefficient of linear expansion and contraction. Some coefficients are as high as $700 \times 10^{-6}/°C$. Moreover, the thermal expansion curve of waxes is not a straight line and the amount of expansion increases with the temperature. It is also affected by the amount of force restraining the wax whilst it is expanding or contracting.

Softening wax

Uniform heating of wax is essential in order to produce a homogeneous plastic mass. If portions of the wax are hard, it cannot be moulded satisfactorily and stresses will be set up. A bunsen burner is the usual method of heating but in order to achieve as even heating as possible, wax should be held above the flame in the warm rising air. If wax is melted, the temperature at which it flows is raised by 1 or 2°C. Consequently such a wax is more brittle to carve and breaks more easily than the original material.

If warm water is used, a more evenly heated wax is obtained but some of the constituents of the wax may be leached out. Any water incorporated in the pattern causes flaking when the wax is carved.

The ideal method for inlay wax is to use a wax 'annealer'. This is essentially a small thermostatically controlled electric oven which keeps the inlay wax at a constant temperature ready for use.

DENTURE WAXES

Applicable specifications: Amer 24; Austral 1453.

Denture waxes consist mainly of paraffin wax and beeswax and have a melting point of 49–58°C. Manufacturers add small proportions of synthetic or other natural waxes to raise or lower the softening point and to 'toughen' the wax. Some denture waxes are rolled to close up voids and to improve their 'toughness', whilst others are supplied as sheets cut from a block of wax. Rolled sheets often show a change in shape on being softened due to release of the stresses induced by rolling.

It is difficult to combine waxes in the correct proportions to make a material which will remain rigid at mouth temperature, and yet which can be softened and moulded easily in sheet form and carved to shape. Most denture waxes soften if left in the mouth for more than a few minutes and must be strengthened with wire or cotton gauze when used in thin sections.

Denture waxes should be tough rather than brittle as they are frequently drawn over undercuts on the plaster cast. If this is done at the right speed and temperature, then only a minor degree of distortion results. These waxes should have a small solidification and cooling shrinkage. On 'boiling out', they should become fluid without leaving any oily residue.

Sheet casting wax

Another type of wax which is supplied in sheet form is that for denture castings. The small sheets of wax are rolled to a precise thickness and are numbered in accordance with the usual metal gauge used in dentistry. In manipulating a sheet of casting wax, the thickness must be maintained, and it is usual to soften the wax in hot water and adapt it into position with some soft material such as cotton wool or rubber.

BASEPLATE MATERIALS

Applicable specification: Austral 1241.

Frequently, a material stiffer and stronger than wax is required as a temporary denture base. Various thermoplastic baseplate materials are available for this purpose and for making special trays. The most commonly used material is a shellac resin filled with a suitable powder to reduce its stickiness. Sheet polythene, polystyrene or acrylic polymer may also be used. These however are less stiff for the same thickness than shellac baseplate materials.

When moulding any of these thermoplastic materials, they must be softened adequately so that little or no stress is created during moulding. Since their softening points are higher than those of the denture waxes, there is a tendency to mould them at too low a temperature. Then stress relief at mouth temperature will produce a change in shape. Rapid moulding of some materials can be achieved by applying air pressure via a rubber diaphragm to adapt the sheet of material to the cast.

Baseplates and special trays are also moulded from a self-cure methyl methacrylate or a glass-filled polyester resin.

STICKY WAX

Applicable specification: Austral 1583.

This is a yellow wax, which melts at 60–65°C. It consists of a mixture of beeswax and various resins. The resins harden the mixture, making it relatively brittle, so that the position of parts of an appliance stuck together temporarily cannot be accidentally altered. Resins also make the wax adhesive. Sticky wax is often difficult to 'boil out' with boiling water alone and a detergent should be used.

Sticky wax should show the following properties:

Flow. 0·25 N/mm² for 10 min. at 20–25°C.   less than 5 per cent
Coefficient of linear contraction   less than $300 \times 10^{-6}/°C$
Residue after ignition at 500°C.   less than 0·2 per cent

It should adhere well to metals, polymers, gypsum.

INLAY WAXES

Applicable specifications: ISO R 1561; Brit 3508; Amer 4; Austral 1582.

The desirable properties of an inlay wax are:

On softening it should be capable of being moulded into a homogeneous mass without the formation of laminations or flakes of wax.

It should be fully mouldable at a temperature slightly above that of the mouth, so that it will record all the detail of the cavity.

It should be hard at mouth temperature so that the pattern can be withdrawn without distortion and so that the wax will fracture if an attempt is made to withdraw a pattern from a cavity with under-cuts.

It must contrast with the colour of the hard and soft tissues. This makes carving easier as thin sections of wax are more easily seen.

It should not chip or flake on carving to a fine edge at room temperature.

To obtain an inlay wax with the above ideal properties requires a careful blending of various waxes. The exact composition of proprietary inlay waxes is unknown, but they are basically paraffin wax, with carnauba, candelilla, beeswax and dammar resin added. Some inlay waxes are made mainly from synthetic waxes. The composition of these waxes is strictly controlled during their manufacturing processes and their properties are therefore more constant.

Direct Patterns

To take an impression, the softened wax is quickly forced into the tooth cavity, and is held under pressure until it cools. Some authorities suggest that a hot instrument should then be plunged into the thicker sections of the pattern to relieve any stresses that may have been set up. This method should only be used where difficulty is experienced in introducing the wax into the cavity, as in these circumstances, the wax may have cooled a little and large stresses may be present. Though these stresses are removed by the heat of the instrument, smaller ones may be set up by the uneven reheating of the wax. Pressure should be applied after reheating until the pattern cools in order to reduce the effects of thermal contraction.

If molten wax is introduced into a cavity, no stresses will be present initially, but the contraction of the wax on cooling from its melting point to mouth temperature will cause dimensional changes. These will produce stresses, particularly when the wax embraces tooth substance. When the wax is surrounded by tooth structure a pattern smaller than the cavity will be produced.

Inlay wax should therefore be heated to a temperature at which it is fully plastic, yet not approaching the molten state. The exception to this method is where the wax pattern can be held under constant pressure during moulding and cooling. If the tooth cavity can be completely surrounded by a well-fitting matrix, and the opposing teeth used to provide pressure, the wax may be inserted in the cavity in the molten state. Pressure overcomes the effects of thermal contraction by causing the wax to flow, and an accurate pattern is produced. It is obvious that some difficulty would be experienced in filling a cavity in a tooth with molten wax, particularly in the upper jaw.

Carving of the pattern should be done with unheated sharp instruments, so that the wax is cut cleanly and is not distorted. No additions of wax nor reheating and readapting must be carried out. If the pattern is short, it must be removed, and a new mass of wax inserted.

To reduce the possibility of stresses, some writers suggest that warm water should be syringed over the pattern as it cools, so that some annealing can take place. For instance, if the operator starts with a tumbler full of water at 44°C, and syringes the pattern with this water at varying intervals of carving, by the time the pattern is complete, the water and the wax will be at mouth temperature. No attempt need be made to cool the pattern below this temperature as the wax will always return to mouth temperature before it can be removed.

The pattern may be removed by attaching a metal sprue former and then withdrawing the wax in a straight line away from the cavity. Alternatively, pointed instruments may be used to remove the pattern. If only one instrument is used, a danger arises of warping a complicated pattern.

The metal sprue former may be of wire or tubing. A metal tube requires less heat to attach it to the wax and so causes less disturbance in the pattern. Its attachment is also better as wax enters the lumen of the tube.

Shrinkage of a wax from mouth temperature to room temperature may be as high as 0·7 per cent, and this will affect the accuracy of the pattern. As little time as possible must elapse before investing, as in the most carefully made direct pattern, some stresses exist, and these will be relieved in time by a slow distortion of the pattern. If the pattern must be stored, it should be placed in a refrigerator at 5°C or less.

Indirect Patterns

Sometimes, instead of making a wax pattern direct to the tooth, an impression is recorded, a die made, and a pattern waxed up in the laboratory. Manipulation of the wax is much easier in this case, and it can be softened thoroughly and held under pressure while cooling. In this case the pattern is made to fit the die at room temperature and not at mouth temperature. However, when no pressure is applied to the wax, some contraction of the main body of the pattern will occur from the normal hardening temperature to room temperature. For this type of pattern, there is an advantage in using an inlay wax which hardens at 28–32°C, that is, slightly above room temperature, just as the wax for direct patterns hardens just above mouth temperature.

Changes in wax patterns during investing are discussed in the next chapter.

Typical properties of a good inlay wax are, therefore:

Ash residue after vaporizing at 500°C; less than 0·1 per cent (carbon only).

Flow under a stress of 0·25 N/mm² for 10 min:

Temperature	Direct pattern wax	Indirect pattern wax
30–34°C		Less than 1 per cent
37°C	Less than 1 per cent	
40°C	Less than 20 per cent	50–85 per cent
46°C	70–90 per cent	

Some hard waxes soften at higher temperatures of 50–52°C.

The linear expansion from 20–38°C should also be known, so that the investing and casting techniques may be modified accordingly.

Chapter 18
Casting investment materials

When the pattern is to be reproduced in an alloy, a mould is made in a material which will withstand the temperatures at which these alloys melt. Making such a mould is called 'investing' the pattern.

Castings vary widely in size, and range from a small filling, or inlay, for one tooth, to a denture. When an inlay is to be cast, dimensional accuracy is essential, and compensation for the dimensional changes which take place during the making of the pattern, investing and casting must be carefully controlled. When casting a denture the accuracy of reproduction of the pattern need not be quite so perfect, as small surface imperfections may be removed by filing and polishing. Nevertheless, dimensional accuracy is still important and a good surface to the casting reduces the amount of finishing which has to be done.

Ideal properties

The ideal properties of an investment material are:

The constituents should not segregate in the container during transit, nor when they are mixed.

The investment should mix to a smooth consistency.

Its particle size should be sufficiently fine so that the surface smoothness of the casting will be the same as that of the pattern. But the investment must have sufficient permeability to allow the gases in the mould to escape when molten metal enters it.

It should not crack or decompose on heating.

It should have sufficient setting, hygroscopic, and/or thermal expansion to compensate for the shrinkage of the cast metal on cooling.

The temperature of maximum thermal expansion should not be critical and should be within the range of normal dental practice.

It should have sufficient compressive strength at the casting temperature to withstand the forces applied when the molten metal enters the mould.

CASTING SHRINKAGE

All casting alloys shrink on cooling from the molten state to room temperature. This shrinkage may be divided into three separate parts:

Contraction of the molten metal to the temperature at which it begins to solidify; that is, to its liquidus temperature.

Contraction while solidifying.

Thermal contraction from the solidus temperature to room or mouth temperature.

The first contraction is of no practical importance as it is compensated by more metal entering the mould.

If the dimensions of the mould at the casting temperature are the same as those of the original pattern the second and third contractions will have the effect of making the casting much too small when it is cooled to room temperature. In order to produce a casting of the same size as the pattern, the mould must be expanded at the casting temperature to the same degree that the cast metal contracts on cooling.

It has been found that the average linear casting shrinkage of gold alloys from the molten state to room temperature is 1·25 to 1·5 per cent when cast into an investment mould. For base metal alloys the shrinkage is 1·8–2·3 per cent. These figures are less than the sums of the two linear contractions which occur when these alloys cool freely in an open crucible. It is probable that this difference in the amount of contraction is due to two factors. First, the alloy and the investment material interlock at their surfaces and hold the outer borders of the metal apart while it is cooling. This is possible during the initial stages of cooling when the metal is still hot and in a plastic state. Secondly, the thinner sections of the casting will solidify first, and on contracting will draw molten metal from the thicker areas. If the sprues are attached to these thick areas and are of sufficient bulk to remain molten, more metal can be drawn into the mould to reduce the actual contraction.

INVESTMENT MATERIALS FOR USE WITH ALLOYS MELTING BELOW 1300°C

Applicable specifications: Brit 5189; Amer 2; Austral T22.

Composition

These investment materials are composed of a mixture of silica (SiO_2) and gypsum, together with small additions such as NaCl, boric acid, graphite (C) or finely divided Cu.

Silica is the most important constituent as it is refractory and withstands the temperatures used in casting. It also causes the mould to expand on heating. Silica exists in several allotropic forms which are chemically identical, but which have different space-lattices. These are quartz (sand), tridymite and cristobalite. Each of these three allotropes changes to an inversion form when heated. At normal temperatures they exist in the α or 'low' form, which changes to a β or 'high' form when the temperature is raised.

Quartz and cristobalite are normally used for dental investments. Cristobalite is found in only a few locations throughout the world. Tridymite exists as an impurity in cristobalite.

The silica is bound together by gypsum which gives the mould sufficient strength to stand up to the manipulation necessary during the casting procedure.

Setting time and setting expansion

The setting time of investment materials depends upon their gypsum content. The variables which affect the setting time and expansion of gypsum are discussed in Chapter 20. They are as follows:

> Whether α- or β-hemihydrate.
> Temperature of the mixing water.
> Powder : water ratio.
> Spatulation.
> Modifiers.

These variables apply to the investment materials also although their gypsum content is only about 25 per cent. The expansion of this mixture of gypsum and silica is not, however, a quarter that of gypsum alone. It shows a greater expansion than would be expected. The silica appears to weaken the crystal structure of the setting plaster so that the outgrowth of gypsum crystals can continue for a longer period of time and is more effective in causing an expansion.

Temperature of mixing water and consistency

It is not advisable to vary the temperature of the water in order to adjust the setting time of investments, as dimensional changes in the pattern take place.

A thick mix of investment sets more rapidly and expands more than a thin mix. It will be seen later that a thick mix has advantages other than that of a high setting expansion. The limiting factor is the investing technique. If too thick a mix is used, the investment is difficult to adapt to the pattern and air pockets form.

Effective setting expansion

The values for the setting expansion of plasters and investment materials are determined by measuring the change in dimension of a freely movable mass of material. It is doubtful whether this 'free' expansion is all effective in expanding the mould when the investment is confined within a casting ring. Some expansion of the pattern does occur and is called the *effective setting expansion*.

Distortion of a wax pattern occurs when the setting expansion is unduly large. It is probably safer to employ a material with a low setting expansion and to rely upon other expansions to compensate for casting shrinkage.

Expansion of the material of an investment cast will produce one that is slightly oversize and this will compensate partly for casting shrinkage. In some circumstances the water in duplicating materials will cause in addition *hygroscopic expansion* of the investment cast.

Hygroscopic expansion

If water is allowed to come into contact with some investment materials, before or at the stage of initial set, a large expansion of the investment occurs. This expansion may be brought about by the addition of other liquids miscible with water, which also have a low surface tension. Various theories explaining this expansion have been given. One suggests that hygroscopic expansion is caused by the formation of further crystals of calcium sulphate dihydrate. Slightly before the initial set, the dihydrate crystals in setting plasters are in contact with each other in a semi-rigid mass. By pushing each other apart as they grow, they bring about the normal setting expansion. If further water is made available to some plasters, however, additional dihydrate crystals form, which push the original structure farther apart and thus cause an increased expansion. Other investigations suggest that the added water reduces surface tension effects within the setting mass and thus allows freer crystal growth. Gypsums with a high setting expansion also show a large hygroscopic expansion.

As in the setting expansion of investments, the silica again acts by weakening the crystal structure of the plaster. It thus allows more crystal growth to take place on the addition of water. The silica also helps the water to penetrate the investment and cause expansion throughout the whole mass of material. Similarly, an asbestos liner helps to 'feed' water to a large surface area of investment material. In order to obtain the maximum hygroscopic expansion, the water must come into contact with the investment just before the initial set takes place. Before this stage of setting, no effective expansion is produced as the mix is too fluid. If the investment is allowed to set completely before placing it in water, the amount of hygroscopic expansion is greatly reduced.

The following factors tend to increase hygroscopic expansion:

Thicker mix of investment.
Immersion of the investment at or before its intial set.
Length of time it is immersed.
Temperature of water-bath.
Lining the ring with 1·5 mm thick asbestos paper.
Using a split ring or one made of flexible rubber.

Linear hygroscopic expansion may be as great as 2 per cent and could theoretically compensate completely for the casting shrinkage of most alloys. But, as with the setting expansion of investments, their free hygroscopic expansion as measured experimentally may not be fully effective when applied to casting procedures. Both setting and hygroscopic expansions are reduced markedly by even a small restraint applied by a container.

The usual method is to immerse the casting ring full of investment in water at 38°C for about 30 minutes. Some hygroscopic expansion occurs when the investment material absorbs water from the wet asbestos used to line the casting ring. In another method the investment is not immersed in a water-bath. Instead, a measured volume of water is placed on the upper surface of the investment material within the ring. The volume of the investment material must be known to control the expansion.

Thermal expansion

When considering the thermal expansion of investment materials it is convenient to deal with the thermal changes of plaster and silica separately.

Plaster content

On heating a mass of set gypsum, it expands slightly (0·12 per cent) up to 125°C, and then contracts at a slightly faster rate to 320°C. Then a marked contraction takes place which produces a total contraction of 1·9 per cent at 500°C. Beyond this temperature it continues to contract slowly. The first two contractions are due to the chemical changes which occur, resulting in the loss of the combined water. First of all the hemihydrate $CaSO_4.\frac{1}{2}H_2O$ is formed and secondly the anhydrite $CaSO_4$.

Fortunately these severe contractions can be entirely eliminated by the incorporation of a small percentage of NaCl or boric acid. A similar effect is achieved by adding 10 per cent by volume of glycerol to the mixing H_2O.

Silica content

Both quartz and cristobalite show at first a thermal expansion as the temperature rises. But at 573°C for quartz and 210°C for cristobalite, a large expansion occurs. In both cases this is due to an *inversion change* from the a to the β form. During the inversion change, the bonds between the Si and O atoms straighten and the volume of the material increases. This type of change is illustrated diagrammatically in Fig. 38. The total amount of linear expansion on heating quartz to 700°C is approximately 1·2 per cent. Of this, about half is due to the inversion change. With cristobalite, the total expansion at 450°C is higher at about 1·5 per cent, and over 1·0 per cent is due to the inversion change. Beyond its inversion change quartz contracts whereas cristobalite continues to expand thermally up to 700°C.

When combined with gypsum in an investment material, the inversion changes are smaller, are less clearly marked and are spread over a range of temperature. The range with quartz is 500–650°C and with cristobalite 210–260°C. The total linear expansions are approximately 0·9–1·0 per cent for a quartz investment at 700°C and 1·2–1·4 per cent at 450°C for one containing cristobalite. The amount of thermal and inversion change expansion is affected by the powder:water ratio of the investment mix. A higher ratio produces a greater expansion.

Investment materials which set under water and undergo hygroscopic expansion have in effect a lower powder:water ratio due to the water taken in during setting. They show a lower thermal expansion than materials which set in air.

On cooling an investment mould after it has attained the casting temperature, a large contraction takes place which is greater than the original expansion. The mould may be as much as 1 per cent smaller than its original room temperature dimensions. This contraction has no effect upon the completed casting as the metal is sufficiently strong to withstand any contraction of the investment.

However, if the mould is not cast, but allowed to cool down, and then reheated, the same amount of expansion as originally took place does not recur and a casting in a reheated mould will be undersize.

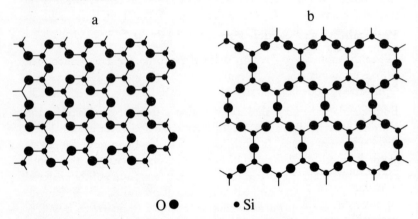

O ●   ● Si

Fig. 38. Bond straightening at the inversion change from α to β quartz. No bonds are broken. (a) Atom centres below 573°C. (b) Atom centres above this temperature

Compressive strength

The greater the percentage of gypsum in the investment, the stronger it will be. This strength is an advantage in a technique which employs a cast made of investment material upon which the denture is waxed up, as the investment cast is not so friable and can be handled more easily.

In some techniques a temporary flexible casting ring is used to mould the investment before it sets, thus allowing greater setting and hygroscopic expansion. Before heating the mould the ring is removed, leaving the investment unsupported. An investment material for this technique should have a high strength.

When an investment mould is heated and molten alloy forced down the sprue the investment material is subjected to quite high pressures. In a complicated casting, the investment may be present in thin sections, and sufficient strength is necessary to prevent fracture of parts of the mould.

The compressive strength of investments at elevated temperatures is not as great as at room temperature. There are two ranges of weakness in a quartz investment, one from 100–125°C and the other from 500–650°C. The former is connected with the dehydration of the gypsum content, and the latter with the α to β inversion change of the silica. With a cristobalite investment, the latter range is 210–260°C. Consequently casting should not take place within these ranges of temperature.

Permeability and particle size

When the molten metal is forced down the sprue, the gases which then fill the mould cavity must escape before the casting can be completed.

In order to obtain a smooth surface on the casting, the investment powder must be composed of fine particles of silica and gypsum. The smaller the particle size, the less will be the surface irregularities on the metal cast against the investment. It might at first be thought that when a fine particle size is used the investment would show little permeability, and that the addition of large silica particles would assist in making pores for the gases to escape. Permeability of the investment is, however, greatest when the particles are all of the same size, and preferably almost spherical in shape. A mixture of grain sizes and shapes produces a more solid mass of investment. Generally speaking, the gypsum-bonded materials have the highest permeability of the dental investments.

Decomposition of the investment

Calcium sulphate itself does not decompose until heated above 1200°C. In the presence of carbon, however, the following reactions occur rapidly above 700°C:

$$CaSO_4 + 4C \rightarrow CaS + 4CO$$
$$3CaSO_4 + CaS \rightarrow 4CaO + 4SO_2$$

Carbon is frequently present as a residue from burning out the wax pattern. It may also be included in the investment material in the form of graphite. Sulphur dioxide may also arise from the decomposition of impurities in the silica between 400° and 800°C. It may pass off as a gas, or be reduced to H_2S or organic sulphides. Cast alloys are discoloured by these products of decomposition. In some cases the mechanical properties of the cast alloy may be reduced by the formation of silver or palladium sulphides within the grain boundaries. This intergranular deposit causes a reduction in the strength of the metal. When decomposition of investment has taken place, the casting is black and discoloured, and is difficult to clean in the pickling acid. In a sound casting, a yellow gold alloy shows a matt yellow surface on removal from the investment, and a white gold alloy a similar grey surface. Some manufacturers suggest that the mould be heat-soaked at the casting temperatures for an hour, so that any decomposition can occur and the products pass out of the investment.

Any boric acid in an investment, besides counteracting the initial contraction of plaster, acts as a flux, and assists in the removal of oxide from the cast metal.

When casting the lower-fusing Co–Cr alloys into a gypsum-bonded mould, the latter may, with advantage, contain an oxalate. On heating, this liberates CO_2 and reduces the attack of the molten alloy by the products of gypsum decomposition.

Typical properties of gypsum-bonded materials:

| | Inlay | | Denture |
	Hygroscopic	Thermal	Thermal
Setting time	15–18 min	10–15 min	10–12 min
Setting expansion, linear, in air	—	0·4 %	0·3 %
Hygroscopic and setting expansion, linear, in water	1·3 %	—	—
Thermal expansion, linear	0·5 % (450°C)	1·3 % (700°C)	1·2 % (700°C)
Compressive strength (N/mm²)			
Wet	4·9	3·9	7·3
Dry	7·8	6·8	12·8
Particle size, pass 100 mesk sieve		95 %	

INVESTMENT MATERIALS FOR USE WITH ALLOYS MELTING ABOVE 1300°C

Applicable specification: Brit 5189.

Normal gypsum-bonded investments are unsuitable for casting many Co–Cr alloys as the bonding decomposes and fuses on to the surface of the casting. Similar difficulties arise with the very high fusing gold alloys. Above 1200°C, the gypsum and silica react:

$$CaSO_4 + SiO_2 \longrightarrow CaSiO_3 + SO_3$$

Rapid gas evolution causes porosity and corrosion of the casting.

Sufficient strength in the investment materials for high fusing alloys is therefore achieved either by silica or phosphate bonding.

Silica bonding

The investment is composed of silica in the form of quartz or cristobalite which is bonded together by silica gel. The silica powder must be of a porous nature and should present an irregular surface. Moreover, a gradation of particle sizes must exist so that the small grains fill in the spaces between the larger grains. If all the silica particles are of the same size, too much space is left between them, and this cannot be filled by the silica gel. Similarly, the amount of bonding must be kept to a minimum or cracking of the investment will occur. A very thick, almost dry mix of investment is used, and it is vibrated for several minutes in order to condense the silica particles into a tightly packed mass and so produce as strong an investment as possible. Because of this dense packing however, silica-bonded materials are generally the least permeable of the dental investments.

The silica gel is usually produced by precipitation from a hydrolysed solution of ethyl silicate. Ethyl silicate is a yellow oily liquid. In the presence of water, and at a suitable pH, it will form silica gel with the liberation of ethyl alcohol.

On heating, the silica gel turns into ordinary silica so that the completed mould is a tightly packed mass of silica particles. During the first stage of heating, a small 'green' shrinkage occurs, probably due to loss of alcohol and water from the gel. This is followed by thermal and inversion change expansion of the silica.

Some sintering of silica occurs on heating the mould. In the presence of fluxes such as the oxides of Na, Ca, Zn and Fe recrystallization of silica occurs. On casting base metal alloys into such a mould, Mn, Co and Fe may react with the investment surface to produce less refractory materials. This effect at the interface between alloy and the mould may reduce permeability of the investment and thus cause microporosity or back pressure effects in the casting.

Ethyl silicate will gel at a low or a high pH. To prepare the binder solution the ethyl silicate is hydrolysed by adding H_2O, HCl and industrial spirit to it. Water will not mix directly with the ethyl silicate and industrial spirit is added as this is miscible with both of them. The hydrolysis is complete in about 12 hours and results in a thin yellow liquid. During the reaction some heat is liberated. This solution will slowly become more viscous, and in time will gel completely at room temperature. It usually has a shelf-life of 3–4 weeks. Hydrolysed ethyl silicate solutions should be stored in a dark bottle, away from sources of heat and light. There is some danger of ignition due to the large percentage of alcohol within the mixture. On adding the hydrolysed solution to the silica powder, gelation proceeds at a quicker rate. This is usually due to the presence of MgO mixed with the silica which produces a suitable alkaline pH for gelling to take place. Both the hydrolysed solution and the setting investment mixture should be handled with care. No attempt should be made to remove air from the investment by evacuation.

Rapid hydrolysis of ethyl silicate can be promoted by amines such as piperidine. Previous hydrolysis is then unnecessary as both hydrolysis and gelation take place together on mixing the binder solution and refractory. A strong gel is produced by this method. Unfortunately hydrolysis is accompanied by a shrinkage, and this together with shrinkage of the gel increases the difficulties in producing a casting of accurate dimensions.

Binding of the silica refractory can also be achieved by precipitating a silicic acid gel from an acidified solution of sodium silicate. This type of investment is, like the gypsum-bonded materials, more suitable for the lower fusing alloys. A fine grain refractory bonded in this manner is sometimes used as a preliminary coating on the wax pattern, thus giving a smooth surface to the casting.

A similar refractory bonded by a silica gel from an aqueous suspension of colloidal silica may also be used.

All these binding agents change to silica on heating, so that the mould is composed almost entirely of silica when it is ready for casting. Typical properties:

Linear expansion (setting and thermal)   1·5–1·7 per cent
Transverse strength 2 hours (green)   0·5 N/mm²
         at 1000°C   0·2–0·5 N/mm²
Fineness   Less than 5% should be
    coarser than 300 × 10⁻⁶m

Phosphate bonding

Other investment materials consist of a powder which is mixed with water or with a liquid supplied. This type may be a mixture of silica with a metallic oxide and phosphate. On adding water, the oxide and phosphate combine.

$$NH_4H_2PO_4 + MgO + 6H_2O \longrightarrow MgNH_4PO_4.6H_2O + H_2O$$

This reaction is the basis of the 'green strength' of the set investment. At about 300°C, the following reaction occurs:

$$2(Mg\,NH_4\,PO_4.6H_2O) \longrightarrow Mg_2P_2O_7 + 2NH_3 + 13H_2O$$

There is always present an excess of unreacted phosphate, which on further heating, reacts with the silica present to form complex silico-phosphates and so increase the strength of the investment. The use of a silicate solution in place of water creates favourable conditions for the formation of silicophosphates and thereby increases both the strength and the thermal expansion.

The setting expansion can vary widely between different materials. It is affected by powder/liquid ratio and spatulation time. Moisture affects the material on storage and the tin should be kept dry and closed when not in use. Setting expansion of phosphate-bonded investments is also increased markedly by water uptake from a duplicating material, particularly if its surface is wet.

Typical properties:

Linear expansion (setting and thermal)   1·5–1·7 per cent
Transverse strength   24 hours (green)   0·4 N/mm²
         at 1000°C   0·4 N/mm²

Heating the casting ring

Either gas or electrically heated muffle furnaces are used to heat the casting ring. Gas heating is a little faster than electricity. A pyrometer is essential to ensure the correct casting temperature.

The furnace door is left open until all the alcohol has evaporated or ignited and then the ring is heated quickly to the casting temperature. When using phosphate-bonded materials, ammonia is given off at 200–250°C. Suitable ventilation is necessary.

With a quartz refractory mould, temperatures of 1100°C are suggested. There is, however, little further expansion of the mould above 850°C, and successful castings can be made with a mould temperature of 900°C. But consideration must be given to any cooling of the mould which takes place whilst melting the alloy. A furnace temperature of 1000°C is often used, therefore, so that the refractory has passed its temperature of maximum expansion by 100–200°C. With a cristobalite refractory slightly lower temperatures may be used. With a lower mould temperature the grain size of the casting is finer, giving a casting of higher strength.

Chapter 19

Variables in casting techniques.
Defects in castings.

From the previous chapter it will be appreciated that there are many variables which affect the accuracy of a dental casting. These must all be controlled in order that a sound and accurate casting may be produced on each and every occasion.

Most of the discussion in this chapter relates to gold alloy castings for inlays, crowns, etc. The technique of making small gold alloy castings has been developed to a high degree of accuracy whereas casting of other alloys particularly those used for dentures, is not such a precise procedure.

COMPENSATION FOR CASTING SHRINKAGE

The wax pattern

A direct inlay pattern is of the correct size at the temperature at which it hardens (38–40°C). For dimensional accuracy of the wax, therefore, a direct pattern should be invested at a temperature only slightly below this. A pattern made on a die by the indirect method is accurate at room temperature if a continuous heavy pressure is maintained on the wax whilst it cools to room temperature. Heavy-pressure 'swaging' the wax into position causes it to flow and cancels out its cooling contraction. This pattern should be invested at the room temperature. Without this continuous pressure, the pattern is accurate at the hardening temperature of the wax. It should be invested at a temperature just below this. At room temperature such a pattern is undersize. A greater compensating expansion of the investment mould will be necessary if we invest a pattern at a temperature at which it is too small.

On reheating patterns from room to mouth temperature, however, there is some danger of distortion due to different expansion of the various thicknesses of wax in a complicated pattern. Then it is safer to invest at a lower temperature and allow for greater compensation later.

The Investment Cast

The setting expansion of the investment material forming the cast or model on which a wax pattern is built up compensates partly for casting shrinkage. Expansion is often affected by the duplicating material and by the shape of the duplicating flask. It is important that relatively unrestricted expansion is allowed.

THE INVESTMENT MOULD

There are four possible types of expansion which investment materials undergo. These are setting, hygroscopic, thermal and inversion change expansions. Combinations of these are used to compensate for casting shrinkage (Fig. 39).

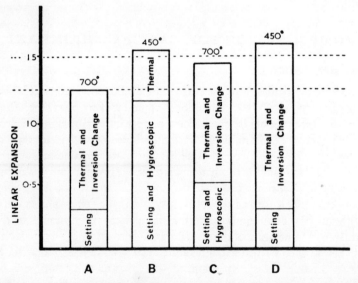

Fig. 39. Expansion of gypsum-bonded investments. (A) Quartz refractory. (B) Quartz refractory; mainly hygroscopic expansion. (C) Quartz refractory; all expansions employed. (D) Cristobalite refractory

Usually a casting ring of Ni–Cr alloy containing some Fe is used, as ordinary mild steel rings corrode rapidly at the temperatures used for preheating and casting. Another method is to make a tube of coarse mesh stainless steel gauze. This is placed inside a split ring of brass or other suitable metal which is of slightly greater diameter. The pattern is then placed within the gauze tube. Investment material is vibrated in to fill the outer split ring. When the investment has set the outer ring is removed. The gauze acts as a reinforcement embedded within the investment and allows very free expansion. In addition, the gauze is protected by the investment, and does not corrode even after being used on several occasions.

In general, the accuracy of castings made in base metal alloys is not yet as high as those cast in gold alloys. When making denture bases, distortion of the investment cast may arise from restriction of its setting expansion by the duplicating material. Dimensional inaccuracy of a casting due to thermal contraction of the thick sprues is not uncommon, particularly of a lingual or palatal bar type denture.

Control of dimensional accuracy

By reference to the values for the various expansions given by the manufacturer of the investment material, a technique can be evolved. When once accurate castings have been produced, the technique should not be varied.

> Use investment materials at a temperature to reduce wax contraction.
> Use constant powder : water ratio.
> For hygroscopic expansion, immerse the investment before it reaches initial set and control time and temperature.
> Allow free expansion either by lining the ring, by using a split ring or no ring at all.
> Cast into the heated mould whilst it is still at the correct temperature.

Surface finish

Before starting to invest a direct wax pattern, it should be washed in water at mouth temperature to remove debris such as mucus, blood, etc.

The contact angle between water and wax reduces at mouth temperature and a surface active or wetting agent may also be used to ensure wetting of the pattern by the investment material. Too much wetting agent, however, will inhibit the setting reaction of the surface layer of investment and so produce a rough surface to the casting.

Double-investment technique

The double-investment technique is sometimes used to ensure that the investment is well adapted to the pattern. In this method, a thin layer of fine investment material is painted on the pattern by means of a camel-hair brush. Before this layer has set, investment powder is dusted on until a more or less spherical and porous mass of investment surrounds the pattern. By this means, any excess water in the first mix is soaked up by the dry powder, and the resultant thick consistency of investment is said to ensure a high setting expansion. This lump of investment with the pattern in its centre is embedded in a further mix of investment of normal consistency. Some hygroscopic expansion of the initial layer of investment will take place when it is wetted by the new investment material.

Uneven expansion may occur and may lead to distortion of the wax pattern because of the uneven thickness of the investment round the pattern. Also, the two different mixes of investment may not have the same thermal expansion, and cracking of the inner layer may occur.

Hand painting

It is preferable to use one measured mix of investment and to paint the pattern with a portion of this to ensure the elimination of air bubbles. Then complete the investment procedure using the same mix of material.

With care, all the air bubbles can be eliminated by the above methods, but great care in working is required. Most of the air bubbles are formed where two portions of soft investment meet on coating a pattern. Therefore, the investment should be applied at one point and worked over the surface of the wax.

Mechanical spatulation and applying a reduced atmospheric pressure to the mix reduces the amount of air incorporated within the investment.

Vibration of the investment mix when pouring it round the pattern will cause air to rise to the surface of the mould. It may also bring air up to the under-surface of the wax pattern and so increase the air-blows near the pattern, while reducing the number of them in the surrounding investment. Some writers have suggested that no vibration is better than just a little.

'Vacuum' investing

An alternative method of avoiding 'air-blows' is to remove the air by subjecting the investment to a reduced atmospheric pressure, either before or after it has been poured round the pattern. The method has one disadvantage in that a thick mix of investment cannot be used, as free bubbling of the mix is essential to remove completely the enclosed air. Careful proportioning of the powder and water eliminates the possibility of using a mix of too thin a consistency.

The degree of evacuation required is to a pressure of $0.006N/mm^2$ (45 torr, or 28–29 inches Hg). This degree of evacuation can be produced by a motor driven pump or by a water pump when connected to a water supply of good pressure.

Even with 'vacuum' investing some air-blows may remain. Any surface of the pattern which is horizontal and which faces downwards will tend to collect a large air bubble underneath it during evacuation. This is particularly true if vibration is used. The air bubble will reduce in size when the pressure returns to that of the atmosphere, but a small bubble will remain to spoil the casting. The pattern must be placed in the casting ring so that the bubbles can flow past it and rise to the top of the investment to burst.

There is some danger of cooling the wax pattern and causing shrinkage if the reduced pressure is held for more than 15–20 seconds. If reduced pressure is applied for too long, setting will commence, and the bubbles will fail to burst. Also, the subsequent degree of hygroscopic expansion will be less as the initial set will have taken place.

Cracks in the investment—'finning'

These occur when the investment is heated up too rapidly in the furnace, or when two different mixes of investment are used.

There are two methods of heating a mould. It may be carefully dried at a temperature of 100–150°C and then heated within three-quarters of an hour to its casting temperature. Alternatively the soaking wet mould, on removal from the hygroscopic expansion bath, can be heated up without preliminary drying-out. The principle behind the last method is that the heat can only penetrate the mould as rapidly as the water is evaporated; water being a poor heat conductor in the absence of convection currents.

A damp investment material, as opposed to one which is soaking wet, will explode if heated too rapidly, as its thermal conductivity is too high.

Too rapid heating of any mould causes the outer layers to expand, due to the silica inversion change. This may lead to cracking of the investment since the outer layer has expanded, whereas the inner portions have not yet done so.

When casting a complete denture, it is common practice to employ an investment cast which carries the pattern. This is usually soaked in a wax or resin to facilitate the adhesion of patterns. In order to obtain good union between this cast and the remaining part of the mould, its surface should be trimmed round the pattern to expose unaffected investment material. The cast should be of recent construction, preferably the same day. A gypsum-bonded investment cast should be soaked in water before investing it. With this technique it is also preferable to cast the mould on the same day as it is made, as this reduces the possibility of cracking. In addition, all investment materials used should have similar thermal expansions.

Any cracking of the mould produces 'fins' on the casting, and if these lead to the outside of the mould, some alloy will be lost, giving an incomplete casting.

DEFECTS IN CASTINGS

Speed of casting: Completeness of the casting

The variables concerned in filling the mould are:

> Casting force.
> Size and number of the sprues.
> Back pressure.

Casting Force
The force necessary to drive the molten alloy into the mould cavity may be applied either by gas pressure or by centrifugal force.

Air, steam or inert gas pressure may be used. In the case of air, compressed air may be used. Alternatively atmospheric pressure can be utilized by creating a reduced pressure at the base of the casting ring. The use of gas pressure has some disadvantages. A blast of cold gas may cool the alloy slightly and chill it prematurely. Also the gas pressure is not all applied to the alloy. Some of the gas passes through the investment material on either side of the alloy and is released at the base of the casting ring. Some casting machines are available which enable melting of the alloy to be carried out in a controlled atmosphere either of an inert gas, or at greatly reduced air pressure, followed by casting under gas pressure.

Centrifugal casting

The great advantage of centrifugal casting is that the casting force is constant for a given mass of metal. Moreover, the casting force is applied directly to the molten alloy and cannot be dissipated as in the case of air or steam pressure.

Centrifugal force is proportional to the square of the speed of rotation of the arm, and directly proportional to the mass of alloy and length of the arm of the casting machine. As filling of the mould by any casting technique is complete in one twenty-fifth of a second, the initial acceleration of the mould is the most important factor in determining the casting force. The arm is rotated either by a spring, or by means of an electric motor.

With a rapid sideways acceleration of the crucible, the molten alloy is, by its own inertia, thrown against the side of the crucible. In one machine, the crucible is built up on this side, and the molten metal runs along the wall of the crucible and into the mould. Other machines have a 'cranked' arm which is placed at right angles to the main arm while the alloy is being melted. On releasing the machine it swings into line and throws the metal into the mould. The subsidiary pivot in this type of machine should be freely moving.

Other centrifugal machines rotate in a vertical plane. The crucible and mould move upwards, and the alloy is forced against the base of the crucible until projected outwards by centrifugal force. This type of machine usually has a stronger spring than the horizontal type and applies a greater casting force.

Size and number of the sprues

as pressure, When casting by gthe alloy must be melted, or placed after melting, in a curved hollow or crucible cut in the top of the investment mould. At the lowest point of this hollow, the main sprue leads into the mould cavity. Application of gas pressure then propels the alloy down the sprue. The diameter of the main sprue leading from the crucible is therefore limited to 3 mm. Beyond this diameter the molten alloy falls down the sprue under the influence of gravity, and freezes before it enters the casting proper. With centrifugal casting, the sprue diameter is unlimited since the alloy is melted away from the mould.

In any casting the greater the number and thickness of the sprues, the more easily will the metal fill the mould. Against this, the sprues must be severed from the completed casting and an excessive number of sprues creates more work in finishing. Also a larger weight of alloy is required for the casting and this presents difficulties in melting. It will be seen later that the point of attachment of the sprues is a common site for porosity and therefore an excessive number should be avoided. Sprues are attached to the thick sections of the casting so that the flow of metal into the mould is as smooth and rapid as possible.

The diameter of the sprue should be greater than the nearest section of the casting. For inlays a sprue of 2 mm (14 swg) diameter is advised.

The shape of the crucible or hollow in which the metal is melted for air or steam pressure affects the casting force. Its sides should be straight, and should present an angle between them of 90–120°' A shallower crucible reduces the 'head' of metal over the sprue and the investment surfaces resist some of the casting force. In centrifugal castings, the walls of the main sprue may be almost parallel. The path of the molten alloy

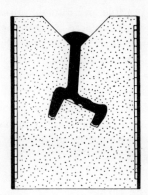

Fig. 40.   Back pressure effect. Pattern invested too far away from the base of the ring

flowing through the sprues to the mould cavity should be continuously away from the main sprue. At no time should the alloy be expected to flow 'uphill' against the effect of centrifugal force.

The length of the sprue, in itself, is not important, but it controls the position of the casting within the investment. It is more important to place the pattern near the base of the ring and so avoid *back pressure*, regardless of the length of the sprue.

Back pressure

As the molten metal enters the mould space, the gases contained therein must escape, preferably through the bottom of the mould. To assist the escape of gases, the investment material between the casting and the end of the ring should be as thin as is consistent with strength. Also, the end of the ring should not be completely covered by any part of the casting apparatus. In all cases the plate of metal which supports the end of the ring must be perforated.

Permeability of investments varies with their grain size distribution, but generally it decreases in the order of gypsum, phosphate, and silica-bonded. Often a rather dense layer of investment material is created at the base of the ring. This is particularly so when the base of the ring has been closed temporarily by a sheet of metal or glass. This dense layer should be scraped away to facilitate the escape of gases. When using silica-bonded or fine-grained phosphate-bonded refractories, a vent $\frac{1}{2}$ mm in diameter should be provided to allow escape of gases towards the crucible end of the mould.

A casting which has been subjected to back pressure is rounded at the edges and lacking in detail.

Porosity

Porosity may be seen as a surface defect on the casting, or may be revealed within the cast metal on filing and polishing.

It may be due to three causes:

Occluded gases.
Cooling shrinkage.
Flux, dirt or investment particles embedded in the metal.

Occluded gases

Copper, Au and Ag will dissolve oxygen in the molten state, and Pt and Pd dissolve both oxygen and hydrogen. On cooling, alloys containing these metals liberate the adsorbed gases. If this occurs when the metal is within the mould, porosity of the casting occurs. This type of porosity affects any areas of the casting and may involve the entire piece. The use of an efficient flux, particularly a reducing one containing carbon will lessen the degree of gaseous porosity. Overheating the alloy must be avoided. Adsorbed gases could also be reduced by degassing the alloy either before it is supplied to the dentist or on melting. If melting and casting is carried out in an atmosphere of an inert gas, adsorbed gas porosity is reduced. If the alloy is melted in a cylindrical carbon crucible, the amount of gas inclusion is reduced. At the melting temperature of most alloys the atmosphere in such a crucible is CO or CO_2.

Gaseous porosity due to the occlusion of the gases within the mould is frequently seen at the rounded ends of a casting which is incomplete due to back pressure.

Cooling shrinkage

On solidification, the alloy contracts but the outer portions of the casting remain in contact with the internal walls of the mould. Voids or secondary pipe will be formed unless more metal can enter the mould.

The thinner sections or those portions which are less effectively insulated against heat loss by the investment material, freeze first. As they solidify, they contract and draw molten metal from the remaining portions. Local shrinkage defects are found, therefore, in the thicker sections (Fig. 41). They are commonly seen in the casting at the base of a sprue. It is preferable, therefore, that the casting should freeze by a wave of solidification traversing its mass, moving towards the sprue. A reservoir of metal is then present within the sprues if these are of sufficient thickness. One method is to thicken up a section of each sprue as near to the casting as possible. These round *sprue reservoirs* should freeze last of all and any shrinkage porosity will be found in them, and not in the casting. Reservoirs should be twice the bulk of the nearest portion of the casting and should be only 1–2 mm along the sprue from the casting. They should also be in the centre of the mass of the casting ring so that they freeze last. Continued heating of the 'button' of alloy assists in preventing a wave of solidification travelling in the wrong direction, and thus producing porosity of the casting.

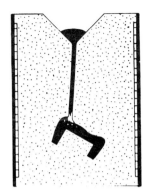

Fig. 41. Contraction porosity at the attachment of a thin sprue

A finer contraction porosity occurs under the surface layer of the casting if the alloy or the mould is overheated.

Embedded foreign matter

In centrifugal casting, oxide from the alloy, or an excess of flux, may be carried along with the molten alloy and become incorporated in the casting. Similarly, any broken pieces of investment, or particles of dirt which have fallen down the sprue, will be embedded in the casting and produce pitting of the surface. For this reason all casting moulds should be handled with the sprue downwards.

Grain structure of the casting

A fine grain structure gives the casting its optimum properties. This is achieved by cooling the casting rapidly when once the mould is filled. A metal temperature 50–100°C above the liquidus temperature should not be exceeded and the mould temperature should be no greater than that necessary to allow the running of thin sections and afford adequate thermal expansion. The bulk of investment material should be kept as small as possible so that cooling is not delayed.

Section D
General non-metallic materials

Chapter 20
Gypsum products

In dentistry the amount of plaster and stone used is greater than that of any other material. Both materials are used to make casts or models, and they also appear as ingredients of investment and impression materials.

PLASTER

Manufacture

Plaster is manufactured from the mineral gypsum; $CaSO_4.2H_2O$ (calcium sulphate dihydrate). The name plaster of 'Paris' arose during the Renaissance period from the fact that a particularly good plaster for the sculptor was made from gypsum mined at Montmarte, near Paris. Gypsum is quite a common mineral. It occurs naturally in a relatively pure state, either as an opaque white mass, or in a crystalline, translucent form known as 'alabaster'. $CaSO_4$(anhydrite), carbonates, and a little SiO_2 are usually present as impurities.

Plaster is made by heating the gypsum to $110-120°C$ causing a loss of water:

$$2(CaSO_4.2H_2O) \longrightarrow (CaSO_4)_2.H_2O + 3H_2O$$

On heating the gypsum in 'kettles' in the open air, rather irregular crystals known as β-hemihydrate are formed. When the reaction is complete the resultant powder is dried at $150-165°C$.

If the gypsum is not heated sufficiently, some unchanged gypsum remains, whereas, if it is overheated all the water is driven off and anhydrite is left. The latter substance appears in three forms; at temperatures between $130°$ and $200°C$ as a soluble or quick setting material, and secondly, if the temperature rises higher during manufacture, as a dead-burnt, slow setting material. Even greater heating than this produces a non-setting anhydrite.

Composition of dental plaster

Normally, freshly made dental plasters contain some soluble anhydrite. This gradually changes to hemihydrate on storing by combining with atmospheric moisture. Plaster also contains some unchanged gypsum. This is often added to the hemihydrate by the manufacturer to assist the setting reaction. Dental plasters as supplied to the dentist, consist mainly of hemihydrate—approximately 75–85 per cent by weight, with 5–8 per cent of unchanged gypsum and a similar amount of a mixture of fast setting and dead-burnt anhydrite. Other minerals are present as impurities up to 4 per cent.

The plaster is ground after heating and the fairly large porous grains are broken up to give fine dental plaster. Microscopically, grains of dental plaster vary in size from small bundles of crystals to small portions of a single crystal which have been broken off in grinding. The large surface area of the grains after grinding gives a quick reaction between the plaster and water and a short setting time.

Setting

On mixing plaster with water, the reaction which occurred during manufacture is reversed:

$$(CaSO_4)_2.H_2O + 3H_2O \longrightarrow 2(CaSO_4.2H_2O)$$

and heat is liberated.

The hemihydrate is slightly soluble in water, and on mixing plaster for use, a saturated solution is quickly produced. While in solution the hemihydrate reacts with the water to form dihydrate. However, the solubility of this is only a quarter of that of the hemihydrate, so that a supersaturated solution of dihydrate arises. Monoclinic crystals of dihydrate grow out mainly in the direction of orientation of the dihydrate crystals present which act as nuclei of crystallization. They meet and form a rigid complex crystal mass.

Setting of plaster takes place over a short period of time. Soon after mixing, a thickening of the mix is apparent but the plaster can still be moulded. After some further thickening, any moulding or cutting becomes impracticable, as the plaster crumbles, At a slightly later time the plaster can be cut readily with a knife, but this becomes more difficult after it has been standing for an hour or more.

Initial and final set

Setting is usually described as occurring in two stages. The 'initial set' corresponds roughly to the stage when the plaster loses its surface gloss and no longer crumbles but can be cut with a knife, and the 'final set' is reached when it is rather too hard to trim easily. These setting times are usually measured by Gillmore or Vicat needles. Initial set is indicated when the lighter of the two Gillmore needles applying a stress of 0·3 N/mm² fails to mark the surface. The heavier Gillmore needle applying a stress of 5 N/mm² similarly indicates final set. The Vicat needle is a form of penetrometer and indicates initial set when it fails to penetrate to the bottom of a mix of plaster 50 mm thick.

Effects of storage

The dental surgeon has no control over the properties of the plaster he purchases except by changing his supplier, although a slight variation is noted between successive batches from the same manufacturer. The treatment of plaster during transit from the manufacturer, via the wholesaler, to the consumer, and its method of storage in the laboratory has a considerable effect upon its properties.

In the details of manufacture, it was noted that some quick setting anhydrite is present in newly made plaster. On exposure to the atmosphere during the first few days after manufacture, this anhydrite absorbs water and turns into hemihydrate. Thus a sack of very new plaster will set much more quickly than one which has been stored and is said to have 'matured'.

Exposure to an excessive amount of moisture in the atmosphere produces a film of dihydrate round each grain. This makes the plaster slow setting, as, on mixing, the water has to penetrate this layer before it can react with the unchanged hemihydrate beneath. The growth of crystals upon setting is also retarded and a weaker crystal mass is produced.

If the plaster is kept in a hot, dry atmosphere, some of the dihydrate grains will change back to hemihydrate and by reducing the number of nuclei of crystallization, will lengthen the setting time, provided the plaster is cooled down before use.

In the dental laboratory, plaster should be kept in metal containers. If stored in bags on a concrete floor, they should be raised to provide a circulation of air beneath the bags.

Consistency of mix

From the equation giving the setting reaction of plaster 100 g of powder need be mixed with only 18·6 cm³ of water in order to convert all the plaster into gypsum. Such a mix of plaster would be too dry to use in the laboratory, and 2–2½ times this amount of water is usually added to produce a smooth, workable mix. The plaster grains themselves soak up water because of their porous structure. The excess water remains in the set plaster, which consists, therefore, of a network of dihydrate crystals, with the spaces filled in by excess water.

When a thin mix of plaster is used, the formation of a supersaturated solution of dihydrate is delayed, and the centres from which crystallization occurs are scattered wide apart. Such a mix takes longer to set than one of higher plaster to water ratio. The dihydrate crystal structure formed from a thin mix is less dense than that from a thick mix. The crystals are not closely packed and more spaces appear between them. Such a structure can be fractured more easily than one which is a dense mass of crystals. Therefore, a thin mix produces a weak mass of plaster on setting, and a thick mix produces a strong material. The limiting factor in the consistency of a plaster mix is that it must be workable. It is not possible to make a workable mix of plaster which contains too little water for complete setting to take place.

Setting expansion

The volume of a set mass of gypsum is greater than that of the mix of plaster and water from which it arose. The increase in volume is due to crystal growth. As the crystals grow out they meet others. During further growth of the crystals, the mass of plaster is expanded.

The linear expansion varies between 0·15 and 0·40 per cent under normal working conditions. Under unfavourable conditions of manipulation, the expansion may be as great as 1·15 per cent. It occurs mainly in the first hour after setting, but continues slowly for a further 24 hours.

In a thick mix of plaster, the crystals quickly meet and expand the setting mass, because the grains of plaster are packed closely together.

Whereas in a thinner mix the crystals have farther to grow before they meet and do not push against each other so strongly. Therefore a thick mix expands more than a thin one.

Linear expansion can be measured by placing a mix of plaster in a V-shaped trough lined with grease or rubber dam, the lining allowing the plaster to expand with some freedom. One end of the plaster is fixed and movement of the other end is recorded on a dial gauge. A more accurate method is to measure the expansion of the plaster while it is floating on a bath of mercury. By this means, the effect of friction upon the expansion is reduced to a minimum. Two vertical metal markers are placed in the plaster and the change in distance between these is measured.

Heat of reaction

The reaction between plaster and water is exothermic. The thicker the mix of plaster the higher the temperature produced. In a large bulk of setting plaster, the internal temperature may rise 20–30°C due to the insulating effect of the outer layers. This property is often made use of when flasking dentures, as the heat softens the wax of the denture and enables it to be removed quite easily from the mould.

Spatulation

The usual method of mixing is to measure into the bowl a volume of water roughly equal to that of the bulk of the mixed plaster required and then to sift in the powder. If sifting is carried out slowly, the dry plaster becomes completely soaked with water, and little spatulation is required to produce a smooth mix. When large amounts of plaster are added at a time, the outer layers of powder are wetted, but lumps of relatively dry plaster remain. More spatulation is then required to produce a smooth consistency. When a small bulk of plaster is being mixed, time is available for slow sifting before the plaster begins to set, but where a large bowlful is needed, the addition of powder must take place at a faster rate and lumps tend to appear. Spatulation should be limited to the minimum necessary to produce a smooth mix. With fine dental plasters, the time of spatulation should seldom exceed $1\frac{1}{2}$ minutes.

No advantage is gained in continuing spatulation beyond the point where plaster and water are smoothly combined. In fact, several disadvantages occur. The crystals of gypsum are broken off as they grow, and these become extra centres of crystallization. As soon as mixing stops, setting starts from a large number of centres and takes place very quickly. At the same time the expansion is increased, since rapid crystallization occurs throughout the entire mass of plaster. The strength of the set plaster is reduced, however, due to the weaker crystal structure which is produced.

Air bubbles cause weakness of the plaster and produce surface imperfections of a cast or impression. Spatulation by a mechanical mixer reduces the amount of air incorporated in the mix and produces a stronger cast with a smoother surface. A mechanical spatulator may be hand or motor driven. In either case the speed of the mixing paddle should be fairly slow or air will be incorporated in the mix.

Mixing the plaster under a reduced atmospheric pressure reduces markedly the number of airblows in the set plaster. When combined with suitable vibration, excellent compaction of the mix can be achieved. Due to settling of the plaster within the impression, the tooth or ridge portion of the cast is stronger than the remainder. This portion is at the lowest level when pouring the cast. The technique of 'boxing in', by creating a greater depth of plaster over the impression surface, assists in this effect.

Most dental vibrators work at a frequency twice that of the AC electric supply and at an amplitude varying between 0·2–0·8 mm. Light pressure applied when holding the impression against the vibrator prevents undue damping of the amplitude of the oscillation. Amplitude and frequency of movement together control the acceleration applied to the gypsum grains and this is the major factor in effective condensation by vibration.

For accurate and reproducible results, the plaster should be weighed and the water measured. When the quantities of plaster and water are not measured before mixing, a too-thick or too-thin working consistency is sometimes produced. The temptation to add more plaster or water to bring the consistency within workable limits must be resisted. Addition of further plaster to a thin mix produces a heterogeneous mass which sets unevenly. The addition of water to a thick mix weakens the crystal formation.

Temperature of mix

The time taken for plaster to set decreases as the temperature of the mix is raised to 30°C; small changes in setting time occur from 30–50°C but above this latter temperature the plaster sets more slowly until at 100°C no setting is apparent.

In the dental laboratory, setting of plaster may be speeded up if necessary by the use of lukewarm water instead of cold tap water. The latter is usually at 14–18°C.

After setting

Note has already been made of the fact that plaster expands for 24 hours after its initial set. During this time, also, part of the excess water evaporates leaving a porous network of dihydrate crystals.

Strength of set plaster

The strength of set plaster is normally measured under compression. As noted previously, a thick mix of plaster forms a dense crystal structure which has a high compressive strength.

The method of adding the plaster to the water, and of mixing, affects the crushing strength. If a large amount of air is incorporated in a plaster mix, it weakens the plaster.

After the final set, the strength of the plaster increases gradually over a period of $\frac{1}{2}$–2 hours, by which time hydration is complete. Strength increases greatly on the evaporation of *all* the excess water present in

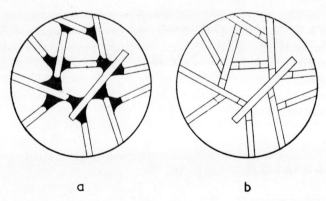

a   b

Fig. 42. Diagrammatic representation of the drying out of gypsum materials. (a) Water causing solution of the surface of dihydrate crystals in contact. (b) More rigid crystal structure after drying out

the spaces between the dihydrate crystals. The crushing strength of plaster containing excess water, or, as it is called, the *wet crushing strength* is only half of the strength after drying. It is probable that the excess water dissolves the surface of the gypsum crystals and thus lubricates their movement over each other when a force is applied. On drying, this solution of dihydrate forms small crystals which bind the main crystals together (Fig. 42). At room temperature and humidity, it would take a long time to dry out a bulk of plaster, and only the outer layers are affected at first, giving a higher surface hardness. A warm atmosphere, up to 100°C, causes more rapid drying out. This should be done with care, however, since the dihydrate decomposes slowly above 45°C, and rapidly above 110°C.

Wet plaster flows or creeps under a load near its compressive strength, whereas dry plaster is brittle but resists a greater force.

Dimensional changes after setting

Set plaster is fairly stable in dimension under normal laboratory conditions of temperature and humidity. As the plaster dries out a slight shrinkage occurs, and similarly an expansion on wetting again. These changes do not appear to be of practical significance. In thin sections, however, drying of the plaster may be accompanied by a slight warpage. On rewetting plaster, it soaks up water and the compressive strength falls until it is dried out again.

Set plaster is slightly soluble in water. If hot water is poured over a plaster surface, as in 'boiling out' a denture mould, a portion of the surface is dissolved and the plaster becomes slightly roughened. This effect is particularly noticeable when the plaster mix was thin and has just set. Frequent washing of a plaster cast is therefore not advised.

To remove remnants of gypsum products from dentures, an aqueous solution of 30 per cent ammonium citrate at about pH8, together with ultrasonic vibration, is recommended.

PLASTER AS AN IMPRESSION MATERIAL

Applicable specifications: Brit 4598; Amer 25; Austral 1651.

The desirable properties of plaster when used for recording impressions are:

Passes 200 mesh	90 per cent
Powder/water ratio	100/45–50
Setting time (initial)	$2\frac{1}{2}$–5 minutes
Linear expansion (2 hours)	0·05–0·10 per cent
Compressive strength, wet	
(10 minutes)	2–5 N/mm^2
Clean fracture after initial set.	

These requirements are not apparent in a plain mix of plaster and water. Additions must be made in order to reduce the expansion and the strength and to achieve a more rapid set.

Control of setting expansion and time

Potassium sulphate reduces setting expansion to a marked degree when added in concentrations of about 4 per cent. The addition of K_2SO_4 to a plaster mix causes rapid initial crystal growth of syngenite, a complex crystal of potassium calcium sulphate. This inhibits further growth and thus limits expansion of the plaster. Together with other metallic salts, it reduces the setting time also.

The most effective accelerators of plaster are K_2SO_4, NaCl, KCl and $K_2SO_4.Al_2(SO_4)_3$ (potash alum). Of these, K_2SO_4 accelerates the setting of plaster in all concentrations, while the others act as accelerators in low concentrations, but may retard the set when present in large amounts. The precise mechanism of the action of accelerators and retarders is unknown, but it is probable that they affect the rate of solution of hemihydrate and so control the speed of the reaction. Accelerators may also provide more centres for crystallization or supply sulphate ions to the solution.

Unfortunately, the amount of K_2SO_4 necessary to reduce the expansion, causes a normal plaster to set too rapidly, and a retarder such as $Na_2B_4O_7$ (borax) must be added.

There is an advantage in having a relatively weak and brittle plaster for impressions. The impression will break cleanly and without the application of undue force when difficulties arise in removing it from the mouth. If necessary the plaster can be broken into two or three large pieces so that an impression of an undercut shape may be taken. Potassium sulphate reduces the strength of the set plaster, as does NaCl.

A pigment is added to an impression plaster so that when a model is cast to the impression in white plaster or stone, the junction between the two materials can easily be seen. Alizarin S (sodium alizarin sulphonate) is a pigment of the madder group, and forms an insoluble 'lake' with calcium salts. This material ensures that the dye remains only in the impression plaster and does not wash over into the cast. Impression plasters are available which are homogenous mixtures of K_2SO_4, $Na_2B_4O_7$, and Alizarin S with plaster, and they require only the addition of water.

Plaster is an unpleasant material to have in one's mouth, and flavouring is added to the commercial products to make the operation of impression-taking more pleasant for the patient.

At one time, plaster was the most frequently used material for impressions of edentulous ridges. Its main advantages are a relatively constant consistency during a short manipulation time, so that it can be moulded by the soft tissues of the mouth. At the end of this short manipulation period, it sets rapidly, and, after only a short waiting

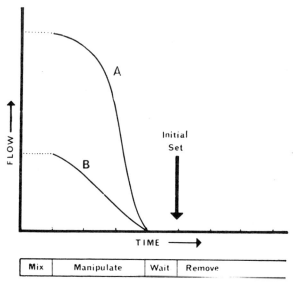

Fig. 43. Change in consistency of plaster and relation to setting time. (A) Thin mix. (B) Thicker mix

period, has achieved initial set and can be removed from the mouth (Fig. 43) A thicker consistency shows a less clearly marked set point and an attempt might be made to mould a partially set material. This, however, produces a rough and obviously incorrect impression surface.

After the initial set, the impression cannot be distorted to any significant extent. Distortion during or after removal from the mouth is seen as a fracture. Imperfections of the impression are also readily seen. Assessment of the accuracy of a plaster impression is therefore easy.

When used for recording impressions of soft tissues only, it is probable that the good working properties and general dimensional stability of plaster are more important than precise control of its dimensional accuracy. The errors produced by expansion of a plaster mix are small in relation to the other dimensional errors which accompany the construction of complete dentures. They are also small in relation to the amount of error which can be detected clinically and which will produce symptoms.

Soluble plasters

In some impression techniques, only a thin layer or 'wash' of impression plaster is used. After the cast has been made, some difficulty is experienced in removing this thin layer without damaging the cast beneath. If starch is incorporated in the dry impression plaster, the thin layer of set plaster can be removed by pouring boiling water over it. The hot water causes the starch grains to swell, and they break up the set plaster which washes away as a fine powder. The addition of starch gives the impression plaster a little more body and enables the operator to mould it in the mouth a little easier than with plain plaster. Other additions, such as gum tragacanth, ZnO or 0·2 per cent polyvinyl acetate have been suggested to improve the 'plasticity' of impression plasters.

Pouring the cast

A plaster impression will not change its shape over a short period of time after removal from the mouth. The cast should, however, be poured into the impression within a few hours to avoid distortion due to uneven drying out.

The surface of a plaster impression must be treated to prevent the impression and cast sticking together. The materials used for this purpose are called *separating media*. These may be of two types. The first type are varnishes such as sandarac, or colloidin, or alginate mould seal. These form a thin film over the plaster and introduce a slight inaccuracy in the cast. The second type, such as soap or dilute water-glass solutions, combine chemically with the surface layer of plaster and cause little or no dimensional change.

PLASTER AS A MATERIAL FOR CASTS

Applicable specifications: Brit 4722; Amer 25; Austral 1652.

The properties of an ideal cast material differ in many respect from those required in an impression plaster. A mix of plaster and water of medium consistency is too weak for making casts as, during the moulding of a denture, large forces, particularly of a compressive nature, are brought to bear upon the cast. A thicker mix vibrated into the impression gives a stronger cast, but its large setting expansion would introduce an inaccuracy.

Ordinary fine dental plaster is used for general purposes in the laboratory and would show the following properties:

Passes 100 mesh	98 per cent
Passes 200 mesh	90 per cent
Powder/water ratio	100/40–50
Initial set	5–10 minutes
Linear expansion (2 hours)	0·2–0·3 per cent
Compressive strength wet (1 hour)	10 N/mm²
Compressive strength dry (24 hours)	24 N/mm²
Tensile strength dry	1·3 N/mm²
Transverse strength dry	0·6 N/mm²

Casts for record purposes may be made in plaster as they are not subjected to large forces. All working casts should be made of a harder material.

ARTIFICIAL STONES

Applicable specifications: Brit 4796; Amer 25; Austral 1616.

Gypsum heated in air produces β-hemihydrate or plaster of Paris. If it is heated under different conditions the same chemical $(CaSO_4)_2.H_2O$

is produced but in single crystals known as α-hemihydrate. When ordinary plaster is mixed with water, a working consistency is obtained only when sufficient water is present both to saturate the porous grains of plaster and also to lubricate the movement of the grains over each other. With artificial stones, little water soaks into the grains at first, and most of it is available to produce a workable mix. Hence, for a given working consistency, a mix of stone contains a higher ratio of powder to water than does a mix of plaster. With some stones, a powder: water ratio as high as 100:20 can be used.

Several forms of α-hemihydrate are available, since the crystals vary with the method of manufacture. Dehydration in a closed container under steam pressure at 120–150°C produces unit crystals of moderate size commonly known as *hydrocal*. If organic acids are added to the water a slightly larger grain size material known as *crystacal* is produced. By boiling the gypsum in a 30 per cent aqueous solution of $CaCl_2$ the largest crystals are produced which form the basis of *densite (improved)* stones. The smaller the surface area of a given weight of α-hemihydrate, the less the volume of water required to make a workable consistency.

The setting reaction of α-hemihydrate is the same as that of plaster. The setting expansion of artificial stones is controlled by the addition of K_2SO_4, Rochelle salt, and the setting time is adjusted by incorporating either $Na_2B_4O_7$ or a mixture of sodium citrate in silica. The chemicals are already in the dry powder bought as artificial stone. To prevent confusion with plaster, artificial stones are usually pigmented. The combined effect of the chemical additives results in a material which has a low linear setting expansion but a relatively long working time. The amount of setting expansion is usually independent of powder:water ratio. Compressive strength increases with the incorporation of more powder up to a maximum, but tensile strength is less affected by the powder:water ratio. Hence the reason why many casts fracture in tension though they are strong in compression. To ensure adequate mechanical properties, the powder: water ratio should be determined by measurement. Where this is not practicable, then a thick putty-like mix should be made which, under moderate vibration, will flow into the detail of the impression. A thin mix gives a weak cast which may not have even the compressive strength of a correct mix of ordinary plaster. A very dry mix which requires heavy vibration to make it flow, usually contains insufficient water to wet the hemihydrate particles and again a weaker cast is produced. Typical properties of artificial stones are:

	Hydrocal and crystacal types	Densite type
Passes 100 mesh	98 per cent	
Passes 200 mesh	90 per cent	
Powder : water ratio	100/25–35	100/20–35
Initial set	5–20 minutes	
Linear expansion	0·1–0·2 per cent	
Compressive strength wet (1 hour)	35 N/mm²	40 N mm²
Compressive strength dry (24 hours)	70 N/mm²	75 N/mm²
Transverse strength dry	15 N/mm²	20 N/mm²

A mixture of plaster and stone does not show a strength proportionate to the amount of stone present in it, unless the volume of water is reduced in the same proportion. Too often a 'sloppy' mix of plaster and stone is made which has relatively poor strength. The powders can be mixed dry, or may be added separately to the water and then spatulated together.

A low powder/liquid ratio with a low compressive strength of only 1·5 N/mm² may be used as the mould for the 'pour technique' for some self-curing acrylic polymers. It is considered that the use of such a material allows less shrinkage during polymerizing than a mould made from an elastomer, whilst allowing easy removal of the denture from the mould.

Densite stones are also used for dies (Chapter 32).

Surface hardness of gypsums is improved by impregnating the surface with a polymer. A cast dried at 40°C can be treated with a solution of a polymer such as polymethyl methacrylate or polystyrene, or by the application of a monomer which polymerizes after soaking into the surface. Epoxide monomer and accelerator, or methyl methacrylate monomer containing 2 per cent benzoyl peroxide are both suitable. This treatment improves tensile strength and abrasion resistance. The effect of impregnating gypsum with a polymer is greater on β than α hemihydrate due to the higher porosity of plaster. After impregnation, the tensile strength of plain plaster mixes is the same as that of densites.

Casts for special purposes

Although dimensional accuracy is essential in a master cast, duplicates for special purposes are sometimes produced which are oversize and which may compensate for the shrinkage of another material during denture construction.

When methyl methacrylate is polymerized, a shrinkage occurs and an expanding stone can be used for casts on which these dentures are to be made. It is doubtful, however, whether any accurate compensation can be achieved.

Joint between two mixes of gypsum

For reasons of economy and simplicity of working, the tooth or ridge surface of the cast is frequently poured in α hemihydrate to which a base of β hemihydrate is added. The joint between the two mixes of gypsum is probably one of attachment only. The strength of joints between any two gypsums is only one-sixth to one-tenth of the tensile strength of the material on either side of the joint.

Chapter 21

Non-elastic impression materials

IMPRESSION COMPOUNDS

Applicable specifications: Brit 3886; Amer 3; Austral T6.

These are thermoplastic materials, that is, they soften when heated and harden on cooling down again to mouth or room temperature.

Requirements

An impression compound should:

Soften at a temperature which will cause no discomfort to the patient.
Have sufficient flow at this temperature so that it will record an impression of the detail of the teeth and soft tissues.
Be cohesive and not adhesive at this temperature.
Harden at a temperature slightly above that of the mouth.
Be cut or trimmed easily with a sharp knife, without distortion, flaking or cracking.
Show no dimensional change on hardening, nor on storage subsequent to its removal from the mouth.
Be capable of being sterilized without loss of properties.

Ingredients

The precise ingredients of impression compounds are not known. They consist essentially of some thermoplastic material which is modified by the addition of resins and fillers in order to give it suitable properties.

The thermoplastic constituent may be stearin, stearic acid, paraffin wax, beeswax, gutta-percha, or a combination of these materials.

Synthetic or natural resins are added in order to increase the hardness of the compound when it has set. These may be shellac, copal resin, Kauri resin, or a resin of the coumerone-indene type. A mixture of thermoplastic materials and resins is made which softens at 50–70°C. To give body to this mixture, and to reduce its stickiness, fillers such as pumice, french chalk, or similar powders are added. The particle size of the filler is important as it affects the detail of the impression which can be achieved with the material. The filler should bond to the thermoplastic matrix, thus forming a composite structure.

Compounds deteriorate after storage for 4–5 years due to changes in the shellac.

The impression compounds or *compositions* available may be divided into two types:

Type 1—These are the lower fusing materials and are usually coloured green, red, brown or grey. They are used for taking copper ring impressions for inlays and crowns, and also for recording 'functional' or 'compressive' impressions prior to the construction of complete and partial dentures. These materials soften at 53–60°C and do not reproduce undercuts. One or two 'elastic' impression compounds exhibit visco-elastic properties at 30–40°C. These may be used for taking impressions when small undercuts are present.

Type 2—Tray compounds. These are relatively tough compounds with a higher softening temperature, and are strong enough to act as a support for other impression materials. They soften above 70°C and may be black or white in colour.

Flow of compounds under a compressive stress of 0·25 N/mm² for 10 min. should be:

	37°C	45–50°C
Type 1.	Less than 6 per cent	More than 85 per cent
Type 2.	Less than 2 per cent	70–85 per cent

Impression compounds generally show a near-Newtonian stress/strain relationship when fully softened. Flow is, however, very temperature dependent. A drop of 5°C in the temperature of the material can cause a tenfold increase in its viscosity.

Softening impression compounds

The thermal conductivity of all types of compound is very poor and softening or hardening of the material in any bulk takes time. For this reason, compounds are sold in sheets about 5 mm thick, or in stick form. The use of too little heat for softening causes a rough surface to appear on the material when it is manipulated. This is due to the lack of flow of the thermoplastic components and the exposure of grains of the filler on the surface. Too much heat makes the compound sticky and difficult to handle. When softening compound in water, a napkin or piece of cloth should cover the inside walls of the bath to prevent the material sticking to the sides. Compound may be softened in a flame but if too much dry heat is applied, some of the more volatile constituents may be driven off and this will spoil the properties of the material.

Softening in water produces the most evenly heated mass, with the best control of temperature. The water also improves mouldability by acting as a plasticizer. New compound which does not contain water is not as easy to manipulate as a similar material which has already been softened in water and has been used recently for an impression. For large impressions, the compound should be 'kneaded' with the fingers during softening in order to incorporate water in it. After such a treatment compound shows up to ten times as much flow as it did at the same temperature in the dry state. For small impressions in a copper ring, this increased flow is undesirable, and softening by dry heat in an oven or above a flame is preferred.

After softening compound several times in water, however, some of the thermoplastic constituents leach out, leaving the material rather dry and difficult to mould. A similar effect is produced by leaving the material immersed in hot water for several hours.

Impression compounds cannot be sterilized by chemical agents. Even after prolonged immersion in an antiseptic only the surface is affected. Heat sterilization can be carried out without causing too great a deterioration in the properties of the compound, if it is heated in an autoclave for some 10 minutes at 0.1 N/mm^2 (15 psi).

Manipulation

To record an impression, the softened compound is placed in a warm dry tray and roughly conformed to the shape of the mouth. Then the surface of the compound is passed through the flame in order to make it a little softer, A smooth, shiny surface layer is produced which is softer than the underlying material and this records the finer detail of the mouth tissues.

Hardening of compound takes place slowly in the mouth, and

except for Type I materials for inlay and crown impressions, the impression is often removed before it is completely rigid. When taking an impression of a single tooth within a copper band, however, perfect accuracy is essential. The compound must be hard at the time when the impression is removed or it will distort.

The cooling curve for compounds indicates a transition temperature as in waxes. All compound impressions should remain in the mouth until they have cooled at least to this temperature. At this temperature, the compound is not completely set, but is capable of much less flow than before crystallization occurred (Fig. 44). In impressions for

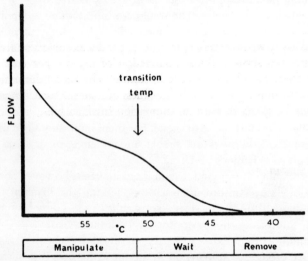

Fig. 44. Flow of impression compound against temperature. Note reduction in flow after transition temperature

dentures when undercut areas are present, the material is removed at a temperature below the transition point, but before it hardens completely. At this stage, the 'elastic' compounds show a slight elasticity. When large undercuts are present, or if the impression is removed before it cools to the transition temperature, the undercut areas are 'dragged', causing a distortion of the surrounding impression.

Distortion after removal from the mouth

Stresses may be set up within a compound impression either during its adaptation to the mouth tissues, or on its removal from the mouth.

Compound must be moulded while fully soft, that is, above its transition temperature. After removal the impression should be chilled immediately, in order to reduce the possible distortion from stress-relief. An impression should be cast within an hour to avoid any change of shape at room temperature.

An accurate compound impression can only be achieved, therefore, when no undercuts are present. The material should be used in thin sections, which cool quickly in the mouth. It must be manipulated in the fully softened condition, and should not be removed until it has hardened completely.

Inaccuracies in a compound impression are not immediately obvious on examination. However, an impression can be replaced in the mouth to check its accuracy, and also portions of compound may be added or trimmed away where necessary in order to produce a correct impression.

Compounds show a linear contraction of 0·3–0·5 per cent upon cooling from mouth to room temperature. The actual dimension of their contraction depends on the thickness of material used. Therefore, care must be taken to keep an impression small in bulk, and also to ensure that it is uniform in thickness throughout.

Making the cast

No separating medium is necessary with compound. The surface of the impression is simply washed free of saliva.

When the gypsum has set, the compound should be softened by placing it in a small amount of water at 60–70°C. Wetting of the entire cast should be avoided, as it will take longer to dry out and achieve its maximum strength. Also, the surface of newly cast stone or plaster is dissolved slightly if it is placed in water. Overheating the compound at this stage will cause it to stick to the cast and discolour the stone or plaster.

ZINC OXIDE IMPRESSION PASTES

Applicable specifications: Brit 4284; Amer 16; Austral T18.

The zinc oxide-eugenol (ZOE) pastes are used for taking 'wash' or 'rebase' impressions of 'edentulous' or non-tooth-bearing portions of the mouth. They are always used in thin sections of 1–2 mm. Like the impression compounds, they will not record accurately an undercut shape. Though many of them show thermoplastic properties, their setting is brought about by a chemical reaction and not by thermal changes.

These materials are generally available as two pastes which on mixing set in a few minutes.

Constituents

The two pastes provided are usually of different colours to ensure even mixing. One contains ZnO, usually mixed with amorphous gums and oils to make a paste. The other contains eugenol together with rosin and oils and often contains a filler such as kaolin or talc. The presence of rosin makes a more cohesive paste.

Zinc oxide and eugenol probably harden by two mechanisms. One is the absorption of eugenol by the oxide, and the other the formation of zinc eugenolate by a chelation reaction between the oxide and the eugenol. This is the attachment of a molecule, ion or group to a metal atom at more than one point, thus producing a ring structure. The term is derived from the Greek word meaning 'crab's claw' indicating a two-pronged attachment.

The actual setting mechanism which predominates depends upon the source of oxide used, and the conditions under which it was manufactured.

The initial reaction is the hydration of the ZnO to give $Zn(OH)_2$; for this, water must be present. On the subsequent formation of zinc eugenolate, water is formed, so continuing the reaction. In general terms, the set material consists of grains of ZnO loosely bonded to a matrix of long thin crystals of zinc eugenolate, together with some free eugenol.

Various accelerators are added to one or both of the two pastes to speed up the setting time to 3–4 minutes. A large number of metallic salts accelerate the setting reaction, but those of Zn appear to be the

eugenol   zinc oxide   eugenol   zinc eugenolate most effective. Zinc sulphate, zinc or magnesium acetate and $CaCl_2$ act as accelerators.

Patients may complain of a mild tingling to a hot burning sensation during impression recording due to the eugenol content of these pastes. The use of oil of cloves instead of the purer eugenol may assist in reducing the amount of irritation. The added oils also help to mask this effect. The patient's reaction is not always the same, but the taste of these materials cannot be considered to be ideal.

Alternative non-eugenol materials are probably based upon the reaction between ZnO and a carboxylic acid, such as orthoethoxy-benzoic acid, to form an insoluble soap. The carboxylic acid may be present as a liquid or as a powder dispersed in a medium such as ethyl alcohol.

After some dental surgical procedures, an intra-oral 'bandage' is required to protect the cut surfaces and to prevent infection of the tissues. ZOE pastes with a long setting time may be used. The phenol group in eugenol is antiseptic in action, but the chelation reaction causes it to be released only slowly. If there is an acid exudate at the operation site, then the ZnO in the paste can absorb and neutralize it. The continuing liberation of eugenol from these pastes may, however, cause the patient some gastric upset. Non-eugenol pastes containing medicaments are an alternative.

Setting time

The accelerator may be present in either of the two pastes, so that before any control of the setting time can be achieved, a test should be made to find out which contains the accelerating chemicals. Sometimes one paste is specifically marked 'accelerator'. In some materials accelerators may be present in both pastes and little control over the setting time can be achieved.

The proportions of the two pastes cannot be varied very widely, as too high a ratio of eugenol to oxide in the mix will cause a slow set, besides affecting the viscosity of the mixed paste.

Water accelerates the setting reaction; but it is difficult to combine water with the oily pastes. If it is incorporated with the oxide paste it reduces the shelf-life. When taking an impression, the saliva in the mouth accelerates the set. Water vapour in the atmosphere speeds the setting reaction, as does the use of damp mixing instruments.

On a warm day the paste sets quickly, as usually the humidity is high under such conditions. The warmth of the mouth also assists in speeding the setting reaction.

Most of the impression pastes available show a suitable setting time when mixed according to the manufacturer's instructions, and it is not advisable to vary the recommended proportions. There are several materials available and if one sets too slowly, another type should be tried.

Flow

The various brands of impression paste differ in consistency and in their properties when set.

A paste of low viscosity produces an impression of minimum thickness and the choice of material depends upon the technique being employed.

On setting, some pastes are hard and brittle and resemble plaster, while others show a less precise set point and appear only to increase in viscosity. The harder materials will break if any alteration in the shape of the set impression is attempted, while the softer variety will continue to flow slowly even when 'set' (Fig. 45). Materials with a definite set point are preferred to prevent distortion on removal from the mouth.

On removal of the impression from undercut areas, some distortion of the less rigid materials occurs. ZOE pastes should only be used where small undercuts of the soft tissue are present.

Dimensional stability

Impression pastes are stable in dimension after removal from the mouth, particularly those materials which set hard. In a warm atmosphere, the less rigid materials flow slightly under pressure. There appears to be no distortion due to any stress-relief within the material. Dimensional stability of the paste impression is, of course, dependent upon the stability of the material which supports it.

Practical points

Mixing is carried out on a waxed paper pad. A glass slab may be used but it is rather difficult to clean afterwards, whereas the used paper is simply thrown away after use. The pastes are extruded, usually in equal lengths, so that proportioning is quite simple. They are mixed

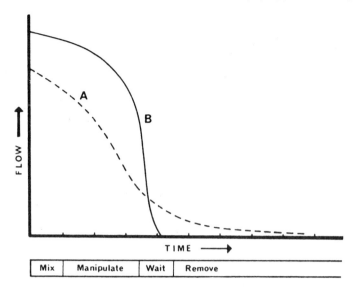

Fig. 45. Changes in consistency of ZOE pastes. 'A' shows a less clear setting point than 'B'

together with a broad-bladed spatula until the two colours of material blend.

Zinc oxide pastes will not adhere to a wet surface. The surface of a denture, record block or compound impression must be dried thoroughly before coating its surface with impression paste. Unfortunately the material sticks extremely well to dry skin and instruments. It is advisable to coat the lips of the patient lightly with petroleum jelly. This enables any excess impression paste to be wiped away. To clean instruments, they should be warmed slightly, when the paste softens and can be wiped away with a dental napkin.

As with impression compounds, additions of new material can be made to an impression which is slightly imperfect.

No separating medium is required when making the cast, and the impression paste can easily be removed by softening it in water at about 60–65°C.

IMPRESSION WAXES

In some impression techniques for dentures, a material is required which flows freely and continuously at mouth temperature. Impression compounds have a limited period of flow depending upon their bulk and degree of preheating outside the mouth. The flow of ZOE pastes is limited by their speed of setting.

Various mixtures of waxes with low softening point synthetic resins are used therefore as impression materials. These materials flow well at mouth temperature and due consideration must be given to this property when recording and handling the impression. It is particularly important to store impressions in these materials at or near 0°C if they cannot be cast immediately. Care must also be taken to avoid distortion of the impression material while pouring the cast.

These impression materials are usually more viscous than ZOE pastes but more fluid at mouth temperature than impression compounds are at 50–60°C. Thus we have a range of materials to suit the various impression techniques.

The flow of these waxes, tested by compression of cylindrical specimens, varies between 2 and 85 per cent at mouth temperature (37°C). Their coefficient of linear thermal expansion is often relatively high, being $350–700 \times 10^{-6}/°C$. Whilst this contraction seems rather large, it is probable that the actual dimensional change it produces is within the normally accepted accuracy of fit of a denture against soft tissues.

TISSUE CONDITIONING MATERIALS

After complete dentures have been worn for some years, they become ill-fitting and traumatize the tissues on which they rest. This is particularly so in the lower jaw. Before impressions for replacement dentures are recorded, it is important to allow the tissues to recover from this trauma. Materials are therefore available for 'tissue conditioning'. These can be left in the mouth for relatively long periods of time.

These materials are usually supplied as a powder and a liquid which are mixed and then applied to the fitting surface of the denture. The powder is a synthetic polymer of relatively low softening point, such as butyl or ethyl methacrylate. It is frequently a copolymer. Ethyl alcohol is present in the liquid to a proportion of 6–20 per cent. This swells the polymer and renders it more readily dissolved by the solvent, which is usually a benzoyl ester. Plasticizers such as dibutyl phthalate or dialkyl tin octoate are present to promote flow of the mixture. On mixing the materials, a viscous solution of the polymer is formed.

Whilst this may be relatively fluid at first, its viscosity increases rapidly until a viscoelastic gel arises. This eventually hardens by loss of solvent and plasticizer.

Since the intention of using these materials is to allow full tissue recovery to take place, the material should exhibit plastic properties for some time, preferably several days. On the other hand, it should possess some elasticity, though limited, otherwise it will soon be expelled from beneath the denture during chewing. Hence a visco-elastic material with low elasticity would be ideal. It would flow gradually and yet would resist elastically the relatively short duration stresses imposed on a denture during mastication. The materials available, however, do not conform to this ideal concept and usually become more elastic and harder with time. Repeated application of the material is therefore necessary to allow complete tissue recovery.

These materials may also be used to record functional impressions. For this purpose, flow is the more important property and the elastic recovery should be almost negligible. Some materials show satisfactory properties during the first hour or so after mixing.

In general, recent impressions recorded with tissue conditioners produce a well-detailed, yet smoothly contoured impression surface, similar to that recorded by the impression waxes. The materials are compatible with gypsum products. Nystatin, a fungicide, may be incorporated in some materials without undue loss of properties.

Chapter 22

Elastic impression materials. Hydrocolloids

Rigid impression materials such as plaster, and the plastic impression materials discussed in the last chapter, have suitable properties for recording impressions of non-undercut shapes. It is possible to record moderate undercuts of the oral soft tissues with these materials, since these tissues will change shape elastically and so allow the release of an impression out of an undercut area. An impression of undercuts of the hard tissues, such as teeth, necessitates the use of an elastic material.

HYDROCOLLOID IMPRESSION MATERIALS

Colloids

A colloid consists of large molecules or aggregates of molecules which are dissolved or dispersed in a dispersing medium. The molecules each possess a similar electrical charge, and therefore repel each other within the dispersing medium. In this way they do not settle out, but remain evenly distributed throughout the dispersing medium. The type of material used for dental impressions employs H_2O as the dispersing medium, and is called 'hydrocolloid'.

Sol and gel state

When aggregates of molecules are dispersed within water, the material is in the *sol* form, and behaves like a fluid of high viscosity. By a reduction in temperature, or by chemical reaction, the aggregates of molecules in a colloid can be made to join together to form a network of chains or 'fibrils'. This fibril network encloses the dispersion medium (in our case—H_2O). After the molecules have joined together to form fibrils, the consistency of the colloid becomes that of a jelly and it is in the *gel* form. The greater the concentration of fibrils in an impression material the tougher it will be in the gel state, and the thicker will be the consistency when it is a sol. This effect is apparent on comparing the toughness of the flavoured gelatin bought from the shop to make a jelly with that of its diluted result when prepared for the table. Indeed, if pure gelatin is purchased, it is brittle, and only upon soaking in water do its jelly-like properties become apparent.

Irreversible and reversible hydrocolloids

Colloids may be reversible or irreversible. If an impression colloid in the sol state can be changed easily into the gel form, and then back again to the sol, the material is known as a reversible hydrocolloid. Such a series of changes is usually brought about by heating to form a sol and by cooling to the gel state. As the temperature rises, the energy of the molecules in the fibrils increases and they separate from each other. When their thermal energy is reduced by cooling, secondary intermolecular forces once again come into play and the molecules join together to form fibrils again.

In other hydrocolloids, the change from a thick colloidal solution to a tough elastic gel is brought about by chemical action. Then the resultant gel cannot easily be changed back to its original state. Such an impression material is an irreversible hydrocolloid. The molecules in an irreversible hydrocolloid are joined together to form fibrils by primary valence bonds. This type of bond is not affected by the application of heat except at temperatures at which decomposition takes place.

Drying, imbibition, syneresis

Since the hydrocolloid gel consists largely of water enclosed rather loosely within the gel fibrils, a completed impression in either of the two types of hydrocolloid will lose water on standing in an atmosphere which is not saturated with water vapour. Loss of water is accompanied by shrinkage of the gel and distortion of the impression.

On the other hand, if a hydrocolloid is placed in water, it sometimes swells and 'imbibes' more water. This phenomenon is known as imbibition. The reversible hydrocolloids imbibe water to replace that which they have lost by drying. However, some distortion of the gel may take place during drying and imbibition and this will produce an inaccuracy of the impression. Irreversible hydrocolloids will continue to undergo imbibition if they are placed in water. They will swell until their water content is much greater than that of the original sol.

On standing, an exudate of some of the more soluble constituents of the material appears on the surface of the impression. This effect is known as *syneresis*. A similar effect may be seen in the separation of a serous exudate from a clot of blood. Syneresis is not necessarily accompanied by loss of water and even when the impression is kept in a saturated water vapour atmosphere an exudate forms.

The degree of syneresis and imbibition of all hydrocolloids is reduced by using as high a concentration of the colloid as possible.

IRREVERSIBLE HYDROCOLLOIDS

Applicable specifications: ISO R 1563; Brit 4269; Amer 18; Austral 1282.

These are based upon alginic acid which is obtained from the stalk of brown seaweeds. Some salts of this acid are soluble in water; for example, those of Na, K and NH_4, whereas those of Ca, Mn, Pb or Fe^{2+} are, like the acid itself, insoluble. The molecular weight of the alginate salts varies considerably between 18,000 and 150,000. When a soluble alginate is dissolved in water, it swells and a viscous sol is formed. As may be expected, the greater the concentration of the alginate in solution, the higher will be the viscosity of the sol. However, the molecular weight of the alginate also affects the viscosity of a solution in that the higher the molecular weight, the stiffer will be the impression material.

Constituents and setting reactions

Alginate impression material is purchased as a fine pink or white powder which is mixed with a measured quantity of water. This forms a sol of fairly thick consistency which is loaded into the tray and inserted into the mouth. The material flows round the teeth and into the detail of the soft tissues and then changes into a tough, insoluble, elastic gel by chemical reaction.

Sodium, K or NH_4 alginate may be used. Some materials may be based on the triethanol amine salt. To change the sol into an insoluble gel, it is cross-linked by reaction with a slightly soluble divalent salt such as $CaSO_4$, either dihydrate or hemihydrate. This is incorporated in the powder. It forms insoluble calcium alginate by a double decomposition reaction:

$$(1) \quad 2Na_nAlg + nCaSO_4 \longrightarrow nNa_2SO_4 + Ca_nAlg_2.$$

Metallic salts other than those of calcium may be used to produce slightly tougher gels. Lead and manganese salts are present in some materials, but the toxic properties of the former cannot be disregarded and many alginates now contain no lead.

It is essential that the above reaction does not take place until the impression material has been thoroughly mixed, placed in the tray and seated in the patient's mouth. When once it is in position, the material should set as rapidly as possible. The simplest way of preventing the formation of calcium alginate, and thus inhibiting the setting reaction, is to remove the Ca^{2+} ions from the mixture. Then the solution of soluble alginate remains unchanged. Fortunately $CaSO_4$ dissolves very slowly in water, and if a small amount of sodium or potassium phosphate, carbonate or oxalate is included either in the powder or in the mixing water, the following type of reaction takes place in preference to (1).

$$(2) \quad 2Na_3PO_4 + 3CaSO_4 \longrightarrow Ca_3(PO_4)_2 + 3Na_2SO_4.$$

Calcium phosphate is insoluble in water and does not react with the soluble alginate. In this way, the soluble alginate remains unaffected until all the Na_3PO_4 is exhausted. Then calcium alginate is formed as in equation (1). The amount of Na_3PO_4 added, is adjusted to give a suitable working time. It is essential that this chemical is evenly distributed together with the $CaSO_4$ throughout the mixture, or setting will be irregular. Thorough mixing of the ingredients by the manufacturer, shaking the tin before use and vigorous spatulation help to produce a homogeneous mix.

Silicofluorides and fluorides may be added to create slightly acid conditions on gelation and improve the surface of the plaster or stone cast.

Alginate impression materials taste slightly of the added chemicals, and flavours such as peppermint or spearmint are incorporated.

The powder as received from the manufacturer also contains a high proportion of inert fillers and colouring matter. The filler may be diatomaceous earth and is often present up to three-quarters of the total bulk of the powder. It is added to stiffen the mix and to reduce its stickiness, besides increasing the strength of the resultant gel.

Some materials show a well-defined gelation point and obviously cannot be moulded when once a certain stage has been passed. If this gel point is followed quickly by the development of suitable elasticity A, Fig. 46, then the material cannot be mishandled without the resultant errors being obvious. Other materials, however, show a more gradual change in consistency and pass slowly from a mouldable to an elastic condition B, Fig. 46. During the intermediate viscoelastic stage the material has developed some elasticity. If it is moulded at this time, the resulting impression will be inaccurate.

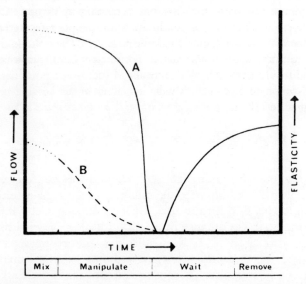

Fig. 46. Changes in viscosity and the development of elasticity in alginates against time

The chemical reactions taking place change the pH of the mixture. Indicators such as phenolphthalein and thymolphthalein, incorporated in some materials, show the stage of reaction which has been reached. For preference there should be a colour warning of the imminence of gelation, and a second colour change when gelation is complete, i.e. when elasticity is almost maximal.

Structure of the alginate gel

Pure calcium alginate is a brittle material with a consistency similar to that of a set mass of very weak plaster. To obtain an elastic material, some of the alginate must remain in the soluble form. What happens in practice is that only the surface layer of each particle of powder changes to calcium alginate, and the centre remains soft. The toughening effect of the outer skin of insoluble alginate produces an elastic material suitable for impressions.

The rigidity of calcium alginate is due to the attachment of Ca between molecules of adjacent fibrils as well as between the molecules of the same fibril. The cross-linkage between fibrils prevents the movement of one fibril over another and thus resists permanent deformation of the gel. The soluble alginate remaining in the centre of each granule prevents the material becoming too rigid. Calcium sulphate produces Ca^{2+} ions in solution at the proper rate, so that only the outer layer of each alginate particle is changed to insoluble alginate, by the time the hydrocolloid has set in the mouth. On standing, after removal from the mouth, the reaction continues slowly and penetrates towards the centre of each powder grain until the whole impression is changed to calcium alginate.

Storage

If any moisture comes in contact with the dry powder during storage, both of the above reactions will take place and, on using the material, a lumpy mix will be obtained. The commercial products are dispensed either in tins with well-fitting lids, or in metal-foil packets which exclude moisture. Care should be taken to replace the lid of any tin after use. Frequently, the last portions of powder in a large tin have a longer setting time. This may be due to the settling of particles of retarder, or moisture contamination. To obtain mixes with similar setting times, the powder in a tin should be shaken well before use.

On storing alginate powders above 37°C for prolonged periods, they depolymerize slowly. At higher temperatures of 50–60°C deterioration is more rapid and the materials soon show poor strength and a variable setting time.

Manipulation

All the above chemical reactions are speeded up by heat and, therefore, an increase in the temperature of the mixing water, of the powder, or of the bowl and mixer, causes a faster set. Adjustment of the temperature of the mix is the only simple means by which the dental surgeon can control the setting time. Manufacturers suggest temperatures of 18–24°C (65–75°F) and care should be taken to see that all materials and tools are approximately at this temperature.

Variations in the powder: water ratio occur when measures or scoops are used to measure the quantities. While the volume of water can be measured with moderate accuracy, the weight of powder obtained depends upon the degree of compaction achieved when filling the measure. Some powders are dispensed in separate weighed portions, in foil or plasticized polyvinyl alcohol packets, so that variations in consistency do not occur.

Within a moderate range of consistencies, however, the effect on setting time and elasticity of the resultant gel is only small. Very thick or very thin mixes cause practical difficulties in manipulating the material. A very dry or very fluid mix shows poorer elasticity. A correct mix of alginate shows a smooth, shiny surface on standing for a few seconds after spatulation.

For general use, a technique of filling the powder measure should be rehearsed until a mix of suitable working consistency is achieved. Weighing the powder is advisable.

The time taken to mix irreversible hydrocolloids does not affect the setting time to any marked degree, as the completion of equation (2) allows a certain length of time to elapse before setting commences. Provided mixing does not continue for too long the only effect of too much mixing is to shorten the time available for loading the tray and inserting the material into the mouth. The efficiency of spatulation, however, affects the properties of the elastic gel to a considerable extent. Poor mixing gives a lumpy mix which sets unevenly and distorts upon removal from the mouth as no uniformity of gel exists. The usual mixing time suggested by the manufacturers is $\frac{1}{2}$ to $1\frac{1}{2}$ minutes, and this time must be fully employed in vigorous and thorough spatulation against the sides of the bowl. Mechanical mixing is preferable.

Since the setting reaction involves $CaSO_4$, the mixing bowl and spatula must be free from any trace of plaster, artificial stones or investments.

Retention to trays

Adhesion of the hydrocolloids to smooth metal trays is poor, and perforated metal trays in stock sizes are available. Similarly, when using special trays made from other materials, holes are made in the tray. The impression material flows through the holes to the outside of the tray and 'rivets' itself into place. If the holes are too small, the 'shank' of the 'rivet' is weak and may break when removing the impression. Whereas if the holes are too large, impression material leaks out and insufficient alginate remains inside the tray to record a complete impression. For alginate impression materials, the holes should be 2–3 mm in diameter and not more than 5 mm apart. If the holes are widely spaced, the portion of the impression between the holes may come away from the tray and cause an inaccuracy.

Retention can also be obtained by flowing sticky wax on to the tissue surface of a metal tray and loading the impression material while the wax is still molten. This method speeds up the setting of the alginate slightly, since there is a rise in temperature from the heat of the tray.

Instead of sticky wax, an adhesive may be used. The strength of the bond between alginate and an adhesive depends upon the pH of the materials. Generally speaking the bond is better between an alginate and the adhesive prepared for use with it. Adhesives resist tensile forces but perforations provide better attachment when shear forces are applied. Good retention is also achieved by using trays with a rim projecting inwards to hold the impression in the tray. Such trays, however, are less convenient to use clinically.

Possible sources of inaccuracy

During impression taking

The sol state of the mix is maintained until the retarder is exhausted; then the alginate begins to gel. An impression taken in a partly gelled mix will be inaccurate due to stresses set up within the gel as it is moulded. It is therefore important to complete the seating of an impression before the gel stage commences.

Since the oral mucosa is warmer than the tray, an alginate impression sets at the tissue surface first; the last material to set being any thick sections. Movement of the tray while setting is taking place will set up stresses in the first gel layer.

Pressure on the tray by the operator, in an attempt to compress the tissues, or to force the material further into place, will, if the first gel has formed, cause stresses to be set up. If the operator does not hold the tray, the effect of gravity upon an upper tray will have a similar result. When a stressed impression is removed from the mouth, the stresses are relieved by distortion of the impression.

The elasticity of many alginate materials improves for a few minutes after initial gelation. It is usual, therefore, to hold the impression in the mouth for at least a minute after it is 'set to touch'. This is particularly important when large undercuts are to be recorded.

Too early removal of the impression is shown by portions of alginate material adhering to the tips of teeth, and by a rough, torn surface to the impression. This effect is commonly seen round the anterior teeth, and is due to the lower temperature of this portion of the impression. The remainder of the impression is warmed by the cheeks, lips and tongue, while that portion near the front of the tray is cooled by the surrounding air. A similar rough impression surface is seen where setting has been irregular due to insufficient spatulation.

Alginate materials will also adhere to the teeth if these are dried before an impression is recorded.

During removal of the impression

The impression is removed with a sudden pull, so that undercut areas are swiftly strained and rebound immediately to their correct shapes. Slow and careful removal of hydrocolloid impressions causes permanent deformation of the material by rupturing the layer of calcium alginate which surrounds the softer soluble alginate. This double alginate structure is elastic to a sudden force, but not to a force applied over a period of time.

Most of the force required to remove an impression is to overcome atmospheric pressure, since at first a reduction in air pressure occurs between the impression and the oral tissues. The use of compressed air has been suggested to blow the impression away from the tissues and thus prevent the setting up of large stresses within the hydrocolloid. During removal it is essential that the alginate adheres well to the tray.

After removal

After removal from the mouth, changes occur which affect the accuracy of the resultant cast.

Where moderate undercuts have been recorded, the material rebounds quickly to an accurate reproduction of the tissue shape and the cast should be poured as soon as possible within the next 15 minutes. If it is subjected to large strains on removal from deep undercuts, then recovery of the strained areas is a little slower and the impression should be left for 5 minutes to recover. It is then poured within the next 10 minutes. The greater the degree of undercut being recorded, that is, the greater the strain on removal, the more the alginate will change shape on subsequent storage beyond this time.

In a dry atmosphere, the alginate gel loses water and contracts. The water lost into the atmosphere cannot be accurately replaced by subsequently soaking the impression in water. The simplest way to maintain a saturated atmosphere round the impression is to wrap it in a damp dental napkin and place it in a closed container. The impression should not be kept for a long time in such a container, but should be cast as soon as possible if a high degree of accuracy is required.

Shrinkage and the production of an exudate also occur on standing, even when there is no H_2O loss. The gel contracts by further reaction and squeezes out an exudate. Linear dimensional shrinkage from syneresis alone can be as high as 0·4 per cent in one hour. The exudate slows the setting of any gypsum in contact with it, and produces a weak surface on the cast. To obtain a good surface after syneresis has occurred, the impression should be washed in a minimum of cold water. Then, if the manufacturer suggests it, the impression should be dipped in a solution of an accelerator for gypsum materials.

Perhaps the question of accuracy may best be assessed by relating it to the type of dental appliance for which the impression is required. If a denture of simple construction is to be made to the cast, then a slight inaccuracy, due to a short period of storing, passes unnoticed. If a cast skeleton denture is to be made, particularly in one of the Co–Cr alloys, a slight distortion will result in a denture which fails to fit the mouth perfectly.

If required surface disinfection of the impression can be achieved by immersion in sodium hypochlorite (1% Cl) or a 2% glutaraldehyde solution. Both, however, cause shrinkage on prolonged immersion.

When pouring the cast

Distortion of elastic impression materials during casting can easily be caused if pressure is applied to the impression via the cast material. Too thick a mix of stone forced into the impression, or excessive vibration, must be avoided. All hydrocolloid impressions should be filled with stone level with the edges of the tray and then left to set. The tray should be held by the handle, away from the bench. Otherwise, portions of the impression which extend beyond the borders of the tray will be distorted by contact with the bench. A base is added when this first portion of the stone has set. An impression should never be inverted on to a partially set mass of stone on the bench.

While the stone cast is setting, the impression material continues to change into hard calcium alginate. This is accompanied by a contraction which is due not only to the chemical reaction, but also to loss of H_2O. A large shrinkage takes place when the impression and setting cast are left on the bench in a relatively dry atmosphere. This shrinkage may cause fracture of weak portions of the cast, such as individual teeth. Similar breakages may occur when attempting to remove the hard calcium alginate from the cast after several hours have elapsed.

The impression and cast should therefore be stored in a humid atmosphere (covered by a damp cloth) until the gypsum material has reached its final set. Then the impression is removed.

Hardness of the cast surface

The hardness of the cast surface is extremely important in the construction of accurate dental appliances.

A strong cast with high strength can readily be cast in an artificial stone, but sometimes it displays a superficial layer of weak powdery material particularly on the surface of standing teeth. Abrasion of these areas will quickly lead to inaccuracies. Surface weakness is seen as a whitish zone on drying, and may be due to several causes.

Substances of high molecular weight retard the setting of gypsum materials. Mucin from the saliva which adheres to the impression causes weakness of the surface. Water on the impression surface dilutes the cast material and weakens it. The use of too thin a mix of gypsum causes a rough surface, as its long setting time enables exudation to take place from the hydrocolloid. If the impression is left on the cast overnight, the exudate which accompanies shrinkage of the hydrocolloid etches the plaster surface and roughens it.

The quality of the surface of the cast is also affected by the relative pH of the alginate and the artificial stone. If the pH of the alginate is high, e.g. 9–10, the surface of the cast is poor since the pH of setting gypsum materials is usually 6–7. Most alginate materials show a stable pH value 10 minutes after setting. Some, however, become more alkaline on standing.

SUMMARY OF THE USE OF ALGINATE MATERIALS

Shake the tin of powder.
Use mixing water and instruments at the correct temperature.
Measure the water and the powder carefully.
Mix vigorously according to the instructions.
Support the material well and see that the tray is properly prepared for retention of the hydrocolloid.
Insert before any gelation is apparent.
Hold the tray and impression material lightly in position. Do not move when once in position.
Remove 1 minute after it is 'set to touch'.
Remove with a sudden pull, not by gentle manipulation.
Wash quickly. Shake and blow out the water.
Cover immediately with a damp cloth, or place in a closed, humid container.
Cast within 15 minutes. Fill impression level with the edges. Support it out of contact with the bench and cover with a damp cloth. Add a base when the first part of the cast has set. Remove the impression 1 hour after casting the first part.

Typical properties of alginate impression materials:

Setting time 20–22°C	2–5 minutes
Elasticity. Permanent set after	
10 per cent compressive strain	2–4·5 per cent
Compressive strength at 30 minutes	0·5–0·8 N/mm²

REVERSIBLE HYDROCOLLOIDS

Applicable specifications: ISO R 1564; Amer 11; Austral T16.

Some years ago the reversible hydrocolloids were deemed to possess properties which made them superior to those of the irreversible type.

The gel of the reversible colloids was tougher and less liable to distortion during removal from the mouth. Improvements in irreversible hydro-colloids have now produced materials which have similar properties to the reversible colloids. For general impression purposes the mani-pulation of the irreversible type is quicker and simpler than that of the reversible type.

Constituents

The chief ingredient of the reversible colloids is agar-agar. With water, this chemical forms a reversible colloid which will gel slightly above mouth temperature. In the pure state the gel is too friable to resist the forces applied during impression-taking. Cellulose fibres are incor-porated to reinforce the gel. The addition of small amounts of peptone or borates increases the gel strength. Glycerol may also be present to increase strength and improve dimensional stability of the gel. Oil soluble colouring matter and inert fillers such as ZnO, SiO_2, powdered wax, etc., give a better appearance and more body to the material. To prevent growth of mould, a fungicide is usually added.

Manipulation

At room temperature reversible hydrocolloids are gels, and they change to a sol well above mouth temperature. In fact, they change to a sol at a much higher temperature than that at which they gel on cooling. The practical application of this effect is that although it may be necessary to heat a reversible impression material to $100°C$ to convert it completely to a sol, on cooling, gelation does not occur until just above mouth temperature.

Reversible colloids are supplied in collapsible tubes, sealed to prevent the loss of water by evaporation. Since colloids are poor conductors of heat, the tube is placed in boiling water for 8–10 minutes to convert the gel to a sol. It is then either cooled in air, or preferably placed in a thermostatically controlled water-bath, until it is at the correct temperature to be used in the mouth. If the material is cooled in air, constant mixing by squeezing the tube is essential to maintain a mass of even temperature and consistency.

As with the irreversible colloids, the retention of agar-agar materials to metal is poor and a perforated tray is used.

Gelation

The warm impression material is placed in the tray and inserted into the mouth. The sol flows round the teeth and soft tissues, and begins to cool. Just as the heating up of the colloid takes a long time, the cooling of thick sections in the mouth is rather slow. Cold water is syringed over the outer surface of the tray and impression, or the tray may be fitted with small pipes along its tissue surface through which cold water flows.

Unlike the alginate materials, the reversible colloids set from the tray inwards. The last portion of impression to set is that against the warm oral tissues, and a small movement of the tray during gelation can be accommodated by flow of this layer of material. Thus, there is less possibility of creating stresses within the gel. Movement of the tray is to be avoided, but the possibility of error from this cause is not quite so great as with the alginate materials, which gel from the tissues outwards.

Rapid removal of the impression is again essential to prevent tearing and distortion round undercut areas. The reversible hydrocolloids tear more easily than the alginate materials.

Pouring the cast

On standing, syneresis produces a surface exudate. To counteract the retarding effect of this exudate upon the model material, a little $K_2SO_4.Al_2(SO_4)_3$ or K_2SO_4 is sometimes incorporated in the impression material. Alternatively, the impression may be dipped in an accelerator for gypsum.

If facilities for casting are not available at the surgery, a reversible hydrocolloid impression may be stored for some hours in a closed container with an atmosphere of 100 per cent relative humidity. No chemical change takes place, but there is a slight loss of water, and some distortion from stress-relief. For accuracy, impressions should be cast immediately upon removal from the mouth as changes in dimension from stress-relief during storage cannot be avoided.

After casting, the impression should be kept in a saturated water-vapour atmosphere until the gypsum has set.

Whilst the reversible hydrocolloids can be used again by loading them into a special syringe, the elastic properties of these materials deteriorate with frequent heating-gelation cycles. These changes are also accompanied by water loss and by the incorporation of small particles of gypsum from the cast. It is usual, therefore, to discard reversible hydrocolloids after one intra-oral use, particularly when accurate impressions of crown or bridge preparations are being recorded.

For use in indirect inlay and similar techniques, a material of slightly greater fluidity, containing more water, is used. The small amount of material required can be stored in empty local anaesthetic cartridges, from which it is 'injected' through a modified syringe into the tooth cavity. The containers may be kept ready for use for a limited period of time by storing them in a water-bath at 63–65°C. They are then cooled further or 'tempered' to 39–46°C immediately before use. After prolonged storage, however, some deterioration of elastic properties is found.

Typical properties of reversible hydrocolloid impression materials:

    Elasticity. Permanent set after
        10 per cent compressive strain   1·0–1·5 per cent
        Compressive strength   0·25–0·50 N/mm^2

DUPLICATING MATERIALS

Applicable specifications: Amer 20; Austral 1097.

In the construction of partial dentures, of either cast or wrought metal, it is often necessary to duplicate the original cast after it has been suitably modified by additions of wax or plaster. Similarly, in orthodontics, casts are required for record purposes, and duplication of an existing one avoids the inconvenience to the patient of a further impression. The duplicate cast may be poured in plaster or stone, or in one of the investment materials.

More than one cast can be poured to the same polysulphide or polyether rubber impression with only a slight falling off in accuracy, provided that the impression is not detached from its tray or support. Accuracy is less well maintained between successive casts poured to a silicone rubber impression. Pouring more than one cast to a hydrocolloid impression is unsatisfactory when accuracy is required.

Both reversible and irreversible hydrocolloids are available as duplicating materials. Other materials consist of a mixture of polyvinyl chloride and acetate, a material whose basic constituents are gelatine and glue, or a material which is an aqueous acrylamide gel.

However, it would appear that the majority of the modern duplicating materials are based upon agar.

The usual method employed with reversible colloids is to stand the cast on a glass slab and place round it a metal duplicating flask which is designed to allow an even thickness of material all round. The reversible colloids supplied for duplicating are of a thinner consistency than those supplied for recording impressions. If a normal impression hydrocolloid is being used, the consistency should be thinned by adding H_2O. The colloid is heated in a double pan until is it completely fluid and then cooled, until it reaches approximately 50°C. The material is then stirred and poured through a hole in the top of the duplicating flask until it overflows through a further hole. The colloid should be poured as cool as possible and to prevent contraction away from the cast, the flask should be cooled from the base. When gelation is complete, the master cast is removed with a rapid movement, rather than gently easing it away. Agar duplicating materials show permanent distortion after the application of a strain for more than a few seconds. If the duplicate is poured straight away, little or no syneresis takes place. The agar materials in general show good compatibility with the silica-bonded investment materials and many of them produce a good surface when the phosphate-bonded investments are used. Care should be taken in the latter case to ensure that the mould is dry before pouring in the phosphate-bonded investment. To obtain a good surface with a gypsum-bonded investment or with a gypsum cast material, the surface of the mould should be treated with an accelerator for gypsum products before pouring the cast.

The materials should inhibit the growth of mould on storage at room temperature, otherwise they rapidly lose their elastic properties.

Typical properties:

Gelation temperature	35–37°C
Permanent set after 12 per cent compressive strain	2·5–3 per cent
Compressive strength	0·2–0·25 N/mm^2

After a period of use, besides becoming contaminated, the agar hydrolyses. This takes place rapidly if the material is left for a long time at a temperature ready for use. As hydrolysis proceeds, elasticity and strength fall. It is necessary to discard old material from time to time and to replace it with new material or that which has been used once for an intra-oral impression.

Chapter 23
Elastic impression materials. Elastomers

None of the hydrocolloid impression materials are dimensionally stable on storage, and all require careful handling to produce an accurate impression. Their accuracy of reproduction, however, must be related to that required clinically. Hydrocolloids, particularly the alginates, are quite suitable for recording impressions for complete and partial denture construction. The resilience of the soft tissues and of the periodontal membranes of the standing teeth compensate for small inaccuracies. When making metallic or ceramic restorations which fit to relatively unyielding dentine, perfect accuracy is essential, and a more elastic and more stable material is preferred.

POLYSULPHIDE RUBBER
(THIOKOL, MERCAPTAN, RUBBER BASE)

Applicable specifications: Brit 4269; Amer 19; Austral 1185.

These are synthetic elastomers based on an industrial polymer:

$$\text{HS}(\text{C}_2\text{H}_4\text{-O-CH}_2\text{-O-C}_2\text{H}_4\text{-S-S})_{23} - \text{C}_2\text{H}_4\text{-O-CH}_2\text{-O-C}_2\text{H}_4\text{-SH}$$

If we indicate the group C_2H_4—O—CH_2—O—C_2H_4 by R, polymerization occurs through oxidation of the terminal -SH groups by a dioxide, commonly PbO_2 producing water:

$$\text{HS (R-S-S)}_{23}\text{-R-SH + HS (R-S-S)}_{23}\text{-R-SH + HS (.......}$$

$$+ \text{PbO}_2 \qquad\qquad + \text{PbO}_2$$

$$\longrightarrow \quad \text{HS (R-S-S)}_{23}\text{-R-S-S (R-S-S)}_{23}\text{-R-S-S (.......}$$

$$+ \text{H}_2\text{O} + \text{PbO} \qquad + \text{H}_2\text{O} + \text{PbO}$$

Cross-linking between chains occurs due to the presence of branched -SH terminated groups present at about 2-mole per cent, again with the production of water as a by-product. The presence of S brings about a rapid curing reaction.

Impression materials of the polysulphide type are dispensed in the form of two pastes, one white and the other usually brown. The white (base) paste contains the polymer which is a fluid of low viscosity. Fillers such as TiO_2, ZnS or lithopone are incorporated together with a plasticizer such as chlorinated paraffin or dibutyl phthalate, to improve the working properties. The base smells of low molecular weight thiols.

The brown (reactor or accelerator) paste usually contains the PbO_2 and S, and is made into a paste with the same type of plasticizer as is used in the base. Lead dioxide is a rather dirty chemical to handle and mixtures of white oxides of other metals with PbO_2 lighten the dark brown colour. Manganese or zinc dioxide can be used. If the accelerator paste is not at all brown in colour, then a hydroperoxide accelerator may be in use. Butyl hydroperoxide produces a light colour but affects the type of setting reaction, making it less suitable for dental use as well as producing a rubber of poor dimensional stability due to the volatility of this peroxide. Butyl hydroperoxide also has an objectionable taste and smell. Cupric hydroxide produces a blue coloured material which does not suffer from the same dimensional instability. However, from a toxic point of view, the copper salt would appear to be no better than PbO_2. Zinc oxide or carbonate can also be used as an accelerator but is rather slow in action.

On mixing the pastes, the base material polymerizes initially into long coiled chains followed later by cross-linking between chains. The resultant rubber shows good elasticity and a toughness related to the amount of filler and the molecular weight of the original polymer.

Mixing

A broad-bladed flexible 'artist's' stainless steel spatula is necessary for mixing. Either a large glass slab or a waxed paper pad may be used. Chilling the glass slab gives a slightly longer working time. The two pastes are extruded in the proportions recommended by the manufacturer. A reduction in the amount of accelerator used gives a very slow setting rubber with poor elastic qualities. Increasing the accelerator content causes a slightly faster set.

As the polysulphide base is very adherent, the spatula blade should be placed first in the accelerator paste and covered with a thin layer. Then, to ensure a homogeneous mix, the two pastes are combined, and are transferred to a clean slab or paper pad where mixing is completed. If mixing is continued on the same slab, difficulty is experienced in combining the thin layer of base material which adheres to the mixing slab.

Most of the polysulphide materials are thixotropic, that is, their fluidity increases with the rate of straining. During mixing or whilst injecting the material into cavities, the material appears to have a low viscosity. When left unstrained, however, its viscosity increases. This is of advantage when recording impressions as the greater flow under a large strain enables detail to be recorded. But where the material is under a lesser strain, it will not run out of the tray but will retain its shape even when inadequately supported.

Setting

Both moisture and temperature have a marked effect on the speed of the reaction. Setting can be retarded by the addition of a few drops of oleic acid, and accelerated by adding water. The effect of heat and moisture on setting is an advantage dentally, as the mixed material cures slowly until it is placed in the mouth. A longer time is therefore available for manipulation outside the mouth. Once it is placed in the mouth, the curing of thin layers takes place more rapidly. With thicker layers, the surface cures, but the deeper portions become elastic much more slowly. Polysulphide rubbers are poor conductors of heat and therefore should only be used in thin sections of 2–3 mm. A close fitting tray is advised.

Setting is a gradual process and the material thickens slowly and then becomes elastic. The beginning of elasticity is difficult to define with the more viscous materials. They should be inserted in the mouth before they have become too viscous and should be held in place for 3–7 minutes before removal (Fig. 47). Even then, polymerization is by no means complete and rapid removal of the impression is necessary to reduce distortion of the viscoelastic material. In general, most manufacturer's recommendations for setting time should be increased by a half.

The polysulphide rubbers are rather tough and require a moderate force to remove them from an undercut area. Of all the elastic impression materials, however, the polysulphide rubbers are the most resistant to tearing. Good retention to the tray is essential and an

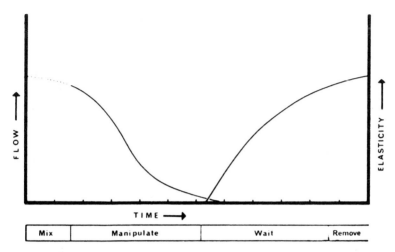

Fig. 47. Slow changes in viscosity and the development of elasticity in a polysulphide rubber against time

adhesive of butyl rubber cement or numerous perforations are used. After mixing, excess material on the mixing slab is easily removed by allowing it to cure fully, when it strips away quite easily. Instruments, etc., should be placed in warm water to speed up curing.

After removal

To allow as full elastic recovery as possible, the impression should be left for 30 minutes before being cast.

On storage, the impressions show a slight shrinkage which, during the first few hours, is probably not of clinical significance even for inlay construction. Shrinkage is due to further polymerization and to the loss of the water produced by the setting reaction. The actual dimensional change is related to the thickness of impression material and its retention to the tray. The general stability of the polysulphides is greatly superior to that of the hydrocolloids, and better than most other elastomers.

Surface of the cast

Polysulphide rubbers are compatible with all cast materials and produce a very smooth surface with artificial stones. Impressions may be electroplated to form dies.

Shelf-life

The shelf-life of the polysulphides is good. The accelerator has the shorter shelf-life and the material should not be stored in a warm place. After prolonged storage, polymerization is slow due to deterioration of the reactor paste.

Use

Materials are usually available in two or more grades of viscosity so that a fluid grade can be injected into the tooth cavities followed by a more viscous mix in a tray. Bonding between the two mixes is satisfactory. Alternatively a close fitting acrylic tray can be made. The use of a compound impression followed by a wash of fluid grade material is not advisable as the plasticizers in the elastomer cause softening of the impression compound and can lead to distortion of the impression.

Thus whilst the polysulphide polymers have a slightly unpleasant rubbery smell and the PbO_2 accelerator is dirty to handle, these materials have a well established place in dentistry. In general they have a fairly long manipulation time with a curing time which is made shorter by their sensitivity to moisture and warmth. Their elasticity is good and they are reasonably stiff, so reducing the possibility of deformation on pouring the impression. As a consequence of their comparatively slow rate of polymerization before they are placed in the mouth, the polysulphide materials produce impressions which are accurate, particularly in inexperienced hands, provided that they are left to cure in the mouth for a sufficiently long time.

When duplicate casts or dies are required, it is possible to pour two or more casts from one impression with only a slight loss of accuracy. Typical properties:

Setting time, 20–25°C	8–12 minutes
Elasticity. Permanent set 2 minutes after setting, after application of 12 per cent strain	3–4 per cent

SILICONE RUBBER IMPRESSION MATERIALS

Applicable specifications: Brit 4269; Amer 19; Austral 1185.

These are polymers based on the siloxane chain of alternate Si and O atoms:

$$-O-\overset{|}{\underset{|}{Si}}-O-\overset{|}{\underset{|}{Si}}-O-\overset{|}{\underset{|}{Si}}-O-$$

The base is a polymer of relatively high molecular weight but which behaves as a liquid. Under the influence of a catalyst, polymerization takes place increasing the chain length. By the incorporation of a cross-linking agent also, a highly elastic polymer is produced.

Setting reactions

The base employed for dental impression materials may be a hydroxy terminated dimethyl siloxane

$$-\left[\, O-\overset{CH_3}{\underset{CH_3}{\overset{|}{\underset{|}{Si}}}}\,\right]_n-OH$$

Polymerization and cross-linking of this polymer is catalyzed by stannous octoate or dibutyl tin dilaurate. Early materials employed organohydrogen siloxane as a cross-linking agent but the reaction with this material evolved hydrogen which caused pitting of the model surface. Alkyl orthosilicate is therefore commonly used as the cross-linking agent. The reaction occurs as on p. 238, uppermost.

$$\left[\begin{array}{c} CH_3 \\ -O-Si- \\ CH_3 \end{array}\right]_n -OH + C_2H_5-O-\underset{\underset{CH_3}{|}}{\overset{\overset{CH_3}{|}}{Si}}-O-C_2H_5 + HO-\left[-\underset{\underset{CH_3}{|}}{\overset{\overset{CH_3}{|}}{Si}}-O-\right]_n + \text{catalyst} \longrightarrow$$

hydroxy terminated dimethyl siloxane   alkyl orthosilicate   hydroxy terminated dimethyl siloxane

$$-O-\underset{\underset{CH_3}{|}}{\overset{\overset{CH_3}{|}}{Si}}-O-\underset{\underset{CH_3}{|}}{\overset{\overset{CH_3}{|}}{Si}}-O-\;\;\;\; CH_3-\underset{\underset{CH_3}{|}}{\overset{\overset{CH_3}{|}}{Si}}-O-\underset{\underset{CH_3}{|}}{\overset{\overset{CH_3}{|}}{Si}}-O- + 3C_2H_5OH$$

$$-O-\underset{\underset{CH_3}{|}}{\overset{\overset{CH_3}{|}}{Si}}-O-\underset{\underset{CH_3}{|}}{\overset{\overset{CH_3}{|}}{Si}}-O-$$

silicone elastomer   ethyl alcohol

$$\left[\begin{array}{c} CH_3 \\ -O-Si- \\ CH_3 \end{array}\right]_n -CH=CH_2 + H-\underset{\underset{O}{|}}{\overset{\overset{CH_3}{|}}{Si}}-CH_3$$

$$\left[\begin{array}{c} CH_3 \\ -O-Si- \\ CH_3 \end{array}\right]_n -CH=CH_2 + H-\underset{|}{\overset{\overset{O}{|}}{Si}}-CH_3 + CH_2=CH-\left[-\underset{\underset{CH_3}{|}}{\overset{\overset{CH_3}{|}}{Si}}-O-\right]_n + \text{catalyst} \longrightarrow$$

Vinyl terminated siloxane   Silane   Vinyl terminated siloxane

$$-O-\underset{\underset{CH_3}{|}}{\overset{\overset{CH_3}{|}}{Si}}-CH_2-CH_2-\underset{\underset{O}{|}}{\overset{\overset{CH_3}{|}}{Si}}-CH_3 \;\;\;\; CH_3-\underset{\underset{O}{|}}{\overset{\overset{CH_3}{|}}{Si}}-CH_2-CH_2-\underset{\underset{CH_3}{|}}{\overset{\overset{CH_3}{|}}{Si}}-O-$$

$$-O-\underset{\underset{CH_3}{|}}{\overset{\overset{CH_3}{|}}{Si}}-CH_2-CH_2-\underset{\underset{CH_3}{|}}{\overset{\overset{CH_3}{|}}{Si}}-CH_3$$

Cross-linked elastomer

The resultant elastomer undergoes shrinkage after polymerization due to the evaporation of the alcohol. Shelf-life of this type of silicone rubber is limited by the fact that the cross-linking agent polymerizes in time. Shelf-life is reduced in humid conditions. If the catalyst and cross-linking agent are both combined in one paste, the shelf-life is shorter than if they are dispensed separately.

A more recent development is the use of a *vinyl* terminated siloxane which cross-links via a silane, by addition polymerization, the vinyl group possessing a double bond. Under the influence of a precious metal catalyst such as chloroplatinic acid, hydrosilylation occurs to produce an elastomer with no byproduct. (See page 238, lower). The fact that there is no volatile byproduct improves the dimensional stability of the resultant polymer.

Silicone elastomers produced by this reaction do not bond to those catalyzed by tin compounds and indeed if the two are used in combination in an impression technique, the tin catalyst affects the rate of addition polymerization and may even stop it completely.

Mixing

The materials are sold in a paste/liquid or two-paste form. Sometimes the catalyst and cross-linking agent are dispensed separately as liquids. Usually one paste or the liquid(s) contains a pigment to ensure good mixing. The different consistencies available range from fluids to stiff putties. This range is achieved by varying the molecular weight of the original polymer and the type and amount of filler which is added. It is generally easier to mix together two pastes than to incorporate a liquid into a relatively stiff paste. The tin catalysts can cause irritation to oral mucosa and skin and should be handled with care. It is common practice, however, to knead putty materials by hand to incorporate the catalyst.

The more fluid grades are mixed in a manner similar to the poly-sulphides. The amount of accelerator is measured either in drops per unit length of extruded base material, or by extruding similar lengths of paste where the cross-linking agent and catalyst are combined in one paste. Greater variations in proportioning occur with a liquid acceler-ator system, causing variations in working properties. For dental purposes, the silicone rubbers are used with a relatively large proportion of accelerator in order to produce a sufficiently short setting time. Consequently an increase in the proportion of the accelerator causes only a slight reduction in setting time. A reduction in accelerator increases the working time but delays the development of good elasticity.

An adhesive of a siloxane and ethyl silicate provides moderate retention to the tray. Retention by numerous perforations is preferred.

Setting

At room temperature the rubber begins to polymerize immediately the accelerator and base are mixed. Consequently a more fluid 'syringe' type gradually becomes more viscous and the manipulation time is limited. The change from plastic to elastic properties is gradual, and a danger exists of trying to record the impression in an already elastic material (Fig. 48). This leads to gross distortion after removal from the mouth.

Techniques with polysulphide and silicone materials

Low viscosity materials are often used to record cavity detail but they must be used in a thin layer. Whilst a close fitting tray can be made out of self-curing acrylic polymer, it is usual to construct the tray by recording a preliminary impression and modifying this. A preliminary impression is recorded with a medium bodied or putty material. A small space within the impression is created either by trimming this impression, by recording it over a spacer between the impression and the prepared teeth, or by recording the impression before preparing the cavities. Then a fluid grade material is injected into the cavities, a small amount is placed in the tray and it is reseated over the preparations. This reduces the thickness of fluid grade material used and also assists in forcing the material into the cavity detail. When using this *two stage* or *wash* technique, care should be taken not to deform the original impression elastically by employing heavy pressure when holding the setting wash impression in place. In addition, sluice-ways should be cut to allow excess fluid material to escape and so reduce the pressure. The putty materials, being very stiff after polymerization, are less susceptible to distortion than the medium grade materials. In some double mix techniques, fluid and medium grade materials are used, the latter having a slightly longer setting time. The fluid grade is injected into place and the medium grade material placed in the tray. The tray

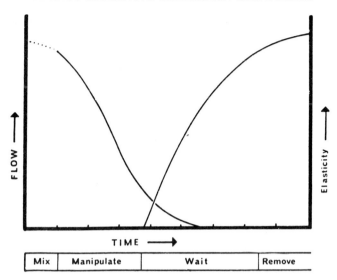

Fig. 48. Changes in viscosity and the development of elasticity in silicone rubbers. Note that the material can still be moulded even when it has some elastic properties

is placed in position before either of the materials has polymerized, thus ensuring good bonding between them.

With care, all the various techniques produce results which are accurate within the limits required for clinical practice. Distortion of an impression is usually due to the placing of a partially polymerized material, the use of too heavy pressure on seating the impression, or a lack of adhesion between two mixes of material.

The silicone rubbers are more highly elastic than the polysulphides. Being slightly 'oily' to the touch, they are easier to remove from under-cut areas.

After removal

As with other elastomers, the impression should be left for 30 minutes to recover elastically. Many of the silicone rubbers show a greater shrinkage on storage than the polysulphides. In general, the low viscosity silicones are less dimensionally stable than the more viscous materials, as the latter contain more filler and this reduces the amount of dimensional change. The actual dimensional change is related to the sectional thickness of material and its adhesion to the tray, but a significant error may appear after storage of an inlay impression for 24 hours. On shrinkage, the impression material moves toward the tray if good adhesion or retention exists between material and the tray. Thus, an impression of a single tooth increases in size due to shrinkage of the impression material. If attachment to the tray is poor, or if complex shapes are recorded, an irregular distortion occurs. Impressions should be cast within the first few hours after removal from the mouth. A moderately fast-setting stone should be used to obtain a good surface. Whilst the lower elastic modulus of silicone rubbers facilitates the pouring of several casts to one impression, the accuracy falls off unless the time interval between successive casts is half an hour or less.

Some difficulties exist in silver or copper plating with the additional problem of continuing polymerization shrinkage if plating is too slow. It is perhaps better to choose other methods for making accurate dies.

Typical properties:

Setting time 20–25°C	5–8 minutes
Elasticity, permanent set 2 minutes after setting, after application of 12 per cent strain	1–2 per cent

POLYETHER RUBBERS

This newer type of elastomer was produced in 1960. It is based on a polyether polymer with a molecular weight of about 4000, which has imino (aziridino) rings at each end:

$$CH_3-CH-CH_2-CO_2-\left[\begin{matrix}R\\|\\CH-(CH_2)_n-O\end{matrix}\right]_m \begin{matrix}R\\|\\-CH-(CH_2)_n-\end{matrix}CO_2-CH_2-CH-CH_3$$

Cross-linking is brought about by the action of an aromatic alkyl sulphonate catalyst which opens up the imino rings and causes addition polymerization with no byproducts.

The base paste contains the polymer together with SiO_2 as a filler and a plasticizer. The catalyst paste contains the sulphonate also with filler and plasticizer. A 'thinner' is supplied to reduce the viscosity of the material for use in a syringe.

Mixing is relatively easy. The setting time is short with a fairly well marked set point. However, almost immediately after mixing, these materials are viscoclastic and show elastic properties at low stresses. The possibility of distortion of an impression is therefore considerable unless the material is seated very quickly into place after mixing. The material is clean to handle and odourless and shows some thixotropic properties.

After setting, the dimensional stability, if the material is kept dry, is excellent. Prolonged contact with water, however, causes the material to swell as the polymer is hydrophilic. This effect is greater if 'thinner' has been added. The coefficient of thermal expansion is relatively high compared with the other elastomers, probably because of the lower filler content.

When polymerized, the resultant elastomer is very stiff and may be difficult to remove from the mouth if large hard tissue undercuts are present. It is often difficult to remove the impression from the cast and thin sections of gypsum may be fractured. However, the stiffness of the polymerized material ensures that no distortion of the impression occurs when it is being cast. Despite this high modulus of elasticity, the tearing energy of polyether rubbers is lower than that of the polysulphides. Tearing of the impression occurs unless care is taken.

The catalyst in these materials can cause sensitization and an allergic reaction. The accelerator paste should be handled carefully.

The surface of gypsum cast into the impression is excellent. The material can be electroplated. The storage life of the material appears to be satisfactory under normal conditions.

Typical properties:

Setting time 20–25°C	3–6 minutes	
Elasticity, permanent set 2 minutes after setting, after application of 12% strain	1–2%	

Thermal properties of elastomers

The thermal conductivity of silicone rubbers is greater than that of polysulphides and polyethers. All the elastomers have fairly high coefficients of thermal expansion though this is affected by the amount of filler which they contain. The error which could occur on cooling an impression from mouth to room temperature could produce a clinically discernible error. For example, in a bridge span of 20 mm an overall error of 0·05 mm could occur. Adhesion of the impression to the tray reduces the effect of thermal contraction to within clinically acceptable limits.

Chapter 24

Non-metallic denture base materials.
Heat-cure PMMA

The materials used in the construction of denture bases may be divided into metallic and non-metallic types. The metals and alloys used in denture construction have already been discussed in Section B of this text. In general, they display excellent mechanical properties, and can be used in relatively thin sections. However, it is easier and cheaper to construct appliances in the non-metallic materials. In addition, the colour and texture of these materials can be made to resemble natural gum tissue, thus making the appliances less conspicuous in the mouth.

There has therefore been a constant search over many years for an ideal non-metallic denture base material. The properties required are as follows:

> High modulus of elasticity with a high proportional limit so that the appliance will be sufficiently rigid against masticatory forces. A strong and rigid material can also be used in thin sections so that the denture is not bulky.
>
> High fatigue strength.
>
> High impact strength. This is important because even the most careful of patients may drop a denture.
>
> Hard surface which is resistant to abrasion, so that the appliance will take and retain a high polish.
>
> The softening temperature should be well above mouth temperature, indeed it would be ideal if a denture could be sterilized by boiling.
>
> Easy to manipulate with accuracy by dental techniques, and must retain its shape permanently.
>
> Easy to repair without any distortion.
>
> Should be impermeable to oral fluids.
>
> Low specific gravity with a high thermal conductivity.

Should be non-irritant to the mouth tissues, non-toxic, tasteless and odourless.

Should resemble gum tissue in colour and translucency, and the colour must be permanent.

It has not yet been possible to discover a material which fulfils all these requirements. Many materials have been tried but have been discarded because they were unsatisfactory from too many aspects. Even the non-metallic denture bases in use at the present time cannot be considered to be perfectly suited to their task.

PREVIOUS DENTURE BASE MATERIALS

Vulcanite

Applicable specification for elastic bands: Austral 1240.

Pure rubber is a polymer of isoprene C_5H_8.

$$CH_2 = \overset{\overset{\textstyle CH_3}{|}}{C} - CH = CH_2$$

Addition polymerization takes place by the opening up of *one* of the double bonds, leaving the other available as a further point of attachment.

Rubber macromolecules consist of a long coiled chain, comprising many thousand isoprene molecules. Such a coiled chain can be extended to a great degree without breakdown of the interchain forces, and this gives rubber its elasticity.

Rubber is used for making orthodontic elastics. These elastic bands are used to promote tooth movement. Most orthodontic elastics are made from surgical latex rubber based on isoprene. Various additions are made to the mix to improve their lasting qualities. When stretched, the load/elongation curve of elastic bands appears to have three main zones. Only in the middle zone does the load remain relatively constant during changes in length. It is preferable, therefore, to use rubber bands for orthodontic purposes at a degree of stretch which falls within this middle zone, so that a constant force is applied.

The addition of sulphur to natural rubber reduces its stickiness and improves its strength and elasticity. A small addition of sulphur affects only a few of the remaining double bonds, particularly those at the ends of the chains. As the amount of sulphur increases, saturation of all the double bonds takes place, and cross-linkages appear between adjacent chains. Complete saturation takes place with 32 per cent of sulphur. In dental vulcanite, this amount of sulphur is present together with pigments which are metallic oxides or carbon. Some addition of sulphur to isoprene takes place at warm room temperature and dental rubber shows a shelf-life of up to 2 years. If old rubber is used, the resulting vulcanite will be weak and will tend to crumble.

Vulcanization

The mould containing the dental rubber is heated in a closed container called a 'vulcanizer' which is full of water vapour under pressure. The steam pressure is raised to 0·63 N/mm² (90 psi) which corresponds to a temperature of 168°C.

Properties

Water absorption of vulcanite is low initially, but continues during the life of the appliance and can reach quite a high figure. The surface is penetrated by bacteria and the denture become unhygienic after a period of use.

Vulcanite is opaque and has no resemblance to gum tissues in appearance. It is still used occasionally as a denture base material when a true allergy to other denture bases has been found to exist and no other denture base is available.

Other materials

Cellulose nitrate, phenol-formaldehyde, polystyrene, polyester, epoxide, nylon, and polycarbonate polymers have all been used as denture bases, but for a variety of reasons, have been found to be less suitable than polymethyl methacrylate.

POLYMETHYL METHACRYLATE (PMMA)

Applicable specifications: ISO R 1567; Brit 2487; Amer 12; Austral 1043.

PMMA or acrylic resin first became available in the form of 'blanks' for moulding. The plasticized polymer was softened by heat and then injected into the mould. However, in 1935, a patent was taken out in Germany by Kulzer, putting forward the idea of moulding fine grains of polymer which were softened by monomer. This method removed many of the difficulties which were inherent in the injection technique. The soft mixture of monomer and polymer could be moulded in a plaster mould without the use of great pressures. Then, on curing, the monomer polymerized, giving a solid mass of polymer.

Methyl methacrylates are available for dental use in the polymer–monomer form, and also as a 'gel'. The latter mode of presentation is not used as widely as the powder–liquid type, as its shelf-life is of much shorter duration. It will be seen that the powder–liquid type pass through a stage similar to that of the gel, and therefore the manipulation of both is similar. Since the powder–liquid type is the more common, this material will be discussed in detail.

Monomer

Acrylic monomer is a colourless liquid consisting mainly of methyl methacrylate. Under the action of ultraviolet light and heat, monomer will polymerize in the bottle and thus become useless. An inhibitor is added in order to prevent polymerization while it is being stored. This is usually hydroquinone, present at about 0·006 weight per cent. The bottle in which monomer is supplied is made of dark brown glass, so that the contents are shielded from ultraviolet light. As a further precaution, the bottle of monomer should be stored in a cool place.

Monomer liquid may also contain styrene, glycol dimethacrylate or other copolymerizing monomers. Glycol dimethacrylate incorporated at up to 2 per cent acts as a cross-linking copolymer, forming cross-linkages between the PMMA chains. This produces a less soluble denture base material and reduces the tendency to surface crazing.

Polymer

This consists of particles of PMMA which are usually spherical and are of different sizes. They are manufactured by heating monomer which is finely dispersed in water. The mixture is stirred vigorously while the temperature is raised to bring about polymerization. The particles of polymer are then filtered off, dried, and sieved for size. Irregularly shaped particles may be produced by grinding or milling a block of solid polymer. Some polymers contain a copolymer such as ethyl acrylate.

Plasticizer

The main reason for adding plasticizer to the polymer is to speed the rate at which the monomer dissolves the polymer. The plasticizer makes the polymer softer and weaker. If present, the amount is limited to a maximum of 10 per cent. Otherwise a highly plasticized polymer may break up in the mouth after it has been further plasticized by absorption of water.

Initiator

An initiator such as benzoyl peroxide is also present in the polymer granules, in amounts varying from 0·2 to 0·5 per cent. This chemical initiates polymerization and also overcomes the effect of the inhibitor.

Pigmentation

Denture base polymers are available in 'clear' and in various shades of pink. Suitably coloured polymers are also available for making teeth. The pink and tooth-coloured materials may be made by mixing together clear particles and pigments in a ball-mill or by making polymer from pigmented monomer. By the first method, the pigments are present only on the outside of the polymer granules, whereas by the second method, the polymer is pigmented throughout. The pigments used must be stable in the presence of the peroxide initiator, and inorganic oxides are usually better than organic pigments. If a large container full of surface-pigmented polymer is examined, it will be found that some variation in pigmentation exists between the upper and lower portions of its contents. Polymer containers should be shaken before use in order to ensure an even distribution of pigment.

Several different shades of pink powder are available, in an attempt to match the colour of the denture base to that of the patient's natural gum tissues. Other supplies of polymer contain fine threads such as nylon, which are coloured bright red or purple. These simulate the mottled appearance of natural gum tissue with its fine blood-vessels near the surface. In both partial and full dentures where the gumwork of the denture is shown when the patient smiles, a natural appearance can be produced by the use of pigmented and 'veined' polymers.

MIXING THE MONOMER AND POLYMER

The ratio of monomer to polymer is important, as the dimensional changes which take place on polymerization are due to the contraction of the monomer. As would be expected the change from free monomeric molecules to polymer chains is accompanied by a contraction. This is over 20 per cent by volume.

The amount of monomer used must therefore be kept as low as possible, but there must be sufficient to have two important effects. First, it must soften the polymer grains and so reduce the moulding pressure, and secondly, there must be sufficient monomer to 'glue' the polymer particles together in a solid mass.

Usually the polymer–monomer ratio is 3 or $3\frac{1}{2}$ to 1 by volume or about $2\frac{1}{2}$ to 1 by weight. This reduces the volume contraction on polymerization to about 7 per cent. This figure still appears to be very high if an accurately fitting denture is to be made, but it will be seen later that other factors reduce the effect of this rather large contraction.

A suitable volume of monomer is measured into a clean, dry mixing vessel, and the polymer is gently poured in. As the liquid is soaked up into the powder, it may be noted that pigment is washed from the surface of the polymer grains and tends to collect in patches. To ensure an even colour, the mixture must be well stirred and vibrated. A well-fitting lid should then be placed on the jar to prevent loss of monomer by evaporation.

Reaction between polymer and monomer

On mixing the powder and liquid together, a material of rather 'sandy' consistency is at first produced. After a short period of time which varies with the different polymers, this mixture changes to a sticky mass. If the mix is stirred at this stage, 'strings' of material stick to the spatula or mixer. After a further period of time, it forms a more cohesive and less adhesive mass which does not stick to the walls of the mixing vessel. This dough-like material is soft, but gradually changes to a tough rubbery consistency. After a further period of time, the material hardens completely.

The stages in mixing monomer–polymer acrylic materials are therefore as follows:

Sandy or granular—stringy—full dough—rubbery—hard.

These changes are due to the solution of the polymer in the monomer.

At first the monomer dissolves the outer layers of the powder grains. Then it penetrates the entire grain of polymer, softening it in a manner similar to a plasticizer. The very small grains of polymer dissolve completely in the monomer, increasing the viscosity of the mix.

The 'gel' form in which acrylic denture base is sometimes supplied corresponds to a stage slightly before the full dough, at which it is maintained by suitable inhibitors for several weeks. During this period of time, the polymer becomes completely dissolved in the monomer and the mix becomes clear instead of opaque.

Doughing time of the mix

The mix is packed into the mould at the full dough stage. The speed with which the polymer and monomer mixture reaches this stage depends upon several factors.

The size of the particles affects the doughing time. Most of the present-day polymers are fine grained and dough quickly.

A polymer of high molecular weight is more difficult to soften than one of short chain length, as the forces of attraction between its chains are greater.

If the powder is a copolymer of PMMA with a softer polymer, the dough time will be shorter.

A similar effect is seen with a highly plasticized polymer. Although, if liquid dibutyl phthalate is added to a mix of polymer and monomer the doughing time is increased, as the oily plasticizer covers the powder grains and retards their rate of reaction with the monomer.

The time available for manipulating the dough before it passes to the tough rubbery consistency, varies with the rate at which the dough stage is reached at normal temperatures. A quick-doughing material can generally be worked for only a short time and only one or two dentures can be packed from the same mix. Some acrylic powders are available, however, which consist of a mixture of low and high molecular weight polymers. The lower polymers soften first and produce a workable mix of a slightly granular texture. The mix remains at this workable consistency until the higher polymers soften. In this way a dough is quickly obtained which has a long working time.

Control of the doughing time

The above factors are not directly under the control of the technician.

He can only speed up or slow down the changes in the dough by adjusting its temperature. If the mixing vessel is warmed before use, or if the atmospheric temperature is high, the material will pass rapidly through the various stages of consistency. When the mixing jar is heated, the mix must be stirred, or an outer layer will dough before the centre. Conversely, a dough can be stored for several hours in a refrigerator, provided cooling commences before it reaches the full-dough stage, as the mix is a poor conductor of heat. During any refrigeration, condensation of water within the jar must be avoided, as the water will be incorporated in the dough and will cause a deterioration in the properties of the polymerized material.

An increase in the polymer–monomer ratio reduces the doughing time, and the opposite effect is obtained by using an excess of monomer. The latter method of increasing the doughing time is to be avoided as the mixture contracts more on polymerizing. As much powder as possible should be incorporated in the monomer. A very stiff mix can be made by stirring and vibrating the mix very vigorously, adding powder at frequent intervals. But care must be taken to see that monomer does not evaporate from such a thick mix. The polymerized material from a thick mix is more opaque than one from a thin mix, as more pigment is present.

Packing the mould

At no stage should the acrylic dough be manipulated with the fingers. A skin reaction or 'dermatitis' may be produced due to the irritant action of the monomer. Irritation may also be caused by continuous contact with the fine polymer granules. All manipulation of the dough should be effected with glass or stainless steel instruments. If the fingers must be used, a sheet of cellophane or polythene placed over the dough will protect the skin and also prevent dirt contamination of the dough.

The volume shrinkage which takes place has little effect on the dimensions of the denture after curing. Its main disadvantage is in creating 'shrinkage voids' or 'porosity'. Therefore, a slight excess must be provided within the mould in order to obtain a sound polymer. The actual contraction volume is proportional to the mass of dough being cured. This varies widely between one denture and another, so that it is difficult to measure accurately the excess volume which is required. There are, however, several methods by which a slight excess can be provided.

Elasticity of the gypsum mould

Gypsum is capable of a small elastic compressive deformation, and therefore a small excess of dough can be forced into the mould. The amount of elastic deformation of the mould is dependent upon its strength. The mould should be left to harden for at least 1 hour after final set. Then, after 'boiling out' it is advisable to leave the open mould in a warm, dry place for several hours so that a greater surface hardness is attained. During packing, then, both the dough and the mould are compressed, but the pressure is reduced when the monomer contracts on polymerization. The disadvantage of this method of overcoming shrinkage is that too great a compressive force will distort the mould permanently, it will break and the teeth may move. Also, the actual increase in volume of the mould is small, and will not compensate for the contraction of a large bulk of dough.

Silicone-lined mould

A mould consisting of an internal layer of self-curing silicone rubber supported by gypsum enables one to cure more bulky sections without internal porosity. To make such a mould, the pattern, i.e. the waxed-up denture, is coated with a thin layer of silicone rubber and then invested in the normal way. Such a mould has a relatively large increase in dimension when the dough is packed into it and this can compensate for a large volume change on polymerization. Separation of the polymerized denture from such a mould is cleaner and the denture requires less finishing than when a gypsum mould alone is used.

However, dimensional accuracy may suffer as a consequence of elastic distortion of the rubber mould. The fitting surface of a prosthesis should therefore be moulded against a gypsum surface whilst polished surfaces can be moulded against silicone rubber.

Trial closure

The mould is usually filled and a 'trial closure' carried out using a sheet of cellophane or polythene as a separator over the cast. By this means the amount of excess left in the mould can be controlled. On opening the flask after a trial closure, a 'flash' of dough appears on the plaster surface outside the mould cavity. This is trimmed away. If the flash is thick, further slow trial closing of the flask is continued until only a thin flash remains. Excessive pressure must be avoided. The thin flash is removed, leaving the mould slightly overfilled, and the flask is closed *without adding further material.*

Pressure applied in closing the flask

Pressure is applied to the dough within the flask in order to fill every part of the mould and also to remove the air which is incorporated within the dough on mixing the monomer and polymer. Without suitable pressure, this air remains and causes porosity of the cured material.

A minimum load of 1800–2500 N (180–250 kg) appears to be necessary to ensure that the dough fills small spaces in the mould. The maximum force which can be applied is related to the strength of the mould. A weak, freshly made, plaster mould limits the packing pressure to a low value. A stronger stone mould enables one to use high loads up to 8000 N (800 kg). By making the more highly stressed portions of the mould in stone, and the rest in plaster, one can combine strength with ease of deflasking.

The load applied when closing the mould depends on the type of press which is used. A flask press with a fine thread works at a better mechanical advantage than one with a coarse thread. Therefore, with a fine thread less force need be exerted by the operator on the arms of the press, and a finer control of the pressure is obtained. During curing, the mould must be compressed by a force similar to that which was used in closing the flask in the bench press. If a lesser force is used, the two halves of the mould will spring apart, giving a change in the occlusal relation of the denture, or a *raised bite.*

Injection moulding

A further method of packing is to 'inject' the dough into the previously closed mould. Suitable sprues are formed in the investing plaster leading into the mould cavity. The dough is injected by a variety of methods. When using the injection moulding technique, it is not necessary to produce a two-part gypsum mould. The wax pattern within a closed mould can be removed by heating and by pouring boiling water down the sprues. With a one-part mould, the denture requires less finishing but there are difficulties in removing the polymerized denture from the mould. Though this method is theoretically ideal, it fails to find a wide application. Even if a two-part mould is used, the two halves are in their correct relationship and the difficulties of raised bite should not occur.

POLYMERIZATION

The application of heat to the dough causes the initiator to decompose rapidly and form free radicals:

Benzoyl peroxide

These activate the monomer molecules, forming further free radicals. This is the *initiation* or *induction* phase:

methyl methacrylate

INITIATION

In turn, further molecules are activated and a polymer chain grows by *propagation*:

PROPAGATION

The energy necessary for initiation is fairly high. Hence the small amount of inhibitor present is sufficient to prevent initiation. Benzoyl peroxide dissociates rapidly at 60–65°C and sufficient energy is then available to initiate polymerization and to overcome the effect of the inhibitor. Less energy is required for propagation and when once it is initiated, it proceeds very rapidly. Polymerization can also be accelerated by adding a very small percentage of an activator to the monomer. This causes breakdown of the benzoyl peroxide initiator at a lower temperature. Activators are present in the self-cure materials dealt with in the next chapter.

Cessation of chain growth or *termination* occurs when the growing chain attaches to an impurity or to a free radical or when it joins to a further growing chain.

Dimensional changes during curing

In the closed mould, the dough expands when heat is applied during curing. The coefficient of linear expansion of PMMA is high, being 81×10^{-6} per °C. Therefore a marked expansion takes place on heating to 60–65°C. This expansion is probably the main factor which compensates for the polymerization shrinkage. If the flask is held in a spring clamp, the latter allows the flask to open slightly as the dough expands and then closes the mould again when polymerization contraction occurs. In a mould which is not under spring pressure, the pressure of the expanding dough added to that already existing within the mould may be sufficient to crack the plaster, or to force the teeth into the plaster. Fracture of porcelain teeth may also occur due to the large compressive stresses which are set up.

The volumetric contraction is about 7 per cent. Provided the mould is full of dough under moderate pressure, this contraction has little effect upon the dimensions of the cured denture. The contraction is overcome by flow of the dough, and also by flow of the resultant polymer at the curing temperature. The denture also adheres to the walls of the mould, particularly if these are of complex shape, and this further reduces dimensional change.

Gaseous porosity

Polymerization is an exothermic reaction, and therefore when a large mass of dough within a flask is heated, the temperature at the centre will rise above that of the flask and the investing plaster. Both the polymer itself and the plaster mould are poor conductors of heat, and the heat evolved is only slowly dissipated throughout the flask. The boiling point of pure monomer is 100·3°C. When a large mass of dough is heated quickly the internal temperature rises well above this temperature. The monomer vapour which is produced becomes enclosed by hard polymer and a porous structure is created. As the rate of polymerization increases, more heat of reaction is evolved. If further heat is being added from the outside of the flask by conduction through the plaster mould, the two sources of heat are complementary. The

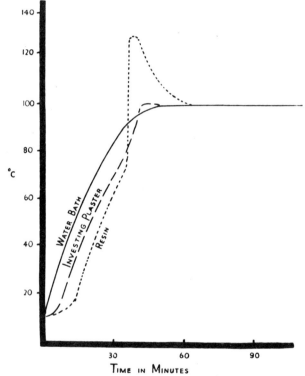

Fig. 49. Thermal changes in a large mass of acrylic dough and in the plaster mould, when heated in a waterbath from room temperature to boiling point

consequent rapid rise in temperature causes a further increase in the rate of polymerization which again liberates more heat. In this way a rapidly accelerating reaction takes place and the internal temperature rises sharply. Figure 49 shows the various temperature changes within a mass of dough compared with those taking place within the plaster and in the heating medium—in this case a water-bath.

The peak temperature in the centre of a mass of dough is reduced somewhat if the packed mould is left for some hours at room temperature before it is heated.

Sites of gaseous porosity

When a flask is heated from the outside, the first portions of the dough to polymerize are those nearest the surface of the flask. These do not show gaseous porosity but their heat of reaction is passed on to the interior portions of dough. It is here that gaseous porosity is seen. In other words, gaseous porosity occurs away from the source of heat.

In lower dentures, the lingual aspect in the premolar region is a common site for gaseous porosity, and in upper dentures a line of porosity is sometimes seen running round the sloping sides of the palate (Fig. 50). The centre of the palate is near the outside of the flask

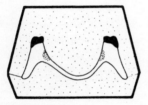 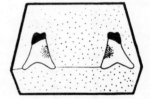

Fig. 50. Sites of gaseous porosity in upper and lower acrylic dentures, showing their position in the flask

and is not usually affected by this type of porosity. It will be appreciated that the lower denture is usually more bulky than the upper and is therefore more prone to gaseous porosity.

Other types of porosity

Contraction porosity arises as a result of the reduction in volume of the dough which takes place on polymerization. If the mould is incompletely filled, voids appear within the hardened polymer. Unlike gaseous porosity, the holes do not appear in any particular portion of the denture. Contraction or under-packing porosity appears in any areas where the dough is not sufficiently compressed.

Granularity is not strictly a porosity, but rather a deficiency of structure. Monomer is added to the polymer grains in order to soften them and to provide a matrix. But monomer is volatile, and evaporates from the surface of a dough which is exposed to the atmosphere. Then there is insufficient monomer left to bond the polymer particles together. A granular structure often arises from exposure of the dough at the trial closure stage. After packing the dough and carrying out a trial closure, the mould is opened for inspection. If packing is adequate, that half of the mould which was protected by cellophane or polythene is coated with a suitable mould seal. While this layer of seal sets, the dough must be protected from the atmosphere. The simplest way of doing this is to leave the separator in position until the mould seal is dry. Then remove the sheet and close the mould. Granularity appears in the thinner sections and at the edges of a denture, as volatilization takes place more readily from these areas.

METHODS OF CURING

Heat may be applied by placing the mould in a water-bath or in a warm-air oven. The resultant polymer is the same whichever method is used. The advantage of a water-bath is that the temperature is self-limiting whilst an oven requires more careful thermal control.

It is perfectly safe to heat the flask containing the dough up to 68–72°C. At this temperature the dough can be left to polymerize under the heating effect of its own exothermic reaction.

One method of avoiding gaseous porosity is to place the cold flask in a water-bath at 68–72°C for at least 1½ hours. After half an hour the contents of the flask are at the same temperature as the bath. During the remaining hour the temperature may rise due to polymerization until it is within a few degrees of the boiling point of monomer. Then it falls again by heat conduction through the flask. The length of time that the flask is heated at this temperature may be increased to several hours, and it is common practice to process overnight, for 12 hours or longer. There are no disadvantages in such a long processing time, but as will be seen later, this low-temperature treatment should preferably be followed by heating for half to one hour in boiling water. Alternatively, curing may be carried out by increasing the time at 68–72°C to 24 hours.

Microwave irradiation has been suggested as a means of heating all the dough evenly in a short space of time.

When only thin sections are present, such a slow curing is not essential, but it is preferable to set a definite processing procedure which will yield a non-porous polymer in all normal thicknesses.

Other methods of preventing porosity involve raising the boiling point of the monomer by the application of increased air pressure.

When an injection method is used, there are advantages in applying heat only to one end of the mould away from the injection mechanism. Then a wave of polymerization passes through the dough and the effect of polymerization contraction is reduced by further dough entering the mould at the site of injection as this is the last area to polymerize.

Degree of polymerization

The degree of polymerization varies to some degree with the temperature and time of curing.

Although polymerization occurs quickly at temperatures of $65-75°C$, a temperature of about $100°C$ produces a degree of polymerization which is near the maximum obtainable by dental processing methods. Only a slight increase in the degree of polymerization is found when temperatures above $100°C$ and up to $145°C$ are used.

Perhaps the most important factor in determining the properties of the resultant polymer is the presence of low molecular weight fractions. These may well act as plasticizer weakening the polymer. It has been shown that the existence of chains with a molecular weight of less than 10^5 can act in this way. Thus the molecular weight distribution is more important than the attainment of a high average molecular weight, provided that the amount of polymer chains with a molecular weight of less than 10^5 is reduced to the minimum.

It has already been shown that when thick sections of dough are heated at $68-72°C$, their internal temperature will rise to within a few degrees of $100°C$ due to the heat of reaction. Therefore, in a denture of uneven thickness, the thick sections will be more fully polymerized than the thinner portions, as the temperature of the latter will rise only a few degrees above that of the mould. A final processing at $100°C$ for at least 30 minutes is preferable in order to complete as far as possible the polymerization of the entire contents of the mould.

Residual monomer

In all acrylic dentures made from monomer–polymer, some residual monomer remains even after lengthy processing. Even after boiling,

0·2–0·5 per cent of monomer remains in addition to short chains of only a few molecules. It is probable that any of this monomer which can be washed out disappears during normal polishing procedures or during subsequent storage in water for 2–3 hours. After correct processing, therefore, leaching of residual monomer in the mouth can be discounted. If processing is carried out at too low a temperature or for too short a time, more residual monomer remains and this can be washed out into the saliva. As the monomer is washed out into the saliva film between denture and tissues, it may affect the latter.

Tissue reaction

Inflammation of the tissues under a denture may be due to primary irritation or to an allergic reaction following previous sensitization. Primary chemical irritation may be from residual monomer, excess initiator (benzoyl peroxide), inhibitor (hydroquinone), or pigment. Whilst these are all possible irritants, it is doubtful whether any of them, apart from monomer, play a part in tissue irritation. Acrylic monomer, besides being an irritant, may sensitize the patient. To be safe, therefore, the amount of residual monomer should be reduced to a minimum.

There are many other reasons for inflammation of oral tissues under acrylic dentures. These include trauma, lack of oral hygiene, fungus infection, occlusion of ducts of mucous glands and the general state of health of the patient. True allergy to methyl methacrylate monomer is a rare occurrence.

Dimensional changes after curing

On Cooling

After the denture has been cured, the flask is cooled slowly to room temperature before removing the denture from the mould. On cooling to 60–70°C, the polymer contracts thermally, but if it is *slowly* cooled, some of this contraction will be made non-effective by flow. Below 60–65°C, the polymer is sufficiently rigid to contract and compress the mould. The coefficient of thermal expansion and contraction of PMMA is much greater than that of gypsum. On cooling below 60–65°C, the denture is stretched over the surface of the plaster cast. Some of this stretching is elastic and will be relieved on releasing the denture from the mould; but some cooling stresses remain. They commonly occur round pieces of porcelain or metal which are incorporated within a denture. The contraction of these materials is less than that of PMMA, and the denture base is stretched round the insert on cooling.

Generally, the lower curing temperature of 68–72°C produces less stress than occurs after boiling the denture. Even at 100°C the polymer does not flow with sufficient freedom to remove completely the stress set up by contraction of the monomer. Nor are all the thermal changes in dimension on cooling from 100°C to 65°C accommodated by plastic flow.

Immediate elastic stress-relief in a denture after removal from the flask produces a denture which is slightly smaller than the cast. A value of 0·5 per cent linear contraction is usually quoted. But this shrinkage is not regular throughout the complex shape of a denture.

In a correctly cured denture, however, these errors of dimension are not of clinical significance. They may be of advantage in providing a slightly 'tighter' denture during the initial weeks of wearing.

Internal stresses

The stress in a denture is related to its shape and size, the pressure applied during curing, the curing cycle used, and the rate of cooling after processing.

A more complex shape, for example, a denture to a bulbous upper ridge, will develop greater stresses on cooling than a bulky denture for a ridgeless lower jaw.

The compressive force used in all methods of packing the mould is not reduced entirely by polymerization shrinkage. Stresses are greater when a high compressive force is used.

The stress remaining within the denture is released at a later stage if the denture is warmed, with a consequent warpage of the denture. An acrylic denture should never be cleaned in water above 70°C— that is, it should never be placed in water which is too hot to use for washing the hands.

Crazing

Small cracks may appear on the surface of a denture after a period of wear. They are often seen to radiate outwards from the necks of porcelain teeth or from metal inserts. They can be produced in the laboratory by exposing the denture to a solvent for PMMA or sometimes to its vapour. Monomer, chloroform (often present in cough pastilles), or ethyl alcohol all produce the effect.

Crazing is caused mainly by drying out of the surface of the polymer. As water is lost, the outer dry skin contracts and tensile stresses are set up across the surface. A solvent reduces the intermolecular attractions and the portions under tension break apart, leaving a narrow crack or fissure between them. It does not occur to the same extent if the denture is completely dry or entirely saturated with water. Crazing is often seen on dentures which have been repaired, when the monomer in the new dough has released the stress present in the older portion of the denture, particularly if this is partly dried.

The alginate or mould seals tend to cause surface stress and so increase the possibility of 'crazing'.

Cross-linked denture base copolymers are less soluble and do not show the same degree of crazing when placed in a solvent.

Water absorption

Acrylic polymers absorb water and expand. The water penetrates between the molecular chains and forces them apart.

The change in dimension depends upon the water content of the denture after curing. Alginate mould seals do not seal the material against moisture. Water enters from the gypsum, and the cured denture is almost water saturated. Little further expansion occurs on wearing.

If tinfoil is used to line the mould, less water enters the denture base in the flask and a greater expansion can be expected on water absorption. With a tinfoiled mould the cured denture is smaller than the cast. After several months' wear the denture approaches the 'correct' size, but this slow change is unnoticeable clinically.

Water acts as a plasticizer and assists in the relief of stress within the denture, so that the swelling due to water absorption may not be measurably the same in all dimensions. For example, if a measurement is taken across the tuberosities of an upper denture, an apparent contraction of the base will be recorded on immersion in water.

This change of dimension with water absorption is important in the storing of dentures and appliances. During all processes in the dental workshop subsequent to curing, the denture must be kept in water until it is placed in the patient's mouth. Subsequently, the patient must place the denture in water whenever it is not being worn. Any denture which has been stored dry for a period of time should be immersed in water for at least 24 hours before it is inserted in the mouth.

There is little or no solution of heat-cured PMMA in water or in the oral fluids.

Properties of PMMA

In the polymerized material, all except the smallest polymer granules can be seen if a section is cut. Due to the penetration of polymer grains by monomer, the resultant structure consists of interpenetrating polymer networks. The two networks are those of the original polymer and that of the polymerized monomer. Greater solution of the polymer by the monomer improves the strength. Indeed the strongest PMMA to impact stresses is produced by complete solution of the polymer in monomer. Hence, speeding up the doughing time may reduce the degree of solution of the polymer, and so reduce the mechanical properties of the resultant denture base. Fracture of the polymerized material occurs through the polymer beads as well as through the matrix.

The mechanical properties of PMMA which are important are transverse, impact and fatigue strengths, hardness and abrasion resistance.

Transverse strength

The load before fracture, the deflection under load and the elastic recovery after removal of the load are important properties. When dry, heat-cured PMMA is a relatively brittle material. Water absorption lowers the strength and increases the deflection under load since the water acts as a plasticizer. The load at fracture is greater when the material has a higher molecular weight. Under clinical conditions, heat-cured PMMA is stiff enough not to flex unduly during function and recovers well from this degree of bending.

Impact strength

The impact strength should be high in case the patient drops the denture, or bites suddenly on a hard object such as a piece of bone during a meal. There is little increase in impact strength with increasing molecular weight.

Fatigue strength

Even the most carefully processed acrylic denture may show a tendency to undergo repeated fracture at a weak point when the masticatory force is high.

Acrylic polymers show *notch sensitivity*. The presence of a notch, crack or deep scratch increases the tendency to fracture. For this reason, overstressing of a denture on deflasking must be avoided. Otherwise a small crack may be produced which later will propagate throughout the material. Similarly, the surface of the denture must be smoothly polished. In an upper denture, stress accumulation during chewing may occur at a point between the central incisor teeth. Here, the facial flange is frequently weakened by a notch to accomodate the labial frenum. Fatigue or 'midline' fracture may then occur if the chewing stresses are relatively large.

Fatigue strength improves with a higher molecular weight and with an increase in plasticizer content.

Hardness and abrasion resistance

Acrylic polymers show a Brinell Hardness of between 18 and 22. Indentation hardness is, however, not necessarily a true indication of the resistance of a material to wear or abrasion. A scratch hardness or abrasion resistance test shows that heat-cured PMMA has an abrasion resistance similar to that of 22 carat gold alloy in the soft condition.

The surface of PMMA is rapidly worn away if it is in contact with a rough surface. When polished surfaces are in light contact, and are lubricated with saliva, little wear is seen.

Density

The density of acrylic resin is $1·18$ g/cm^3 and this is an advantage for upper dentures.

Typical properties of heat-cured acrylic polymers:

Tensile strength	55–65 N/mm^2
Modulus of elasticity in tension	1000–1750 N/mm^2
Transverse strength	
Specimen $10 \times 2·5$ mm over 50 mm span	
Deflection at $3·5$ kg	$1·8$–$2·0$ mm
Deflection at $5·0$ kg	4–5 mm
Fracture at	$6·0$ kg
Water absorption	$0·5$–$0·6$ mg/cm^2
Solubility	$0·02$–$0·03$ mg/cm^2

Strengthening acrylic polymers

The strength of PMMA is sometimes not sufficient to withstand the heavy biting pressure of a person with very strong jaw muscles. Also dentures for young children, may not be strong enough to withstand the rather rough treatment which they receive. Greater strength can be obtained by thickening the denture, but this makes it rather clumsy and heavy.

It is useless to place a piece of thin wire within a denture, and expect it to increase the strength. The wire reduces the bulk of polymer which is present, and this smaller section will break, leaving the wire intact. To strengthen a polymer, fibres must be incorporated which have a high tensile strength and which bond to the polymer. Glass fibre is not readily wetted by acrylic polymers but if the fibre is treated with a silane coupling agent, bonding takes place. Woven glass fabric has been shown to increase the impact strength of acrylic polymers. If short strands of glass fibre are used, a very high percentage is necessary to achieve an improvement in mechanical properties, since not all the fibres lie in the anticipated direction of stress. This creates difficulties in moulding such a heavily filled polymer.

Whiskers or very short fibres of other materials can be grown with care so that they possess near perfect crystal structure with few dislocations. These have high strength values. They may be made of a variety of materials including carbon, sapphire and alumina. Incorporation of about 10 per cent of such whiskers improves the mechanical properties of PMMA, but often reduces the aesthetic qualities. Carbon fibres have a tensile strength of $1 \cdot 7 \times 10^3$ N/mm². The incorporation of these improves transverse strength and stiffness of PMMA but unfortunately spoils the natural pink colour.

Modifications to PMMA to produce 'high impact' materials have been made. The usual methods of copolymerization and cross-linking reduce solubility but do not affect mechanical properties greatly. A copolymer of polystyrene and PMMA has properties similar to that of PMMA. However, by incorporating an elastomer such as polybutadiene 5–10 per cent, a material with higher impact strength is produced. It is probable that the polybutadiene acts as an energy absorber, limiting fracture propagation and so increasing strength. The use of a copolymer of PMMA and hydroxyethyl methacrylate produces a more flexible, though weaker material. It has been suggested that due to the more hydrophilic character of the resultant denture surface, retention and cleanliness are improved. Clinical experience does not seem to support these suggestions.

In general, attempts to improve the strength of PMMA create materials with greater flexibility and sometimes a lower softening temperature. There is some debate as to whether a flexible or a rigid polymer is preferable for dentures. A rigid denture base will resist a heavy load, but may break after a small deflection. On the other hand, a flexible polymer will bend with a moderate load and so reduce the incidence of fracture. But it will apply large forces to small areas of the natural tissues. As far as the denture alone is concerned, flexibility is an advantage, but it may well be a greater disadvantage when we consider the continued health of the patient's remaining teeth and gums.

A lower softening temperature increases the possibility of warping the denture whilst cleaning it as distortion can take place as low as 60°C with some materials.

The attainment of a high molecular weight by boiling PMMA for half an hour, followed by slow cooling and the avoidance of sharp notches and careful polishing of the surface, seem to reduce the incidence of fracture. It is possible, however, that PMMA undergoes biodegradation after some years of intraoral use, and fractures can then be anticipated.

Radiopacity

Acrylic polymers are radiolucent. In an accident, a portion of a broken denture may be swallowed or may lodge in the bronchi, and be difficult to locate by X-rays. Metal inserts such as clasps facilitate location only if the whole denture is swallowed. The incorporation of 1 per cent of amalgam alloy particles or of metal foil strips renders the entire denture sufficiently radiopaque.

The incorporation of 8 per cent $BaSO_4$ or BaF_2 causes a general slight radiopacity. To give sufficient radiopacity, a large amount has to be added but the strength of the denture is reduced to an unacceptable level. Use of organo-iodine or -bromine compounds has been suggested but unfortunately these act as plasticizers. Heavy atoms in the form of bismuth glasses can, however, be incorporated as fillers. An acrylic polymer containing 10 per cent of a powdered bismuth glass has been suggested. The surface of the glass is treated with a coupling agent. The material is said to produce a polymerized denture with adequate strength and good radiopacity.

Surface treatment of the denture

Many chewing gums adhere to denture base polymers. Alternative gums are available but the denture itself may be coated with silica by exposure to silicon tetrachloride. The layer formed enables the patient to keep the denture clean more readily and claims are made that the coating improves retention.

REPAIRS

When a denture is broken, the fragments show a greater degree of internal stress than existed when the denture was complete. This increase is due to the breaking of the molecular bonds at the point of fracture, and an alteration of the intermolecular forces within each new portion. When a highly stressed denture is fractured, a distortion of thin sections of the fragments may create difficulties in reassembling the broken pieces. In fatigue failure, when a small crack has propagated slowly, the two surfaces at the point of breakage may not fit each other, as some permanent deformation has occurred.

The usual method of repairing is to pour a cast to the denture, and then cut away material from either side of the fracture line. New material is then processed between the two halves of the denture in order to join them together.

Preparation for repair

The method of preparation of the edges of the joint has an important effect upon the strength of the repair. These edges should be rounded and of as large an area as possible. If the edges are trimmed to a profile consisting of straight lines meeting at sharp angles, stresses within the old and new polymer are concentrated at the angles and the denture will again fracture at these points of maximum stress.

Union of old and new polymer

A strong joint is produced only if the polymer networks of the previous denture base and the new material interpenetrate. Any dirt, oil or grease present on the old polymer surface reduces the amount of linkage of polymer chains across the joint. A smooth, newly polished surface gives the best joint. On boiling out the repair, a detergent should be used to eliminate all traces of wax. Sufficient monomer must be present to penetrate the surface of the old polymer and then by its polymerization between the old and the new produce a strong joint. The alginate mould seals will not react with PMMA to form a calcium alginate film; but it is possible to leave a thin film of soluble alginate on a surface. This dries out by evaporation of its water content and will reduce the amount of polymerization across the joint. It is, therefore, advisable to paint the mould seal carefully on to the plaster, avoiding any excess.

Processing a repair

There is a probability that stresses in the old denture base were increased at fracture and that these will be released if the denture is reprocessed above 70–75°C. To reduce the amount of warpage and to remove old denture base which has possibly undergone biodegradation, as much as possible of the old denture base should be removed so that virtually a new denture is made. It can then be processed as for a new denture. If a rapid repair is necessary, then a self-cure material should be used.

A denture repaired with heat-cured acrylic polymer shows about 85 per cent of the strength of the original material. For this reason also it is frequently better to make a new denture than to repair it. This is particularly so if the fracture occurs in an area which is subject to high stresses during oral function.

Use of adhesives

Where breakage of a denture produces two well-fitting fracture surfaces, it would seem sensible to join them together by an adhesive. Cyanoacrylate adhesives have been used experimentally. The monomers of several alkyl cyanoacrylates polymerize in a very few minutes by catalysis with weak bases such as water or alcohol, when spread into a thin film. They appear to form a strong bond but the adhesive is not resistant to mouth temperature and humidity and degrades to form toxic products. Another difficulty in use is that the surfaces must be held together accurately while the material cures. It does so rather rapidly as soon as it is compressed into a thin film. No adjustment is possible. In addition, the adhesion to other materials, including human tissues, is excellent and care in handling is required.

REBASING OR RELINING

Rebasing a denture presents problems similar to those which were discussed under 'repairs'. Special reference should be made, however, to the effects of some impression materials on the polymerization of methyl methacrylate. Impression pastes containing eugenol are very difficult to remove from the surface of the denture. If a thin film of oil is left, it acts as a physical barrier, and prevents chemical union. In fact, if much oil remains, some difficulty will be experienced in obtaining a really hard polymer even after prolonged heating. A dilute detergent helps to remove the oil, but it is preferable to cut away a layer of material and thus ensure a clean surface. Removal of a layer is advocated for other reasons. It is difficult to compress a very thin layer of dough, and if a great pressure is used to close the mould, the cast may be fractured. Also a thin layer of dough rapidly loses monomer to the atmosphere, thus producing granularity. The loss of monomer also reduces the quality of the joint between old and new material.

The small mass of new material used in rebasing a full lower denture can be processed fairly quickly. When rebasing upper dentures, it is advisable to remove as much old denture base as possible, leaving only a 'horseshoe' carrying the teeth. In this case a normal denture processing should be given.

Chapter 25
Self-cure acrylic denture bases

Applicable specifications: ISO R 1567; Brit 2487; Amer 12, 13, 17; Austral 1043, T31.

Denture base materials are available which polymerize without the application of external heat. They are called 'self-cure', 'autopolymerizing' or 'cold-cure'. The term 'cold-cure' is not very appropriate as, except in small sections, these materials show a rise in temperature on curing.

In the heat-cured materials, polymerization is started by free radicals from benzoyl peroxide. This chemical dissociates rapidly at 65°C and its radicals activate monomer molecules, so that they form chains. The stimulus which brings about rapid polymerization in the heat-cured material is the external heat which is applied.

The stimulus may also be supplied chemically. A small amount of a tertiary amine such as dimethyl-p-toluidine (DMPT) may be added to the monomer. When this *activator* or *promoter* meets the benzoyl peroxide in the polymer, it starts a chain of events similar to that which occurs when heat is applied.

Tertiary amines continue to react with benzoyl peroxide to form a coloured end-product. Reaction between the hydroquinone inhibitor and benzoyl peroxide also causes discolouration. Both these types discolour therefore after a period of time. Ultraviolet light absorbers are present to reduce this effect. Other chemicals act directly upon the monomer at room temperature and cause it to polymerize, instead of acting indirectly through the benzoyl peroxide. An example of this type is p-toluene sulphinic acid. The polymers produced by this type of reaction appear to be more colour stable, though discolouration may still occur. As in the heat-cure materials, a comonomer which cross-links may be present.

Degree of polymerization

As much as 5 per cent of a self-cure material may still be monomer after polymerization. This compares with only 0·2–0·5 per cent with the heat-cured type. Large variations in residual monomer content may occur in materials polymerized by a tertiary amine/benzoyl peroxide system. An increase in residual monomer occurs if the amounts of activator and initiator are not balanced due to an error in proportioning the monomer and polymer.

Dimensional accuracy

There is no doubt that a denture base which is cured at room temperature is more dimensionally accurate than one cured by heat. If an attempt is made to refit a heat-cured upper denture on to a cast it will show a typical shrinkage away from the palatal area. The self-cured acrylic base will fit much better, though a slight error in adaptation will still be seen. Some thermal shrinkage of the self-curing polymers does take place when a large bulk is present. The rate of polymerization is fairly rapid, and the heat of reaction may raise the internal temperature to 40–60°C.

MECHANICAL PROPERTIES

The presence of a relatively high proportion of low molecular weight fractions plasticizes the material, making it more flexible and weaker. The transverse strength of self-cure materials is about four-fifths that of the heat-cure type, whilst its deflection under a given load is greater, particularly as the load increases. The self-cure materials also take longer to recover from a deformation than those which are heat-cured. They exhibit creep to a greater magnitude than the heat-cured materials.

The fatigue strength of the self-cure polymers is similar to that of the heat-cured type, whilst its hardness is slightly less.

Those self-cure materials which polymerize rapidly produce a weaker structure than those with a slower polymerization rate. Sufficient time must be available for the monomer to penetrate into the polymer grains and on polymerization, produce interpenetrating polymer networks. When this does not occur, there is only weak bonding at the surface of the polymer grains and fracture occurs at this relatively weak interface.

MANIPULATION

In constructing a denture in self-curing material, a similar technique is used to that already described. The mix of monomer and polymer doughs quite rapidly. The time available for trial closure is not very great, and usually only one denture can be packed from each mix unless the mix is refrigerated. During dough formation, polymerization of monomer takes place and this reduces the working time of the mix.

The mould is packed in a manner similar to that already described, except that spring pressure is not essential. The material undergoes only a slight thermal expansion and therefore the pressure within the mould does not rise as sharply as with the heated materials. Injection moulding can be used, and has the advantage of speed over other moulding methods.

Self-cure bases polymerize within 20–30 minutes depending upon the room temperature. Polymerization is speeded up by immersing the flask in water at mouth temperature (37°C).

In the *fluid resin technique* a polymer of slightly coarse grain size and high molecular weight is used together with a self-curing monomer. A mix in the 'sandy' state is poured into a closed mould. The mould may be of hydrocolloid (reversible or irreversible), silicone rubber or of a relatively weak gypsum. The mix is fed into the closed mould by means of sprues. The wet mix is poured or centrifuged in, and a slight excess provided in the sprues. Under air pressure of 0·2–0·35 N/mm^2 (30–50 psi), the mix will cure without contraction porosity. Greater dimensional changes occur when such a high proportion of monomer is included in the mix. Depending upon the rigidity of the mould used, various dimensional changes occur which might be as great as one millimetre in any direction. There is a high proportion of residual monomer remaining (2·5–5·5 per cent) and in addition, the material tends to creep more than the normal self-cure bases. There is little or no adhesion of these materials to acrylic teeth and mechanical attachment should be obtained by preparing the ridge lap portion of the tooth. Alternatively this area of the acrylic tooth can be treated with a solution of PMMA in a suitable solvent which will attack the tooth surface and assist bonding.

It is advisable to leave the self-cure denture for as long as is practicable in order to achieve as much polymerization as possible. As with the heat-cured materials, the thicker sections will be slightly better polymerized than the thin areas due to the greater amount of exothermic heat evolved. In the thickness used in denture construction, the heat evolved is never sufficient to cause gaseous porosity.

Polymerization continues for several days with consequent slight improvement in mechanical properties.

General assessment of self-cure acrylic denture bases

A denture base in self-cure acrylic will fit the original cast better than one which is heat-cured; but on water absorption, a self-cure base will expand and be a little oversize, whereas the heat-cured denture base is usually slightly undersize. It may well be that the retention of a heat-cured denture is enhanced by the fact that it is a tight fit on to the tissues of the mouth.

From the experience gained with heat-cured materials, it would seem inadvisable to use a weaker and more flexible material, particularly for the thinner sections of partial dentures. Self-cure materials have a satisfactory application where they can be used in moderate bulk and when they will not receive large stresses in use. They are satisfactory for use in many complete dentures and in joining teeth to the saddle areas of metal partial dentures. There is some difficulty in securing adhesion between the denture base and acrylic teeth if a full dough is used to fill the mould.

The incomplete polymerization of these materials is an undesirable factor, as it infers some dimensional instability and also increases the possibility of irritation of the patient's soft tissues. In fact, residual monomer is readily washed out of the self-curing acrylic denture bases for several days. It is therefore advisable to store such dentures in water for as long as possible before inserting them in the patient's mouth.

REPAIRS

A self-cure repair has only 55–65 per cent of the original heat-cured denture strength. The bond between old and new base appears to be satisfactory in repairs. This is probably due to the fact that the repair material is applied to the denture in a very 'wet' state, and not as a 'full dough'. Thus there is plenty of monomer available to promote bonding; whereas in heat-cure repairs, a drier 'dough' of material may cause a poor union.

After mixing the monomer and polymer, there is an initial period during which little polymerization occurs. Then the reaction accelerates and the temperature rises rapidly. A better junction is obtained when using a material with a longer initial period. This may be attributed to the better solvent action of the monomer upon the polymer granules and on the denture base.

The structure of the hardened polymer is not always perfectly sound unless pressure has been applied to it; small porosities are often seen. Porosity can be reduced by using a mix of thin consistency, so that air bubbles will rise to the surface. By applying the 'wet' mix in thin consecutive layers, porosity is minimized. A less porous structure may also be obtained with some materials by applying air pressure at 0·07–0·4 N/mm² (10–60 psi). There is some danger, however, of causing solution of air in monomer at this pressure. Water pressure at 0·35 N/mm² (50 psi) seems to be more effective. When applied with a water temperature of 37°C, the strength of a self-cure repair rises to 70–75% of the original strength.

When pressure is not applied, the material contracts away from the free surface. An excess of repair material is therefore used. Monomer is lost by evaporation, but it may be reduced by coating the surface of the repair material with a silicone oil.

Though self-curing repair materials have inferior properties, their speed of use causes them to be selected for most repairs. To avoid repeated repairs, however, their use should be restricted to areas in which little stress will be applied. As with the self-cure denture base materials, some of these materials tend to go brown in colour after a period of wear.

REBASING AND RELINING

The self-curing materials can be used in the normal technique of relining in the laboratory, after an impression has been recorded in a material such as zinc oxide paste. The same precautions should be taken as were given before.

Materials are also supplied for direct relining in the mouth. With care, small areas of a denture which are of thick section can be rebased by this method. A small 'saddle' or tooth-bearing portion of a partial denture may be readapted by applying a dough to its fitting surface, and thus taking an impression.

Two difficulties arise in the use of self-cure materials for this purpose. First, the monomer is a strong irritant to living tissues and must not remain in contact with the gum tissue for more than 20–30 seconds. To reduce the effect, the tissues may be coated with a thin film of Vaseline or liquid paraffin. Secondly, if a large area such as the palate of a denture is to be relined, the monomer will cause stress-relief within the original denture base with its attendant distortion. Crazing may also occur. Various self-cure 'gels' are available for rebasing, but their effect is the same as that of the powder/liquid type.

Frequently, the structure of the hardened polymer is not perfectly sound, and a line of demarcation between the two portions is often visible after a few weeks of wear in the mouth. This type of rebase should be looked upon as a temporary rather than a permanent measure.

Chapter 26
Flexible materials

Soft rubber-like materials are used for artificial replacements such as ears, noses, and cleft palate obturators. They are also used as a 'soft lining', particularly to a lower denture. This lining is intended to absorb some of the forces applied to the denture during chewing and so reduce the trauma to the patient's tissues. Soft materials are also employed in areas of a denture where bony undercuts prevent the insertion of a rigid denture.

Natural rubbers combined with a low percentage of sulphur were used at one time. These *velum rubbers* have a short intra-oral life. They soften, distort, and become foul after 1 or 2 month's wear.

Natural rubber latex has a very short clinical life as it is weak and it turns brown as it dries out. A synthetic latex based on a terpolymer of methyl methacrylate, butyl acrylate and methacrylamide can be made into very lifelike prostheses but again has a short life. It may be used as a 'skin' over a support of foamed silicone rubber.

VINYL COPOLYMERS

Vinyl chloride and acetate were the first synthetic materials to be used. Polyvinyl chloride is relatively brittle, whilst polyvinyl acetate is pliable. A copolymer of the two shows intermediate properties. To achieve sufficient softness, plasticizers are added. The powdered polymers are mixed with dioctyl phthalate to the consistency of thin cream. The softness of the resulting material increases with the plasticizer content. Usually 5 per cent by weight of calcium stearate and 0·5 per cent of zinc oxide is added to the mix in order to improve the flow and appearance of the resultant material. Pigments may also be added at this stage.

The mixture of polymers and plasticizer can be gelled by heating it slowly, or it may be poured into the hot, dry mould, where gelation will take place. If the material is to be joined to methyl methacrylate, a thin layer of acrylic 'dough' is then spread over the surface. Polymerization is completed by closing the mould and heating it to 140–150°C for a period of 1 hour. Dry heat should be used. Curing at lower temperatures produces a very weak material. After polymerization it may be tinted with Waxoline dyes.

Unfortunately, the plasticizer washes out after periods of wear varying between 3 and 18 months As the plasticizer is lost the material hardens, particularly at the edges, and also becomes yellow, even when ultraviolet light absorbers are incorporated.

ACRYLIC COPOLYMERS

Plasticized copolymers of methyl, ethyl and butyl methacrylates are also used. These join well to PMMA but harden in use. Some of these materials show poor abrasion resistance and others discolour after a period of wear. In general, those materials which cure at room temperature (self-cure) appear to be less satisfactory than those cured by heat. Neither type can be considered as 'permanent'. These copolymer materials change in softness between room and mouth temperature. A material which appears to be relatively hard, and can be trimmed and smoothed at cool room temperature, softens appreciably at 37°C. After prolonged use, absorption of water pushes apart the molecular chains and eventually leads to breakdown of these materials. Tartar deposition upon the surface is a frequent problem. Occasional cleaning with a dilute acid is the most satisfactory.

A similar material to which a blowing (foaming) agent has been added is used for maxillofacial prostheses. The blowing agent is added to the copolymer and a small amount of the mixture placed in the mould. On heating, the blowing agent decomposes, releasing a gas which expands and forms a sponge, filling the mould. The resultant polymerized material has a continuous surface skin free from bubbles with a porous structure beneath. It resembles skin more closely than solid materials. Unfortunately the material has poor elasticity and high water absorption.

SILICONE ELASTOMERS

These are probably the best flexible materials available today. In general, they maintain their elastic properties for long periods. Two types are available. The self-curing materials are similar to those used as impression materials, but the amount of stannous octoate catalyst added is much less. It is not advisable to leave excess catalyst in a material which is to be in close contact with tissues for a long time. A curing time of half an hour or longer is necessary to ensure adequate polymerization. Heat-cure materials are processed at 75–100°C and contain dichlorobenzoyl peroxide as an initiator. Dry heat curing for 2–4 hours is preferable. These materials should be used in thicknesses of approximately 3 mm to produce a lining which can absorb pressure without gross distortion. Silicone rubbers absorb water due to the presence of SiO_2 filler.

Invasion of both types of silicone material by fungi occurs (particularly *Candida albicans*), partly because the materials are difficult to clean. A non-toxic fungicide such as 1·5 per cent zinc undecylenate may be incorporated to overcome this. Bonding to PMMA is poor with self-cure materials, but better with heat-cure. Various bonding agents are available based on methoxy-or acetoxysilanes. It is preferable to 'box in' the lining so that all the silicone rubber is supported. A layer of new methyl methacrylate dough should be interposed between an already polymerized denture base and a silicone lining.

This weakness of the joint contributes to the difficulty of polishing and of cleaning the prosthesis. Hypochlorite cleansers cannot be used as they damage the rubber. Swelling and distortion due to water absorption occur with the less satisfactory materials. The heat-cure materials generally show better properties in service than those which cure at room temperature.

When used for facial prostheses, the materials are difficult to colour except uniformly and the material tears readily. Silicone rubbers have a relatively high specific gravity and they are generally stiffer than the patient's soft tissues. Heat-cure materials are preferably processed in low fusing alloy moulds.

HYDROPHILIC POLYMERS

Solutions of hydroxyethylmethacrylate (HEMA) can be polymerized in the presence of small amounts of cross-linking agents such as ethylene glycol dimethacrylate. Polymerization produces a three-dimensional structure. Due to the presence of large numbers of hydroxyl groups, this type of polymer is hydrophilic. It was used initially for body implants where a resilient material was required. The material is now available as a soft lining material for dentures.

Whilst it is dry, the polymer is hard and resembles PMMA. It can, however, absorb water up to 37 per cent by volume when it becomes extremely pliable. Swelling accompanies such water absorption and the linear expansion can reach 20 per cent, most of it within one week. This would cause unwanted dimensional changes in the fitting surface of a denture and additions are made to reduce this dimensional effect. The incorporation of diacetins is said to improve dimensional stability and also to improve the mechanical bond between the hydrophilic polymer and the PMMA denture base. Claims that retention is improved by the addition of this polymer are not substantiated.

When dry, the material has a Knoop hardness of 16 and a modulus of elasticity of 2×10^3 N/mm^2. When wet, the hardness falls to 1·5 and the modulus of elasticity to 1/1000 of its previous value.

POLYURETHANE

This material is formed by the reaction of di- or polyfunctional hydroxy compounds with di- or polyfunctional isocyanates. For dental use the material is supplied as three liquids. The first part is a polyol, the second is an isocyanate and the third a catalyst. Precautions must be taken to avoid contamination of the components by moisture. The mould can be dry dental stone, urethane, silicone or metal, though the latter is preferred.

Prostheses made from such a material have excellent flexibility and good edge strength. The material is not simple to use and there is difficulty in producing a good moulding each time. The material also suffers from colour instability.

Conclusions

It will be realized that the main difficulty with all these flexible materials is the maintenance of shape and cleanliness in use, together with the creation and maintenance of a good bond at the junction between hard and soft materials. None of the present-day materials is really satisfactory and all must be considered as temporary expedients to be replaced at fairly frequent intervals.

Chapter 27
Alginate mould seal

When polymers were first used for the construction of dentures, the gypsum mould was coated with a thin layer of tinfoil. This thin coating of metal kept moisture away from the material, and also prevented monomer from soaking into the mould. If the surface of a mould is not coated with a separating material, it will be found on deflasking, that a layer of plaster impregnated with polymer remains attached to the surface of the denture and is extremely difficult to remove.

Many methods are available to simplify tinfoiling, but at the best it remains a time-consuming and exacting task. It is not essential that all water be kept away from PMMA during polymerization though there are advantages in doing so. The inclusion of water while the dough is polymerizing causes a 'white bloom' which is particularly noticeable in clear copolymer materials. The white colouration or 'bleaching' also causes an apparent lightening in colour of the pigmented polymers. The water can be removed by dry heat, but will return when the denture is again placed in a moist atmosphere. When processing 'clear' materials, tinfoil must be used to produce a glass-like material.

Tinfoil substitutes or mould seals are basically solutions of a soluble alginate, such as that of sodium, potassium or ammonium, together with sodium citrate or trisodium phosphate. The action of the alginate solution with the gypsum is similar to that which takes place during the setting of the irreversible hydrocolloids. By a double decomposition reaction, insoluble calcium alginate is formed. In other types of mould seal, the solution of soluble alginate is painted on the mould and is then treated with a solution of calcium chloride in order to form an insoluble calcium alginate film. The film formed by either method seals the surface of the mould against the monomer, and enables it to be removed easily from the processed denture. Unlike tinfoil, the alginate mould seals do not seal the mould surface sufficiently to stop penetration of water vapour from the plaster into the denture.

Stresses due to mould seals

In addition, the alginate films cause stresses within the surface of the denture and this may lead subsequently to crazing. The stresses are said to be produced by the retarding action of the alginate film on the polymerization of the surface layer of the denture. Tinfoil does not produce this effect to the same degree. Despite these differences, the alginate films are in general use and are satisfactory for pigmented resins.

Film thickness

When using these materials, no attempt should be made to increase the thickness of the film by applying several coats as though it were a varnish. One coat is usually sufficient, although two coats may be applied. Any further additions do not change to calcium alginate, but simply dry out slowly. On packing the dough into the mould, this thick gel may loosen from the plaster and become incorporated within the denture, where it appears as a white lamination.

The addition of an alginate film to a gypsum surface adds approximately 0·013 mm to its dimension. The tinfoil commonly used is 0·05 mm (gauge 40). Therefore, slightly less alteration in the mould dimensions takes place when an alginate mould seal is used.

These alterations in the dimensions of the denture have little practical effect upon its fit, but may theoretically compensate to a very small extent for the thermal shrinkage on processing.

As an alternative to alginate mould seal or tinfoil, the mould may be lined with a thin layer of self-curing silicone rubber. This is painted on to the surface of the waxed-up denture and is retained mechanically by the remainder of the mould as it has no adhesion to gypsum.

Chapter 28
Acrylic teeth, acrylic crowns, temporary crown and bridge materials

ACRYLIC TEETH

Applicable specifications: Brit 3990; Amer 15; Austral 1626.

The natural tooth derives its colouring mainly from the dentine, but the colour of this structure is modified by the overlying layer of enamel. Enamel has little colour, but it gives the tooth a translucency which is greatest where the enamel is thick. For instance, the incisal edge of an anterior tooth is mainly enamel, and is more translucent than the body portion.

Both PMMA and porcelain are used to manufacture artificial teeth, which resemble closely their natural counterparts in pigmentation and translucency. A correctly made acrylic tooth has a close resemblance to a natural tooth, though a high-grade porcelain tooth may be slightly superior in this respect.

A comparison between artificial teeth made of the two materials will indicate the advantages and disadvantages of each type:

	Acrylic	*Porcelain*
Appearance	Good in thick sections	Excellent in the more expensive types.
Retention	Adhesion possible.	Mechanical retention by pins or 'diatoric' holes.
Strength	Good in thin sections.	Brittle in thin sections.
Stresses	Cause little stress in denture base.	Cause stress in denture base due to different thermal expansion.
Adjustment	Can be ground to a new shape and polished.	Can be ground, but not easily polished.
Weight	Density 1·18 g/cm^3	Density 2·35 g/cm^3

| Wear | Tend to lose shape. Wear takes place rapidly when a large force is applied to a small area. | Maintain shape and wear away very slowly. |
| Noise | No noise on contact with opposing teeth. | Some 'clicking' on contact. |

For a more complete discussion the reader is referred to prosthetic text-books.

Acrylic tooth manufacture

Two types of tooth are made—dough-moulded and powder-moulded. The dough-moulded tooth is fabricated in a manner similar to that used for denture bases except that metal moulds are used. The polymer is usually copolymerized and highly cross-linked. This type of tooth shows less internal stress than those which are powder-moulded, but may be subject to gaseous and contraction porosity, due to the rapid cycle of production which is employed.

A powder-moulded tooth is manufactured by moulding polymer in a closed metal mould and then cooling it. The moulding temperature is higher than that used to polymerize a dough and therefore greater contraction stresses are set up. A high moulding pressure is applied and this also increases the stress. There is therefore a tendency towards loss of shape when a powder-moulded tooth is reheated.

USING ACRYLIC TEETH

Certain difficulties attend the use of acrylic teeth. These are as follows:

> Lack of attachment to the denture base.
> Crazing.
> Bleaching.
> Wear.

Lack of attachment to the denture base

In the section dealing with repairs, it was noted that bonding between old and new polymer was obtained only when certain conditions were adhered to. The tooth surface must be perfectly clean. Most acrylic teeth are supplied mounted on a card to which they are attached by a soft, rather sticky wax. This wax is frequently difficult to remove with boiling water, though the addition of 1–2 per cent of detergent to the water will leave a clean surface. Attachment of acrylic teeth to self-curing denture bases packed at the dough stage and to fluid resin materials is mechanical. Bonding does not take place.

Crazing

The application of monomer to acrylic teeth either during denture construction or upon its subsequent repair may release the stress within the tooth and cause crazing. As with a denture base, partial drying out of the teeth produces favourable conditions for surface crazing to appear. Acrylic teeth are therefore made from a copolymer material. Usually a cross-linking comonomer is used which improves the resistance of the tooth to solution.

Bleaching

A lightening in the colour of acrylic teeth sometimes occurs after they have been attached to a denture. Bleaching of dough-moulded teeth is much less frequent than those which are powder-moulded. The effect is due to the incorporation of steam within a stressed polymer at the curing temperature of 100°C.

Another cause of bleaching is heating the surface of the tooth when waxing up a denture. It is usual to smooth the wax by passing a flame quickly over its surface. Care must be taken to direct the flame on to the wax and away from the teeth. Quite often this effect is seen only on the prominent thin portions, such as the incisal edges of anterior teeth and the cusps of posterior teeth.

Sodium silicate Na_2SiO_3, was at one time used as a sealing medium for the plaster mould. This chemical causes bleaching and should be avoided. A dilute solution of water-glass or sodium silicate is commonly used as a separating medium on the surface of the first half of the plaster mould. When used for this purpose, the amount of water-glass solution should be kept to a minimum.

Wear

Acrylic teeth show signs of wear after periods of time which vary according to the conditions under which they are used. When acrylic teeth occlude with other smooth acrylic opponents, and where the force applied to the teeth by the patient is not too great, little wear appears after some 2–5 years. In a patient who chews vigorously and forcefully, obvious signs of wear can be seen after periods of 1 year or less. To reduce the rate of abrasion in full dentures, acrylic posterior teeth may be used on one denture, with opposing teeth of porcelain. Provided the surface of the porcelain is glazed and is not ground, wear appears to be moderate.

There is some advantage to be gained if a slight amount of wear takes place. Small errors in the occlusion and articulation of opposing teeth are rapidly corrected by wearing away of the 'high spots'. When once the teeth meet over broad surface areas, the rate of wear decreases markedly. It is doubtful whether acrylic posterior teeth are suitable in countries where the food is of a coarse nature and must be chewed vigorously before it is swallowed. In 'highly civilized' communities so much of the food requires but little chewing and wear of acrylic teeth is not always marked.

Acrylic tooth wear is also related to the habits of the patient. Anterior teeth are rapidly worn away by some pipe-smokers. Patients who grind their teeth together during physical effort, moments of mental stress, or during sleep, also cause excessive wear. Rapid wear also occurs in the mouths of patients who constantly suck certain types of sweet which may be slightly abrasive in texture, or contain a solvent such as chloroform.

The sharp contours of acrylic teeth tend to become rounded during the finishing of a denture or any subsequent manipulation such as repair, as the teeth can easily be abraded unless care is taken during polishing.

To obtain as great a surface hardness as possible, the polymer used for the manufacture of acrylic teeth does not contain plasticizer. Surface hardness can also be improved by using high molecular weight polymers.

Copolymerization with some monomers creates difficulties in obtaining bonding between the teeth and the acrylic denture base. Others have little or no effect. When using a suitable copolymer acrylic tooth, monomer or other solvent may be applied to the tooth surface without fear of crazing, thus creating good conditions for union between tooth and denture base.

ACRYLIC POLYMERS FOR CROWNS

The physical properties of the tooth-coloured heat-curing polymers and their methods of manipulation are identical with those described for the heat-cured denture base materials, except that everything is on a smaller scale. Though any dimensional changes are therefore small in actual measurement, their effect upon the completed restoration is much greater, as crowns or inlays fit against rigid tooth structure which allows no dimensional inaccuracies.

Acrylic polymers show a lack of permanent retention when cemented with the normal phosphate cements. This is due probably to fracture of the cement lute when the polymer swells on absorption of water from the saliva. To reduce the effect of this dimensional change, small acrylic restorations should not be cemented in place until they have been soaked in water for at least 24 hours. Acrylic cements are available and these ensure that both the crown and its cement undergo similar dimensional changes. It is preferable, however, to make the fitting portion of the crown from metal. Then the difficulties due to dimensional instability of acrylic polymers arise at the metal/polymer interface and not at the surface of the tooth where they could lead to further decay. The acrylic facing on the metal can be replaced at suitable intervals of time when it becomes discoloured due to accumulation of breakdown products in the joint.

Whilst acrylic crowns enjoy a moderate degree of use, they are considered by some to be temporary structures only, with a short useful clinical life.

Highly copolymerized and cross-linked methacrylates are available which can be built up into shape without a mould. Whilst these modifications reduce, they do not overcome the dimensional instability of methyl methacrylate in thin sections. The difference in coefficient of thermal expansion between copolymerized methyl methacrylate and the tooth still creates problems of cementation.

TEMPORARY CROWN AND BRIDGE MATERIALS

It is advisable to protect the preparations of teeth during the interval of time during which the crown or bridge is made.

Self-curing PMMA is used but it has several disadvantages. Its high polymerization shrinkage produces leakage of the temporary structure. Monomer is an irritant to the gingival tissues. If the material is used in any bulk, the exothermic reaction of polymerization brings about a marked rise in temperature.

A self-curing material is available in which the polymer is polyethyl methacrylate (PEMA) and the monomer is principally butyl methacrylate. This monomer is not so irritant and the polymerization shrinkage is less. Polymerization is retarded, however, if any eugenol is liberated by a lining cement. The material offers more working time than the self-cure PMMA. It is, however, a softer polymer and abrades readily though this is not important since its lifespan is intended to be very short. In addition, the material is more flexible than PMMA and this may give rise to problems of non-retention during mastication.

A further material developed particularly for dentistry employs an unusual chemical system. It is supplied as a paste which contains 75 per cent epimine monomer and 25 per cent of a fine polyamide (nylon) filler. The liquid contains a sulphonic acid ester as a catalyst. Addition polymerization occurs in a manner similar to that already noted for polyether impression materials via the imino rings. This material has a low polymerization shrinkage and the amount of heat produced on polymerization is less than with either of the above materials. There is, however, some danger of hypersensitivity to the catalyst and whilst the polymer has similar stiffness to self-curing PMMA, its tensile strength is only about a third.

Typical properties:

	PMMA	PEMA	EPIMINE
Mod. of elast., N/mm²	2·7	1·2	2·3
UTS, N/mm²	55	28	19
Polymerization shrinkage, linear per cent	1·8	1·2	0·6

In addition, temporary crown forms are available in PMMA, polycarbonate and other polymers. These are cemented in place with a temporary cement. Alternatively crown forms can be moulded under heat and vacuum from thin sheet polymers to the shape of the tooth recorded before the cavity is prepared.

GUTTA-PERCHA

Applicable specification: Austral 1258.

Gutta-percha is a polyisoprene with the same empirical formula as rubber, but which is an isomer of that material. Included in this elastic material, are various natural resins which soften the gutta-percha. Most of the dental gutta-perchas contain some 20–30 per cent of resin, in order to lower the softening point to within a range of temperature which can be used in the mouth. The various gutta-perchas vary in properties with their district of origin, but most soften at 60–70°C.

When combined with a large percentage of filler, such as ZnO, waxes, and similar materials, gutta-percha is sold in thin sticks of white or pink colour for temporary 'stopping' or filling. This type of material is used to cover over and protect a completed tooth preparation while an inlay or crown is being made, or to displace gum-tissue from the margins of a cavity. It softens at high temperature and can cause appreciable thermal shock to the tooth pulp when it is placed in position. As it does not seal the margin of the cavity and tends to increase the sensitivity of the dentine, it should be used only as a very temporary 'stopping'. Perhaps its main advantage is that it is simple to use and can be removed in one piece.

As gutta-percha is inert biologically and also radiopaque, it is available in the form of root canal points. These are softened superficially with chloroform so that they may adapt more readily to the inside of the prepared root canal. They may also be cemented in place with a ZOE cement, preferably one containing Ba salts for radiopacity. Sterilization by exposure to propylene oxide at 50°C for 30 min is preferable to heating in a normal sterilizer or autoclave, as it does not cause deterioration in mechanical properties.

Gutta-percha is a viscoelastic material which is extremely sensitive to the rate of straining. To a rapidly applied force, it behaves elastically. The best adaptation to cavity or root canal is achieved when maximum pressure is applied over an extended period of time.

Typical properties:

Tensile strength	$0 \cdot 1$–$0 \cdot 2$ N/mm^2
Mod. of elast.	100–150 N/mm^2
Elongation %	175–475

OTHER TEMPORARY MATERIALS

One type is based on a polymer reinforced ZOE cement. The surface of the ZnO has a layer of zinc proprionate. The amount of finely divided polymer particles may be 20–40 per cent by weight. These materials harden quickly and appear to have adequate abrasion resistance for a service over a period of months.

Other materials are available as heavy bodied mixed pastes which harden on contact with air and saliva. Little is known of their formulation or their properties.

Chapter 29
Abrasives and polishing agents.
Denture cleansers

'Dental plaque' consists of a mixture of exfoliated tissue cells, salivary deposits, mucin, food debris and bacteria. This mixture collects readily on unpolished areas and produces conditions suitable for corrosion of any metals present and for tooth decay. If the surface of all materials placed in the mouth is polished, the cleansing action of the tongue assisted by a toothbrush or denture brush is usually sufficient to prevent any permanent deposit forming on them.

ABRASION

An abrasive is harder than the material which it abrades. Abrasive particles possess sharp edges, and cut shavings from a surface in a manner similar to the action of a chisel in carving a piece of wood.

A hand file is a coarse form of abrasive, as its individual teeth cut away small filings and smooth a surface. Usually, however, the term abrasive is applied only to hard and sharp-edged materials in the form of grains or powders. These grains may be bonded together to form a grinding wheel. Alternatively they may be carried across a surface by the bristles of a revolving brush or 'buff', or bonded to a piece of cloth or paper and rubbed across the surface.

By producing numerous scratches or grooves an abrasive material gradually cuts the surface of a material away. The smoothness which is achieved and the speed with which the material is cut away both depend upon several factors:

> Hardness and shape of the abrasive particles.
> Size of particles.
> Speed of movement.
> Pressure applied.

Hardness and shape of the particles

As already noted, an abrasive must be harder than the material which it abrades, and this relationship must still apply at the relatively high temperatures which are created on a surface during abrading or grinding.

The abrasive must be fairly strong, and it should show no permanent deformation under a load. In other words, its elastic limit should be equal to its maximum strength. When such a material is overloaded by the resistance of the material which is being trimmed, it will fracture cleanly to form a new sharp cutting edge. An abrasive which becomes rounded at its edge soon becomes useless. Fracture of the abrasive grains plays an important part in maintaining abrasive action, as by this means, debris which is clogging the cutting edge is removed with the fractured piece of abrasive material. Those bonded abrasives which are so strong that they do not fracture become clogged after a period of use, and the fragments of abraded material must be removed by washing in water.

A soft material is not always worn away rapidly by abrasive action. For example, a soft metal such as pure gold shows little wear under abrasive action. In such a material, the abrasive particles make a hollow on the surface, but most of the material from this hollow is pushed up on either side of it, instead of being cut away by the abrasive. Materials which are brittle are, therefore, more rapidly abraded than those which are malleable and ductile. This point illustrates the difference between indentation hardness and abrasion resistance which was discussed in Chapter 3, and shows how some materials with a low hardness may have excellent resistance to abrasion.

Size of particles

Large abrasive particles present wide cutting edges and cut large and deep grooves. A fine abrasive removes smaller shavings of materials and leaves a smoother surface. The large abrasive grains remove more material in a given time, but because they leave a deeply scratched surface, are only used where large surface irregularities have to be removed. A coarse abrasive must be followed by a finer one before the surface can be polished.

In taking a large and deep cut, the coarse abrasive is subjected to a large force resisting its progress across the material. Therefore, if such an abrasive is moved slowly over a surface, frequent fracture of the grains of abrasive would be expected.

In a grinding wheel or 'stone', the abrasive particles are bonded together either by porcelain, vulcanite, rubber or electroplated metals. A heavy pressure applied to the abrasive particles will not only cause them to fracture, but will also break them away from the bonding material. Thus the grinding wheel will wear away rapidly.

Speed of movement

The slower the speed of movement of the abrasive, the deeper are the scratches which are produced, and the greater are the forces trying to fracture the abrasive or remove it from its bonding material. When the abrasive moves quickly over a surface, it does not take quite such a large 'bite', and is therefore subjected to less force. But since more particles will be following it in rapid succession, the total amount of material removed will remain approximately the same, the difference being that a slowly rotating wheel removes material in large shavings, while a faster rotating one takes away smaller fragments. Therefore, for a given abrasive particle size, a high rotational speed does not alter the amount of material removed, but reduces the amount of wear of the abrasive. At the same speed, a coarse abrasive still removes more material than a fine one and leaves slightly deeper scratches.

The correct working speed for efficient abrasive action varies with the abrasive which is being used. The speed of an abrasive is measured as its linear speed over a surface. This is simply obtained by multiplying the speed of rotation by the circumference of the abrasive wheel. A linear speed of 1500 m (5000ft) per minute has been suggested as being the optimum speed for most abrasives. A wheel 76 mm (3 in) diameter should therefore be rotated at 6300 rpm to enable it to grind with maximum efficiency. This speed is somewhat beyond the normal rotational speed of electric motors, and most dental 'lathes' run at speeds between 1450 and 3000 rpm. Nearly all grinding is therefore performed below maximum efficiency. Nevertheless, with modern abrasives the efficiency does not appear to fall too greatly when linear speeds of only half the optimum are employed.

When we consider the small abrasives for use in the mouth, these should rotate at a much faster speed; an abrasive 'point' of 3 mm diameter should rotate at 150,000 rpm to work at maximum efficiency.

A dental bur is in effect an abrasive of very coarse grain size, as it usually possesses only five to twelve cutting blades. Its efficiency is related to linear speed of movement in the same way as the bonded abrasives, except that burs appear to reach their peak of efficiency at lower linear speeds than the normal abrasives. For the small diameter dental burs, rotational speeds of up to 500,000 rpm are used, so that efficient cutting of both enamel and dentine is obtained. These ultra-high speeds are achieved with an air turbine or a small high-speed electric motor, instead of the mechanically driven handpiece. The speed of the air turbine falls markedly on increase of load due to the low torque available. To maintain cutting efficiency, the small electric motors held in the hand have electronic systems which automatically increase the power available as the load on the cutting edge increases.

Generally speaking, it is the lower range of vibrational frequencies which is distressing to the patient. These may arise from simple mechanical noise, for example, in the cord-driven engine, or from eccentricity of the cutting tool. A high–speed, true-running cutting tool causes the least discomfort and cuts with the greatest efficiency. To dissipate the heat created during this efficient cutting action, a coolant such as water must be used at all times.

When an abrasive cuts efficiently, the external surface of the cutting tool is reproduced upon the material being abraded. Thus, a crosscut dental bur gives a rougher surface to the walls of a tooth cavity than does a fine-grained diamond-coated abrasive. A plain-cut bur of good concentricity will give the best finish to a cavity wall, if it is used at optimum speed. Chipping of the enamel occurs, however, when the bur cuts from dentine to enamel instead of vice versa.

Other methods of increasing the speed of the abrasive include the use of compressed air to blast an abrasive powder on to a surface. 'Sand-blasting' is commonly used for cleaning metal parts, and is applied dentally in the cleaning and smoothing of Co–Cr castings. It has been further developed for use in cleaning and cutting tooth structure. In the 'airbrasive' technique a suitable abrasive powder is blasted against a surface by carbon dioxide gas pressure.

An alternative way of overcoming the difficulties of high rotational speed is to move a single cutting edge backwards and forwards by vibrations of ultrasonic frequency. By this means, the linear speed of movement of the edge is quite high, as 20,000 vibrations per second can be achieved. The effect of ultrasonic vibration is assisted by implosion (as distinct from explosion) of the fluid behind the vibratory point. As the tool moves rapidly through a fluid, it creates cavities in the fluid along its path.

Pressure

The greatest control over an abrasive tool is achieved when it is applied with only a light pressure. In the mouth, a heavy force should never be used in applying a bur or stone, as fracture of the cutting instrument may occur. If the instrument slips, it may damage the soft tissues such as the lips and cheek.

When using the correct rotational speeds, cutting efficiency is good, and only light guiding pressure need be applied. The large force frequently applied to an abrasive which is working inefficiently only increases both the rate of wear of the abrasive and the frictional heat which is evolved.

Heat generated by abrasives

Any abrasive action is accompanied by a rise in temperature, as part of the energy applied to the abrasive is liberated in the form of heat.

The amount of heat produced varies with the weight of material which is removed. The heating effect depends upon the rate at which abrasion takes place and the method by which the heat is dissipated. Rapid abrasive action will cause a rapid rise in temperature both of the abrasive and of the material being trimmed. Heat can also be created frictionally when a blunt cutting edge is used. The heat may be conducted away in the shavings or can be removed by bathing the cutting material and the abraded surface in a stream of cooling water. This also assists in removing debris from the cutting edges of the abrasive.

Since a rise in temperature always accompanies abrasive action, a limit is imposed upon the rate of abrasion which can be used both in the mouth and in the dental laboratory. If tooth structure is cut too rapidly without efficient cooling, the rise in temperature will cause damage to the sensitive pulp tissue. The rise in temperature at the surface of dentine which is being abraded may be as great as 200°C, and on conduction to the pulp, the heat may cause the temperature of this structure to rise some 15–30°C, with painful consequences. Similarly, in the dental laboratory, heat will cause the relief of stresses and warpage of a thermoplastic material.

It will be appreciated that many dental abrasives are used at less than their maximum efficiency, but that the heat evolved limits the speed of working. The most efficient dental abrasives are those which are extremely hard and strong so that they do not fracture, and also are well supported by a bonding material, so that wear and loss of the abrasive does not take place even at low linear speeds.

Abbrasive materials

Diamond

Diamond dust embedded in a porcelain or other binder is one of the most efficient abrasives for dental use. This abrasive is usually used in the form of a coating on the surface of a metal substructure. Little wear of the diamond particles takes place, as they are extremely hard, and the binder retains the particles very well. In consequence, the cutting edges of the diamond particles become clogged with debris after a period of use. This debris may be removed by scrubbing the abrasive surface with water and a detergent. To maintain the efficiency of diamond instruments over a period of continuous cutting. they should be used in conjunction with a water spray. This cools the abrasive and binder, as well as the tooth, and also washes away the debris.

Tungsten carbide

This material has already been discussed in Chapter 13. Besides its use in the manufacture of burs and chisels, tungsten carbide dust is applied in a similar manner to diamond dust.

Silicon carbide—carborundum

Carborundum is manufactured by fusing sand and coke at 2000°C. It may be purchased as a powder of stated grain size, but is more commonly used in dentistry in the form of stones, 'mounted points' or grinding wheels. In these, the abrasive is embedded in a suitable bond. Carborundum does not adhere well to the bond, and for this reason, when dental stones are used at a low cutting efficiency, they wear away very rapidly, particularly if overheated. A carborundum stone should therefore always be kept wet when in use, though this reduces its speed of cutting. Boron carbide is also used as a similar abrasive.

Both materials can be used as a coating on cloth or on a paper disc.

Emery

This is a mixture of aluminium oxide (Al_2O_3) and Fe, which is found
in nature. The oxide is the abrasive component. In some cases a purer
form of oxide is found naturally and this is a more efficient abrasive
than the mixture with Fe. This form of oxide is called 'corundum', and
is an impure form of the ruby. It should not be confused with the
harder carborundum, an artificial product. A fine corundum powder is
sometimes also known as 'alumina'.

Emery is commonly used as an abrasive coating on a cloth or paper
support, though it can be made into grinding wheels in the same way
as carborundum.

Fused aluminium silicate is used also for making grinding wheels,
the resulting abrasive being light in colour.

Sand

The familiar sandpaper is used in the form of small discs for oral use.
It is also a very suitable intermediate abrasive for removing the coarse
scratches produced by filing and grinding prior to the use of pumice.
Irregularly shaped sand or quartz particles are obtained by crushing
sandstone, and are bonded to paper.

Garnet

There are several garnets. They are all double silicates of Al with either
Ca, Mg or ferrous iron. They are very mild abrasives. Garnets are used
as a coating on paper discs for oral use.

Cuttle fish bone finely ground is used in a similar manner.

Kieselguhr

Commonly known as 'diatomaceous earth', consists of the shell-like
remains of small aquatic plants called 'diatoms'. In addition to its use
as a fine abrasive on paper discs, it is employed as a filler in various
impression materials.

Tripoli

This is often described as being a diatomite. Tripoli is in fact a fine
abrasive obtained from porous rocks in North Africa.

Pumice

This is the commonest fine abrasive used in dentistry. The powder is obtained by crushing pumice-stone, a porous volcanic rock. The grains of pumice powder are not very hard, and this material can only be classed as an efficient abrasive when it is used upon fairly soft materials. Its abrasive action increases with particle size, but the grains of pumice are quickly broken up when it is used to smooth the surface of a hard material, and its abrasive action is reduced. It is an excellent abrasive for denture base polymers, and is suitable for use with gold alloys. For stainless steel, its abrasive power is too slow; a mixture of pumice and fine carborundum powder being much more efficient. Pumice will not abrade the Co-Cr alloys. Because of its moderate hardness, pumice is used by the dentist for cleaning away tartar deposits from the surface of natural teeth. It abrades the tartar, but has little effect upon the harder tooth enamel.

Pumice powder is usually mixed with water and sometimes a little glycerine, and is carried across the surface of the work by a revolving brush or 'mop'. If the brush or mop rotates sufficiently fast to produce the correct linear speed for abrasion, the centrifugal force throws most of the pumice from the brush. Therefore a much slower speed is used, and since pumice is cheap, the wear of the abrasive is unimportant. The water helps to keep the work cool, and so prevent distortion, and together with the glycerine reduces the loss of pumice dust to the atmosphere.

There appears to be little possibility of a chest complaint (silicosis) due to inhaling proper pumice dust, but pumice substitutes often known as 'pummy' can cause this disease in a person who performs a great deal of polishing. For safety, the dust from abrading and polishing should be sucked away by a simple exhaust system, the particles of powder being removed from the extracted air by a suitable filter.

Preparation for polishing

A surface which is to be polished should show only fine scratches from a fine abrasive lightly applied. During abrasion, the direction of movement of the abrasive particles over the surface should be changed constantly. Otherwise deep parallel scratches are made which are difficult to remove and the surface appears to be finely ridged even after polishing.

When only fine scratches remain, which are barely visible to the naked eye, the surface is well washed to remove all the abrasive, and is then ready for polishing.

POLISHING

Unlike an abrasive, a polishing material does not cut a groove, but causes the fine scratches to be filled in and so produce a perfectly smooth surface. During the polishing of metals, a highly stressed layer is formed on the surface which is called the *Beilby layer*.

It is probable that the rapid movement of a polishing agent across a surface heats the top layer of the material, and causes it to flow and fill in the scratches.

The theoretical optimum linear speed for polishing is higher than that suggested for efficient abrading, and is in the region of 2100–3050 m (7000–10,000 ft) per minute. The harder the material to be polished, the greater must be the linear speed used. For instance, the Co–Cr alloys require a much higher polishing speed than the gold alloys. However, polishing of the softer dental alloys and of polymers can be accomplished at slower speeds provided a light pressure is used in applying the material to the buff.

Little or no material is removed during polishing when the surface has previously been properly prepared with a fine abrasive.

The following polishing agents are used:

Whiting (precipitated chalk). Whiting finds an almost universal use for the softer metals and for polymers. It is moderately clean to use.

Rouge (Fe_2O_3). This material is rather dirty to handle. It produces an excellent shine on gold alloys, but should never be used for polishing stainless steel as it contaminates the surface with Fe, thus providing suitable conditions for corrosion.

Chromium oxide (Cr_2O_3). Green chromium oxide is also dirty to use, but produces an excellent polish on stainless steel.

Use of these materials

Whiting is mixed with water for use, in a manner similar to pumice; while rouge and chromium oxide are generally available in the form of a 'cake'. This consists of the respective polishing agents mixed with a wax. The cake is applied to the surface of a revolving buff, which becomes impregnated with the polishing agent. The material to be polished is then applied to the buff.

Tin oxide (SnO_2), or 'putty powder', is used for polishing glass or porcelain. It is not used in the mouth. Tin oxide is not a constituent of glazier's putty, which consists of a mixture of boiled linseed oil and chalk.

Toothpastes

Applicable specification: Brit 5136.

Prepared chalk is the purified natural material. Both precipitated and prepared chalk are used in dentifrices. Other frequent constituents of these products are MgO, (magnesia), zirconium silicate or oxide, PMMA granules, NaCl, and Na or Ca phosphates. To these are added soap or other detergents, and flavouring.

Dentifrices should not contain any material which is abrasive with respect to enamel, dentine or cementum. A simple test is to place a portion of dentifrice between two clean microscope slides. If a powder is being tested it is moistened with water. The slides are rubbed together vigorously by hand, then washed and dried. If scratches occur on the glass, the dentifrice is too abrasive.

Burnishing

The surface of a metal can be smoothed by rubbing it with another small, highly polished, harder metal surface. This action disturbs deeper layers of the metal than are affected by polishing, and also work hardens the metal surface.

It is commonly used to smooth and adapt the edges of gold inlays. The metal used for the burnishing instrument should not be capable of combining easily with the metal or alloy being burnished, or some metal may be conveyed either on to the filling or the instrument. Usually stainless steel or chromium-plated instruments are used either by hand, or in the form of smooth, rotating engine burnishers.

DENTURE CLEANSERS

To clean their dentures, patients may use proprietary cleansers, or household cleaning materials. Dentures should be kept free from any oily deposit as this reduces their wettability by saliva and so reduces denture retention. Denture cleansers are of four types, powders and pastes, alkaline hypochlorite, alkaline peroxide or dilute HCl. Denture powders and pastes consist essentially of finely divided chalk, zirconium compounds, or pumice, together with flavouring and, in the pastes, a suitable base. Some of the denture powders and pastes are quite abrasive and if used vigorously over a period of time, cause marked wear of acrylic polymers. It is preferable that pastes do not contain essential oils or antiseptics based on phenol. Both these soften or craze PMMA, and cause deterioration of soft lining materials. Irritation of soft tissues and an allergic reaction may follow the use of a eugenol-containing cleanser which is not removed completely on washing the denture after cleaning.

Dilute hypochlorite solutions render mucin and other proteins soluble. The loss of organic components from tartar deposits makes them friable, and the remaining inorganic matter is brushed away. Hypochlorites also remove tobacco and other stains by the bleaching effect of their available chlorine. These solutions attack base metal components of the denture. Severity of attack by denture cleansers is reduced by adding excess alkali, sodium silicate, or sodium hexametaphosphate to the hypochlorite solution. Attack is particularly severe if much stronger household 'bleach' solutions are used. These will also bleach the surface layer of acrylic dentures if they are immersed regularly in a strong solution.

Peroxide cleanser is sold as a powder containing sodium perborate or percarbonate with a detergent, flavouring, etc. From this powder, a solution is made and the denture immersed for a period of time. The solution is in effect an alkaline solution of H_2O_2. In the presence of organic matter, oxygen is liberated and assists in the mechanical removal of small amounts of debris and deposits on the denture.

Dilute HCl is also sold as a denture cleanser. This dissolves calcified deposits and is applied locally to heavily contaminated areas of the denture.

After the patient has 'soaked' his denture in a cleansing solution, it should be well rinsed before inserting it again into the mouth. Retention of a strong solution of denture cleanser between denture and mucosa will cause an irritation of the tissues.

The most satisfactory method of maintaining denture cleanliness is regular cleaning with a stiff brush. Soap, salt, dentifrices and denture powders are also suitable. Coarse abrasives such as household scouring powders cause rapid wear of denture base polymers, and patients should be advised against their use.

Dentures with soft linings should be cleaned gently with a softer brush, using $NaHCO_3$ mixed with a little water. The occasional local use of dilute HCl will help to remove hard deposits.

All dentures should be inspected annually so that they may be cleaned and polished by the dentist.

To reduce the incidence of fracture, dentures should be held over a bowl of water while they are being brushed.

Where the denture covers a large area of natural tooth substance, e.g. where onlays cover the whole occlusal surface, the fitting surface of the denture may be coated with a flouride toothpaste before inserting it into the mouth. This reduces the possibility of carious attack of the covered teeth.

Chapter 30
Dental porcelain

Fused porcelain has long been used in the construction of works of art. It can be produced in almost any shade or tint, and its translucency imparts a depth of colour unobtainable in other media. The technique of porcelain fusing is exacting, but the material can be shaped by hand before fusing, and additions or alterations can be made at various stages of the work. The finished material is almost indestructible chemically, though highly susceptible to damage by force.

It is not surprising, therefore, that dentistry turned to porcelain for the production of artificial teeth, crowns and inlays.

Composition

True porcelain consists of china-clay (kaolin), silica, and a flux, usually feldspar. The china-clay gives density of colour and strength to the porcelain, while the silica also imparts strength and gives the material a translucent appearance.

China-clay is hydrated aluminium silicate $Al_2O_3.2SiO_2.2H_2O$. It is formed by the decomposition or 'weathering' of igneous rocks.

Silica, SiO_2, exists as quartz, tridymite or cristobalite and has already been discussed in relation to the dental casting investments.

Flux. In order to bind these materials together, a lower-fusing material is added. The flux reacts with the outside of the clay and silica grains forming a vitreous mass which joins them together. Feldspar is the common flux used in commercial porcelain and pottery manufacture. It consists of mixtures of Na, K, and Al silicates.

The fusion temperature of the feldspar may be reduced by adding to it low-fusing materials such as Na, Ca, or K carbonates, or $Na_2B_4O_7$.

Porcelains used for the manufacture of tableware and ornaments consist of 50 per cent of clay with 20–25 per cent of silica, the remainder being feldspar. Dental porcelains, however, do not conform to this composition and can hardly be described as porcelain. They are really glasses. They are still obtainable in two types, high- and low-fusing, though the low-fusing porcelains are by far the more common.

High-fusing

These porcelains may contain a little clay (up to 4 per cent), some 15 per cent of silica and 80 per cent of feldspar. They fuse at 1300–1400°C (2372–2552°F).

Low-fusing

These fuse at 850–1100°C (1562–2012°F). They do not contain china-clay but consist of about 25 per cent of silica with 60 per cent feldspar; the remaining 15 per cent being low-fusing fluxes, such as borosilicate glass.

Small alumina crystals 10–25 μm across are now added in a proportion of 40–50 per cent to many low-fusing porcelains. This increases the rupture strength of the procelain at least twofold.

There is less shrinkage on firing and the material is much less susceptible to thermal shock. Unfortunately, its appearance is unsatisfactory, being too opaque, and the core of alumina porcelain is usually veneered with non-alumina material.

The powders supplied to the dentist are not just mixtures of these substances. During manufacture, the constituents with the exception of alumina, are mixed together and then fused to form a *frit*. This is broken up, often by dropping it, while still hot, into water. It is then ground to the fine powder which the dentist receives.

In the fusion process during manufacture the flux reacts with the outer layers of the grains of silica and clay (if any) and partly combines with them. This process takes a long time to complete and since the mixture does not show an obvious fusion temperature it requires careful control. When the technician fuses 'porcelain' powder, he simply remelts the fluxes already formed without causing any great degree of further reaction between flux and silica. This second fusion is fairly rapid and takes place at a well-defined temperature, thus making the task of the technician easier.

Pigments

Some of the porcelain powders supplied fuse to basic tooth shades, while others are heavily pigmented and are used for producing stains or particular areas of colour on the tooth or crown. The pigments used to colour porcelains are metallic oxides which will withstand the fusion temperature. Oxides of Ti, Cr, Ni, Co and Fe are used. The use of uranium compounds in dental porcelains to simulate fluorescence of natural teeth is inadvisable as the performance of such fluorescing agents is unsatisfactory in ultraviolet light and they are unnecessary in normal light.

Glazes

A final coating of an almost transparent glass may be fused over the completed body of the crown. Such a glaze consists of a lower-fusing glass. This glaze gives the crown an impervious, smooth surface and imparts greater translucency.

A smooth surface can be obtained, however, without the use of a glaze. By careful control over the furnace temperature, the surface of the normal porcelain will flow and glaze with only a slight rounding of the contours of the crown. Unfortunately any overheating will completely spoil the shape of the crown. This method requires a more precise technique than when a glaze is used, but the appearance of the completed crown is said to be more natural.

Binders

The porcelain powders are damped with water to produce a mass of material which can be moulded and carved, and also to bring the powder particles close together. Porcelain powders do not stick together very well when simply damped with water and, on drying, the shaped crown is rather friable. To improve the working properties before fusion, a binder such as sugar or starch is added to some powders.

Condensing or compacting

In an attempt to reduce the firing shrinkage, the powder particles are condensed together as much as possible so as to reduce the size of the air spaces between them. A damp mix of powder will condense due to the surface tension of the water present, particularly if the amount of water is gradually reduced. A powder consisting of a mixture of grain sizes will compact more easily than one with grains of one size only.

The moulded crown may be lightly vibrated, thus settling the powder grains and bringing excess water to the surface, where it is 'blotted' by an absorbent cloth. Alternatively the powder surface may be 'patted' with a spatula or brush to achieve the same effect.

A large contraction always occurs, but it can be reduced slightly by good condensation. In addition, a well-condensed powder crown is easier to carve, and on firing shows a regular contraction over its entire surface, thus maintaining the original form on a slightly reduced scale. The mass of porcelain powder must be kept damp and not allowed to dry out until carving is completed, not only to obtain condensation by the surface tension effect of the water, but also to keep the powder in a state in which it can be carved.

Porcelain furnaces

A porcelain furnace consists essentially of an electrically heated muffle controlled by a rheostat or by a variable transformer. It should also have a pyrometer which indicates the temperature in that part of the muffle where the crown or inlay is placed.

The furnace windings for the high-fusing porcelains are of Pt or Pt–Rh wire. On the other hand, ordinary Ni–Cr elements are suitable for furnaces in which the low-fusing porcelains are to be used. The windings are usually applied to the outside of the relatively thin muffle, so that they are not contaminated by any materials which are placed inside the furnace.

A pyrometer is simply a millivoltmeter which is in circuit with a thermocouple and is calibrated to read temperature directly. The thermocouple is Pt/Pt–Rh for the high-fusing porcelains, but for low-fusing procelain furnaces can be of the base alloys chromel/alumel. The cold junction of the thermocouple is often placed within the millivoltmeter and care should be taken to see that it remains 'cold' and is not affected by the heat of the muffle, or the pyrometer readings will be incorrect.

Changes on firing

If the wet powder crown is placed in a warm furnace, the rapid evolution of steam will cause the powder to crumble or even explode. A 'wet' crown or inlay can only be placed, therefore, in a cold furnace, and this takes a long time to heat up to the fusion temperature. In order to speed up the making of a crown, the moulded powder should be dried in a warm atmosphere, and can then be placed directly in a hot furnace. For high-fusing porcelains, the furnace may be preheated to approximately 1035°C (1900°F), and for low-fusing 600–700°C (1112–1292°F).

At these temperatures, any organic binder in the porcelain powder ignites, and the surface of the crown or inlay blackens. During this stage, the muffle door should be kept slightly ajar to allow the products of combustion to escape. When the blackening has passed off, the furnace is closed.

Biscuit stage

At first, the fluxes fuse at the points of contact of the grains and the porcelain is 'sintered' into a very porous mass. Little shrinkage takes place. Then the particles join together over large areas and collapse together. The mass is still porous, but a large shrinkage has occurred. Additions are made at this stage before the surface becomes glazed and non-porous. Otherwise large internal voids will appear on further firing due to expansion of entrapped air.

Whenever porcelain work is heated or cooled, the process must be carried out slowly. Rapid cooling causes cracking of the porcelain with loss of strength.

Similarly the furnace must be allowed to heat up and cool down slowly in order to prolong the life of the heating element, and of the refractory material of the muffle itself. Careful use of the furnace is most important when using high-fusing porcelains.

Shrinkage

A volume shrinkage of 30–35 per cent takes place on firing dental porcelain powders. The reduction in volume is brought about by the particles of powder settling together as they fuse. It is really due to the closing of some of the air spaces between the irregularly shaped grains of powder. Firing shrinkage is dependent upon the particle size distribution of the powder. If the powder packs (and is packed) well, then shrinkage is less.

The volume change does not cause as great a discrepancy in the accuracy of fit of a jacket crown as it does in a porcelain inlay.

In a jacket crown, the porcelain powder surrounding the platinum m. :ix appears to contract from its outer to its inner surface by about 25 per cent measured linearly. This causes little or no change of dimensions in the matrix itself. The external shape of the powder crown must be larger in all directions in order to compensate for this shrinkage. On the other hand, when a porcelain inlay shrinks on fusing, it becomes smaller than the cavity within the refractory matrix in which it is formed.

STRENGTH

Porcelain shows less strength to a transverse, shearing, or impact force than it does to compressive stresses. Its compressive strength, under a slowly applied stress may be 350–550 N/mm², whilst its transverse strength is only 30–70 N/mm² and its tensile strength lower still at 20–40 N/mm².

The structure of dental porcelain is that of a supercooled liquid. In the fluid state, each atom has *temporarily* related close neighbours as all atoms are in constant motion. On supercooling to the solid (glassy) state, the disordered arrangement remains but the components are frozen into their positions in the network. The structure is based on SiO_4 tetrahedra (see Fig. 38) in which each silicon atom is surrounded by four oxygen atoms. The oxygen atom at each corner is itself shared with an adjacent tetrahedron, so providing linkage between the groups. The tetrahedra are therefore interconnected in a three-dimensional random network. The network is modified by other metallic ions present.

The incorporation of Al_2O_3 (alumina) forms a composite. It is essential that the Al_2O_3 particles and the glass are bonded at the interface and that their coefficients of thermal expansion are matched. Then, when a stress is applied and there is a possibility of fracture, the energy required to rupture the material is much greater since the crack can propagate less readily through the stronger ionic alumina crystals.

The strength of glasses is also affected by their surface. Small superficial flaws due to thermal stresses can propagate when a further stress is applied. Fracture also starts from scratches or grinding marks which are left in the surface of the fused porcelain. Cracking due to thermal stresses is reduced by slow cooling and the surface of porcelain should always be smoothed after grinding, preferably by further fusing.

The commonest cause of fracture of a porcelain crown is trying to force it on to a die when it is too tight to fit, due to an error in the shape of the matrix. During clinical use, fractures occur when small areas are loaded particularly in tension during incising or chewing movements.

The strength of porcelain is maximal when all the powder grains are completely encircled by fused fluxes. Before this stage, porcelain is weak and porous. On over-fusing a porcelain, the fluxes fuse more of the grains of silica, the porosities increase in size, and the strength falls. Correctly fused porcelain consists, therefore, of islands of silica (and clay if present) joined by fused fluxes.

This structure is achieved when time is allowed for fusion of the flux to take place throughout the entire mass of porcelain. It is better to fuse the crown or inlay for a longer period at its correct fusion temperature than to heat it more rapidly by raising the furnace temperature.

After a low-fusing glaze has been applied, the porcelain displays an improved strength, due probably to the effects of a 'stressed skin' upon its surface, as the glaze may have a lower thermal expansion.

Slow cooling also increases the strength, by reducing the amount of internal stress which remains.

A fine-grained powder gives a more dense porcelain than one of uniform coarse grains. Firing at a reduced pressure also reduces porosity. The pressure is reduced to approximately 50 torr (2 in Hg) during the firing stages before any surface fusion or glazing has occurred. Normal atmospheric pressure is then restored while the porcelain is still soft. When glazing the surface finally, no reduction in pressure is used, or any small air bubbles remaining will expand to form large bubbles within the viscous surface skin. Vacuum-fired dental porcelains are solid in thin sections, but appear porous in the centre of thicker sections. The reduction in porosity may cause a slight improvement in strength. Perhaps the greater advantage is that porosity is not encountered on grinding the surface lightly.

In non-vacuum-fired porcelain, the colour is affected by the numerous small air spaces. These reflect and refract the light, and so make the porcelain appear lighter in colour. On reducing the size and number of air spaces by vacuum-firing, a more translucent, darker porcelain is produced. Porcelains for vacuum-firing are usually more opaque, to counter this effect.

ACCURACY OF FIT

The shape of the prepared tooth must be reproduced in a material which will withstand the fusion temperatures. Two main methods are used. The first employs a Pt or Pd foil matrix of a thickness just sufficient to retain its shape on careful handling. The foil is adapted to the die and a folded joint made where the edges of the foil meet. After fusing the crown on this matrix, the foil is removed. A dimensional inaccuracy of the thickness of the foil (25 μm) is thus always present and the lack of adaptation is greater at the joint. The reduction in section of the crown at the joint can lead to stress accumulation in this area and subsequent fracture. In addition, voids occur at the interface between the porcelain and the matrix, as the latter is not wetted by the fused porcelain. These voids provide mechanical retention when the crown is cemented in place. Thus a crown made on a matrix may not fit with the accuracy normally expected of tooth restorations which are cemented into place. On the other hand, the change in shape of a conical structure produced by a matrix, may not prevent the crown from seating well on to the prepared tooth. The resultant cement film thickness may be clinically acceptable. The second method is to use a refractory die material, usually based on a fine phosphate or silica–bonded refractory. This method is applicable only to the low fusing porcelains but it eliminates the dimensional inaccuracy and possible distortion of shape which occurs when a metal matrix is used.

Due to the dimensional error when using a matrix, the cement lute may be too thick for permanency. Suggestions have been made to improve the life of the cement lute by bonding it to the crown or inlay. In one suggestion, a thin layer of reactive glass powder is applied to the matrix first, followed by normal porcelain powders to complete the crown. This initial layer will bond to a glass ionomer cement if this is used as a lute. Alternatively the surface of the crown or inlay may be treated with a silane coupling agent and a composite cement used.

METHODS OF OVERCOMING
THE WEAKNESS OF PORCELAIN

Two practical methods are at present in use. The first employs a metal base to which a veneer of porcelain is added. The second relies upon a core of fused alumina also veneered with normal porcelain.

The alloys used for the base in metal/ceramic techniques have already been discussed.

The incorporation of rods or sheets of fused alumina offers another method of strengthening thicker sections. For example, a sheet of fused alumina 0·8 mm thick may be placed over the lingual aspect of a crown. Similarly, reinforcing bars, rods or tubes up to 1·5 mm diameter may be used to strengthen anterior bridges. To obtain a good bond between the glass phase and the incorporated alumina, the fusing time is extended. When a section of alumina is incorporated, it is preferable to anneal the fused porcelain at 500°C for one hour after glazing. Gold alloys may be cast on to the alumina–porcelains to attach them to other components.

The main difficulty with crown and bridge construction in porcelain is the small amount of tooth structure which can be removed during preparation. This limits the section of materials which replace it.

A metal base beneath a porcelain veneer reduces the aesthetic qualities of the restoration unless it is covered by an adequate thickness of porcelain. But the metal base to carry a porcelain veneer must itself be sufficiently strong and rigid to resist the stresses applied to it during oral function. A thickness of 0·5–0·8 mm of metal is preferable, though the strength can be modified by increasing the section locally.

The surface of the metal base must be curved and not angular to reduce stress concentrations in the porcelain. The porcelain should embrace the metal on three sides rather than be placed in a recess within the base casting. All these requirements make the total thickness rather great.

When making a metal/ceramic crown, therefore, a minimum space of 1·2–1·5 mm on either side of the tooth is necessary. This frequently means the construction of a crown thicker than usual, that is, outside the normal tooth contour. Besides the aesthetic problems that this brings, the health of the gum tissue may suffer in consequence. A lesser thickness of 0·7–1 mm is practicable, however, with an alumina-reinforced core, provided that the occlusal stresses are not too high.

Glasses can be strengthened by other methods. If metallic phosphates are included as nuclei, a stronger and more opaque material known as devitrified glass is produced by heat treatment for an hour at 600–800°C. Devitrified glass can be shaped in a mould and may prove suitable for artificial teeth.

Strength of porcelain can also be improved by removal of surface defects or by producing a stressed skin effect on the surface. Ion exchange methods enable one to substitute larger ions for those existing in the outer layers of the crown, thus creating a compressive stress. Other methods involve the insertion of interstitial atoms in the outer layer.

COMPARISON WITH ACRYLIC POLYMERS

With the advent of PMMA, the difficulties of fused porcelain were abandoned in favour of the simpler polymer processing techniques. These new materials were used not only for denture bases, but were also applied to the construction of artificial teeth, crowns, inlays and bridges. It was not long, however, before a comparison between acrylic polymer and porcelain revealed the disadvantages of the former for use in crowns and inlays.

PMMA is simple to mould and process, and is good aesthetically. But it is dimensionally unstable in the mouth and is not suitable for the construction of small restorations. Marginal adaptation is soon lost, due to the high coefficient of thermal expansion. Products from the decomposition of foodstuffs collect in the space between the crown and the tooth, and the crown assumes a grey shade. Even when supported on a metal base, this deterioration in appearance frequently occurs.

Porcelain, on the other hand, is an exceedingly stable and permanent restorative material. It has a low thermal expansion, and its surface is impervious to water. The main disadvantages of porcelain are that the finished product is brittle, and the porcelain cannot be moulded with the same precise dimensional accuracy as, for example, the gold casting alloys. The combination of a metal fitting surface with a porcelain veneer, however, overcomes this difficulty.

The joining of porcelain teeth to an acrylic denture is at present by mechanical retention. It is possible, however, to treat the surface of porcelain with a silane bonding agent and so achieve adhesion between the tooth and the denture base. This would prevent seepage and staining round porcelain teeth, though mechanical retention might still be necessary.

Chapter 31
Materials for implants

Applicable Specification: Brit 3531.

The loss of natural teeth is followed inevitably by the continuing loss of their supporting bone over the ensuing years. Since dentures rest and derive their support and retention from the residual ridges, the function and comfort of complete dentures becomes less with age. Yet due to progress in medical science, people are living to a greater age. Attention has therefore been turned to the development of methods of improving the function and comfort of dentures where there has been gross bone resorption.

The use of implants to reduce denture discomfort on ageing is directed in three main ways. First, to provide a better support for a denture than can be achieved by simply placing the denture on the resorbed residual ridge. Secondly, to replace lost alveolar bone and so restore the ridge contour. Thirdly, to provide a 'replacement' for an extracted tooth. The third type of implant may be used as a support for a denture or it may be retained as a functional 'tooth' in its own right.

Transplantation of teeth and of developing tooth buds has been carried out with a moderate degree of success, particularly in the jaw of the same patient. However, such a transplantation is not always available and attempts are being made at present to provide denture support or to replace individual natural teeth by implants.

Some implants are not visible when in position, being entirely covered by mucosa. These are mainly the type designed to increase the size of the alveolar process rather than to provide retention for a prosthesis. Others protrude through the oral mucosa, the buried portion lying between the periosteum and the bone (*subperiosteal*) or within the bone (*endosteal or endosseous*). A denture or tooth can then be attached to the exposed 'post'. A third type starts within the pulp chamber of the natural tooth and extends past the apex into the bone. This is called an *endodontic endosteal* implant.

METHODS OF ATTACHMENT

An implant usually becomes surrounded by fibrous connective tissue and/or oral epithelium. A review of the literature shows that there is disagreement as to which of these two tissues encases the deeper portions of implants. Some reports suggest that implants are surrounded by epithelium whilst others consider that they are surrounded by connective tissue. When the implant is subperiosteal, there is no possibility of it becoming entirely surrounded by bone. Some workers have, however, described direct bony contact with endosteal implants. Thus whether the implant is surrounded by epithelium, connective tissue or perhaps bone, it is attached and not adherent to these tissues.

Implants may be solid, with a smooth or rough surface, or may be as porous structures with definite pore sizes and configurations. Solid implants are designed with holes in them or in the form of a network of metal bars which become surrounded by tissues. Other developments are directed towards the production of porous implants or implants with a suitable surface which will become invaded by bone or by connective tissue and thus held more securely but still mechanically in place. It would be preferable if chemical bonding could be achieved between the implant and the tissues and suggestions have been made that adhesion should be possible between the collagen of bone and a 'bioglass'.

There is some evidence of cessation of plaque at a definite level where the post of an implant projects through the mucoperiosteum. Some adhesion appears to exist, therefore, between the junction of the epithelial cells and the penetrating implant surface. The surface finish of the 'neck' of the implant post is important in enabling the patient to keep the area free of plaque. A smooth, highly polished surface is essential in this region of the implant.

Alloys and metals

Alloys such as stainless steel, Co–Cr and metals such as Ti and Ta have all been used as implants. The Co–Cr alloys may be Co–Cr–Mo or Co–Cr–W–Ni. Of these, only the Co–Cr alloys with Mo can be cast, the remainder are used in the form of prefabricated structures. Titanium and Co–Cr alloys are the most common. The retention of solid metal implants is gained by suitable shaping of the implant. Screws, blade-vent or anchor-like shapes or divergent pins are all employed (Fig. 51).

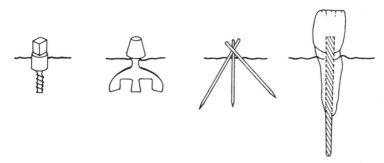

Fig. 51. Types of endosseous implant. Screw, blade-vent, divergent pin and endodontic

The materials used for making metallic implants are similar to those previously described in the chapters on stainless steel and Co–Cr alloys. The mechanical properties necessary are probably similar to those required for alloys used in denture construction. Stainless steel, however, undergoes more corrosion than Co–Cr alloys when embedded in the tissues. Pitting, galvanic corrosion, crevicular and stress corrosion are all observed in metallic implants. This corrosion may be enhanced by the piezoelectric properties of bone which causes the release of metallic ions into the surrounding tissue. A tissue reaction may then occur when the ion concentration reaches a high value. Cobalt chromium alloys containing Be are not suitable for implantation. Should ions of this metal be liberated into the tissues, they will cause an extremely toxic reaction.

All metals and alloys have relatively high elastic moduli in comparison with that of bone which ranges 7–20×10^3 N/mm². It varies rather widely dependent upon the type of bone and the animal from which it is taken. An implant with a high modulus can lead to high stress locally in the bone with consequent resorption. Bone resorbs rapidly under only a moderate compressive stress.

The properties of stainless steel and cast Co–Cr alloys are noted elsewhere.

Wrought Ti appears to have good properties for use as an implant. This metal can be annealed at 765°C and has the following typical properties:

PL	300–500 N/mm^2
UTS	400–600 N/mm^2
Mod. of elast.	120 × 10^3 N/mm^2
Elongation	20–35 per cent
VHN	150–250
Fatigue limit	45% of tensile
Coefficient of linear expansion	9·0 × 10^{-6}/°C

Titanium passivates spontaneously and the passive film is maintained over large potential ranges. The film is probably TiO_2 and causes the metal to be approximately the most inert of implant materials.

Tantalum, on the other hand, in the annealed state, has the properties:

UTS	60 N/mm^2
Mod. of elast.	180 × 10^3 N/mm^2
Elongation	40 per cent

Cobalt–chromium castings for use as implants should be radiographed to ensure that they contain no voids which would lead to mechanical failure of the implant in use. A fine-grain industrial film is used with lead foil screens to improve contrast. Views from more than one angle are necessary to disclose flaws. Eighty to 110 kV at 200 ms exposure is used at a target distance of 0·4 m.

Because of the doubtful attachment of tissues to the surface of solid metals, various porous implant materials have been suggested. Porous Co–Cr alloy can be produced by sintering alloy powder at a temperature of approximately 1200°C. By control of the powder size, the sintering temperature and the pressure, the pore structure can be varied. Alternatively a solid central core can be made from, for example, pure Ti and then an alloy containing 90 per cent Ti, 6 per cent Al and 4 per cent Va in powder form sintered on to the surface of the Ti core in an inert atmosphere. Alternatively some pin implants have been coated with either a porous ceramic coating of aluminium or titanium oxide. This is done to try and isolate the metal implant from body fluids and in the case of the porous ceramic coating, to allow for some tissue ingrowth.

Polymers

Because of the high elastic modulus of metals and alloys, polymers have also been investigated as possible implant materials. Polymers have some attractive properties, including low thermal conductivity, non-corrosion and ease of fabrication, but they have mechanical properties unsuitable for structural applications where large stresses are applied. Some polymers are partially soluble in body fluids and, in addition, their mechanical properties may deteriorate after as little as three years due to biochemical degradation. Products of such degradation may cause toxicity. Whilst the polymer itself may be biologically inert, additives and modifiers may be leached out and cause a tissue reaction. This is particularly so if they have low molecular weights. Small particles of polymer produced by abrasive wear also cause tissue irritation.

The polymer most commonly used is polymethyl methacrylate (PMMA). Initially, solid polymers were used but they appear to have only moderate attachment and are eventually exfoliated. A porous PMMA structure can be formed by several methods. In one, a blowing agent, anorganic bone and n-tributyl phosphate, are added to the normal polymer/monomer mixture. After heat processing at 150°C for 30 minutes, the outer surface is sandblasted to open up the internal pores. The surface then has a lace-like appearance with several large craters to which attachment of connective tissue can occur. Polymethyl methacrylate can also be made porous by mixing with it vitreous carbon balloons at 3–6 weight per cent. This non-toxic addition enhances the porosity of the PMMA as the large carbon balloons rupture and fracture during preparation of the implant. This provides surface pores which are not interconnecting. Their size depends upon the size of the balloons. Alternatively, NaCl can be incorporated in the mix and dissolved out subsequently in H_2O.

In order to improve the properties of plain PMMA, graphite fibres have been incorporated up to 40–60 per cent by volume and so form a composite. This composite material has a modulus of elasticity similar to that of bone, but the fracture strength is only approximately 240 N/mm^2. Porous polytetrafluorethylene (PTFE) implants have been investigated as has the use of porous polyethylene. A composite of porous PTFE and vitreous carbon has been used experimentally. The same material can be used as a coating on a metallic implant

Polyhydroxyethylmethacrylate (HEMA) can be manufactured as a porous sponge which, on implantation, becomes invaded with fibrous tissue.

Ceramics

Ceramics in general have good corrosion resistance, low thermal conductivity and an elastic modulus similar to bone. Whilst their tissue compatibility is generally considered to be good, doubts have been cast on the possible tissue effects of soluble silicates which can be released from some ceramics. In addition, some porous ceramics may concentrate viruses *in vivo*. Unfortunately ceramic materials generally have low tensile and transverse strengths, low impact resistance and are not easy to mould. They tend to vary in mechanical properties unless great care is taken during fusing.

Certain borosilicate glasses are unacceptable as implants due to corrosion. Fused quartz, aluminosilicates, some borosilicates, alkali resistant glass, soda lime glass, titania frit, arsenic trisulphide, lithium and magnesium aluminosilicate glass ceramics and calcium fluorapatite all appear to be possible materials for use in implants.

A biodegradable ceramic (tricalcium phosphate) can be used as an alloplastic implant. It is used to rebuild a resorbed alveolar ridge. It undergoes progressive degradation and replacement by the bone which has infiltrated into its porous structure. Porous α hemihydrate of $CaSO_4$ has been assessed for similar use. Whilst it causes little tissue reaction, it has poor mechanical strength and is soluble in water and in tissue fluids. Coating with n–butyl–2–cyanoacrylate reduces the rate of degradation.

The principal ceramic materials used experimentally at present for implants are $Ca_3(PO_4)_2$, $MgAl_2O_4$, Ca aluminates, $Ca_3(PO_4)_2$-bonded Al_2O_3 and glass ceramics. Implants may be solid, solid with a porous surface or porous throughout. Ceramics may be combined with metals and alloys.

Porous ceramics can be made by the incorporation of calcium carbonate into the powder mix. On firing, this decomposes and gives a porous material whose pores are similar to that of the size of the calcium carbonate particles. Alternatively a porous structure can be made by binding a watery ceramic slurry with polyvinyl alcohol. Hydrogen peroxide is then stirred in and the slurry is allowed to dry. Decomposition of hydrogen peroxide produces oxygen bubbles which form a highly porous structure. After complete drying, the material is sintered.

As a further development, research has been reported on the production of non-porous glass and glass/ceramic materials which have ionic surface activity so that bonding to the collagen in bone is possible. It is thought that the surface of the glass in contact with tissues forms an amorphous gel on its surface. Collagen fibres become attached to this gel and mineralization within the gel layer occurs, forming a bond.

Vitreous carbon

Solid or porous vitreous carbon has also been used. If certain polymers are carbonized under carefully controlled conditions, they yield glass-like carbon bodies. Being pure carbon, this material is highly resistant to oral and tissue fluids and unlike polymers, contains no stabilizers, plasticizers, etc. It has the following typical properties:

UTS	170–240 N/mm^2
Compressive strength	700 N/mm^2
Transverse strength	70–210 N/mm^2
Density	1·47 g/cm^3
Coefficient of linear thermal expansion	2·2 × 10^{-6}/°C

At present, it has a relatively low impact strength.

The shape of the vitreous carbon structure is related to the shape of the polymer from which it arose, thus making it possible to produce a variety of shapes. The manufacture of vitreous carbon structures, however, requires specialized equipment. The material can be used as a surface coating on metals.

Pore size

Generally a pore size of 100–200 μm seems to be the most suitable one for penetration by cells, either of bone or of connective tissue. If the pore sizes are less than approximately 50 μm, then penetration appears to be poor. Pore sizes of larger than 250 μm appear to be inadvisable as they cause considerable weakening of the structure. Whilst surface pores offer the opportunity for mechanical retention between tissues and the implant, continuous interconnecting pores throughout the material enable tissue cells to permeate the entire mass of the implant, thus producing a tissue/implant composite.

Synthetic hydroxyapatite has been converted into a ceramic material by sintering. The crystalline lattice structure is not changed on firing but there is partial dehydration and transformation from apatite to α Whitlockite. The resulting calcium phosphate ceramic appears similar to tooth enamel and is a possibility as an implant material. Porosity of the apatite can be achieved by the addition of cellulose before sintering.

PRESENT POSITION

Subperiosteal implants have been available since 1950 but their use is still limited. The endosteal metal implants of the blade-vent and pin type have found success in the hands of some practitioners, when used in the anterior segment of the upper jaw. The endodontic stabilizing implant shows long term success. The literature is not entirely clear on the life expectancy of subperiosteal implants. These are more satisfactory in the lower jaw. The variation in useful life of an implant is due mainly to the large number of variables, both patient and operator, which affect the length of time during which successful retention of the implant is achieved. There is at present insufficient information on the success rate of implants of porous metal or of solid metal implants coated with a porous ceramic layer.

Polymers have more suitable mechanical properties, but their biodegradation produces a problem. The main advantage of polymers, particularly those based on PMMA, is that a copy of an extracted tooth can be made fairly quickly after its removal so that the implant fits the tooth socket. Otherwise a further disturbance to the alveolar process has to be made at a later stage in the production of a new socket to take an implant of a different, usually regular, shape.

Porous ceramics perhaps offer the best possibility in the future for an implant material, but their mechanical properties are doubtful.

Many questions, therefore, remain to be answered. What specific material or combination of materials is best suited in terms of function and of compatibility? Is porosity, either surface or continuous through the implant, necessary for long-term attachment? If so, what percentage of porosity and what size of pores will allow the best attachment compatible with strength? Is precise tooth root duplication after extraction necessary and if so how can it best be achieved rapidly? Is it feasible to fabricate an implant that includes both crown and root of the tooth, realizing that the appearance of the crown is more important than the appearance of the root? Should the implant be splinted and if so, for how long? Is soft tissue attachment or bony attachment preferable? What is the relationship of epithelium to the implanted material? Is adhesion by chemical bonding preferable to attachment?

Chapter 32
Materials for dies

When making an inlay, crown or bridge by the 'indirect' method, an impression of the prepared tooth is taken and from this, a *die* is made to which the restoration is constructed. Usually the die is extended with a dowel or 'root' which can be located in a larger cast of the patient's dentition. A die must be accurate in dimensions and not particularly subject to wear and tear during subsequent technical operations. Impressions for dies are recorded in elastomers, impression compounds, or hydrocolloids. The materials used for making dies range through metals, gypsums, cements and polymers. Not all die materials are suitable for use with all impression materials.

Metals

Silver–tin or copper amalgams may be packed into rigid impression materials such as compound. The dimensional accuracy achieved depends upon the efficacy of condensation and the dimensional changes of these materials discussed in Chapter 34. Where thin sections of impression compound occur in the impression, these may well be damaged on condensing the amalgam. There is a delay of some 10–12 hours before the die is sufficiently hard to be used. Location of a dowel into the amalgam is not easy; the root extension is usually added afterwards.

When these materials are used, careful Hg hygiene should be practised, not only because of the health aspect, but also to avoid contamination of gold alloys by Hg.

Electrodeposition of metals

Electroplating is discussed in Chapter 16. The method can be applied to most impression materials with the probable exception of the hydrocolloids and the silicone elastomers, because of their dimensional instability. It is possible to plate the hydrocolloids successfully but it is difficult to obtain dimensional accuracy. Some dimensional changes occur with the silicone materials due to shrinkage of the impression material during the time that plating is proceeding. The use of silver plating is not applicable to impression compound as the plating solution reacts with the compound and softens it. Silver plating of polysulphide materials is preferable to copper plating. Polyether elastomers can also be electroplated successfully.

Plating with either metal therefore produces dies whose accuracy is dependent upon the dimensional stability of the impression material. Good detail is reproduced. The surface is resistant to abrasion. It is important that the thin film of metal deposited is supported either by a strong gypsum or a well adapted self-curing polymer. Voids at the interface between the metal and the supporting material should be avoided.

The total time taken to produce a die is 4–8 hours. In the case of silver plating, the bath is poisonous and it should also be stored in a fume cupboard.

Metal spraying

Many alloys or metals can be melted and dispersed in fine droplets within an oxyacetylene or other flame. These fine particles of molten metal or alloy can be sprayed on to many dry materials without burning. Metal spraying of molten Bi–Sn alloy under air pressure is used to form an accurate metal shell in a manner similar to electro-deposition. The method is applicable to the elastomers and with care, to impression compound. Provided spraying is done slowly, softening of the compound does not occur. Dies can be produced in one hour. It is, however, difficult to spray into deep recesses. Special equipment is needed and a face mask must be worn to prevent inhalation of the fine spray of metal. Accuracy is good.

Similar techniques have been used experimentally for building metal structures directly on a cast. The mechanical properties of such sprayed structures are, however, not suitable for intraoral use.

Gypsums

The most frequently used die material is α-hemihydrate in the form of densite stone. The material can be used with any of the impression materials. It is mixed at the correct powder/liquid ratio and vibrated or centrifuged into the impression. Accuracy and detail are of a very high order. If, however, the casting is replaced on the die or if the die is handled carelessly, abrasion of its surface occurs with resultant inaccuracy. Usually the completed dies after final set are soaked in an oil such as liquid paraffin or in glycerine. While this reduces the strength and surface hardness, it reduces the possibility of cutting the die surface whilst the wax pattern is being trimmed. The oil lubricates the surface of the die and the knife slips over this surface. In addition, the oil greatly facilitates the removal of the wax pattern from the die.

Whilst the dies are hard within 15 minutes, they should be dried at a temperature below 100°C to obtain maximum strength. It must be remembered that gypsums are slightly soluble in water and that their wet strength is only half that of their dry strength.

Surface hardness of densite stones and other gypsums is improved by impregnating the surface of the die with a polymer. This may be achieved either by treating the die with a solution of PMMA or of polystyrene, or by the application of a liquid epoxide which polymerizes after soaking into the surface.

Refractory materials

There are advantages if the die, together with its pattern, can be used directly for casting. This eliminates possible errors in the shape of the pattern on removing it from the die. A gypsum-bonded material is available for gold castings. The use of phosphate-bonded investment materials has also been suggested for high fusing alloys.

The gypsum-bonded material is mixed with a liquid containing a large percentage of colloidal silica. It may be used with any impression material but requires a special separator when used with polysulphides. Without the separator, the colloidal silica softens the elastomer and the die sticks firmly to the impression. The disadvantage of the method is the destruction of the master die during the casting process. A duplicate die may therefore be necessary and this may not have the accuracy of the first die poured to the impression, due to subsequent dimensional changes in the latter. In addition, the investment model is more readily abraded than a gypsum die treated with oil. There is a possibility of 'fins' on the casting if the die is kept for several days before it is invested.

Typical properties:

Compressive strength	45–50 N/mm²
Setting time	15 min.
Setting expansion, linear	1 per cent
Thermal expansion, linear	0·3 per cent
Hygroscopic expansion, linear	0·3 per cent

Die materials based on fine grained phosphate–bonded investment materials are available for porcelain work. Some of these can be used without a platinum or palladium matrix.

Cement dies

Silicophosphate cements may be used with all impression materials. They are vibrated or centrifuged into the impression. Dies are ready for use within an hour. Whilst the cement die is hard and relatively strong, it is a rather brittle material and readily fractured in thin sections. It is therefore preferable to make the die and the 'root' out of silicophosphate cement rather than to try and attach a separate pre-formed root. When making a post crown, there is a danger of fracture if the root canal preparation is rather wide in a tooth of small dimensions. To prevent drying out of the die and an increase in brittleness, it may be stored in light oil. Detail is good but the die is usually slightly undersize due to the setting contraction which occurs.

Polymers

Although self-cure acrylic polymers are often recommended for use as die materials, they have several disadvantages. The monomer reacts with all except silicone impression materials. The heat of reaction distorts thermoplastic materials. In the consistency which must be used to adapt these materials into an impression of a tooth preparation, there is a large percentage of monomer and the resultant volumetric contraction makes the material unsuitable as a die material.

Polyester resins filled with quartz flour or metal powder are available. Polymerization is achieved with an amine and an accelerator. The surface of polysulphide impressions must be protected with a silicone oil before forming the die. Many materials harden within an hour and produce well defined sharp margins. There is a polymerization shrinkage producing a slightly undersized die. Many of the dental materials are similar to those which are available commercially for the repair of car bodies. In this form they are very much cheaper.

Section E

Filling materials

Chapter 33
Introduction

The filling materials used today differ widely in composition and in properties. With the exception of pure gold foil, the materials which have already been dealt with are made into a suitable shape outside the mouth, generally in the dental laboratory, and are then cemented in place within the tooth cavity. There remain, therefore, those materials which are placed in the tooth cavity in a condition such that they can be moulded, and which harden or set *in situ*.

Some of these materials are used as a temporary measure, and others comprise only a portion or section of a filling which is completed with another material. For example, some dental cements are used to cover or 'line' the base of a cavity, and also to support weak tooth structure. After the cement has set, the filling may be completed with another restorative material. Cements are also used as a *lute* or cementing medium for retaining inlays or crowns in place.

Because of these variations both in use and in composition of the filling materials, it is difficult to give a list of ideal properties which are universally applicable. However, an ideal filling material should:

Be insoluble in oral fluids.
Adhere to tooth structure.
Set to a hard mass which can be highly polished and which resembles tooth structure in both colour and texture.
Be easily manipulated under mouth conditions.
Set in the presence of a small amount of water or saliva without deterioration of properties.
Not contract greatly on setting.
Have a coefficient of thermal expansion the same as that of tooth structure; and a low thermal diffusivity, so that heat is not readily conducted to the pulp.
Have no chemical action upon the dentine of the tooth, nor must

it damage or irritate the pulp. It should have a neutral pH value during setting and also when set. It should not irritate the soft tissues of the mouth.

Should prevent the multiplication of bacteria; that is, it should be bacteriostatic.

Should prevent further carious attack of the tooth substance in contact with it.

Have mechanical strength and elastic properties similar to tooth structure.

As a comparison for all filling materials, both metallic and non-metallic, the natural tooth structure shows the following properties:

	Enamel	Dentine
Hardness (KHN)	280–360	60–80
Under compressive stress		
PL, N/mm^2	100–240	140–170
UCS, N/mm^2	140–380	280–320
Mod. of elast., N/mm^2	20–70 × 10^3	9–18 × 10^3
Under tensile stress		
UTS, N/mm^2	10	35–50
On transverse loading		
PL, N/mm^2	80	60–70
Breaking stress, N/mm^2	80	270
Mod. of elast., N/mm^2	130 × 10^3	13 × 10^3
Thermal conductivity cal/sec/mm/°C	2·23 × 10^{-3}	1·36 × 10^{-3}
Thermal diffusivity cm^2/sec	4·2–4·7 × 10^{-3}	1·8–2·6 × 10^{-3}
Coefficient of thermal expansion	8–11 × 10^{-6}/°C	

CLEANING OF THE CAVITY

Various cleaning methods are applied to the cavity to try and ensure that it is clean and dry before the restoration is placed within it. In addition, the cavity should be free of bacteria which will cause pulpal irritation if they remained under the restoration. This is particularly so if the restoration does not fill the cavity perfectly. Incomplete filling of the cavity may be due to dimensional changes of the filling itself, either at the time of insertion or later, or to lack of adaptation to the cavity walls when the filling is first placed *in situ*. Since spaces often do exist between the restoration and the tooth tissue, it is important that the dentinal tubules are protected by a cavity lining either in the form of a varnish or cement. Such a lining should be applied as perfectly as possible to the clean dentine surface. The lining should also possess certain mechanical properties.

It is not practicable to dry dentine as it is a semipermeable membrane and tissue fluid oozes from the cut dentinal tubules. Both enamel and dentine contain free H_2O in addition to H_2O bonded to the hydroxyapatite crystal. Drying with air removes some of the superficial H_2O. The use of alcohol or other media in which H_2O is soluble also helps to dry the surface.

After cavity preparation, however, there is always a layer of dentine debris over all the cut surfaces. Cleaning by air, H_2O or alcohol does not remove the layer of debris to any great extent. The debris remains irregularly over the cut surface and plugs of debris remain within the orifices of the dentinal tubules. Treatment with a surface active fluoride solution has been shown to clean the surface but not to remove the plugs of debris. It is suggested that this situation prevents the ingress of bacteria into the dentinal tubules because the plugs of debris remain in their orifices. Yet cleaning of the remaining cut dentine surface provides better attachment for cements placed in the cavity since the layer of loose debris has been removed.

The use of demineralizing solutions such as H_3PO_4 on dentine is inadvisable since the acid will cause pulpal irritation via the dentinal tubules. Acid treatment of dentine is also thought to be inadvisable as it causes an enlargement of the aperture of the dentinal tubules. Then, any bacteria present or any irritants released from the cements applied can more readily penetrate into the tubules.

Chapter 34
Dental amalgams

Applicable specifications for amalgam alloy and mercury: ISO R 1559, R 1560; Brit 2938, 4227; Amer 1, 6; Austral 1581, T2.

An amalgam is an alloy of Hg with another metal or metals. Since Hg is liquid at room temperature, it will combine with many metals to form alloys without the application of heat. An amalgam usually displays a melting-point which is between that of Hg ($-39°C$) and the metals with which it is combined. Therefore, most amalgams are solid at room or mouth temperature, and set by a process which is essentially a peritectic reaction.

Dental amalgam is made by mixing small particles of a suitable silver–tin alloy with Hg. The plastic mass so produced is packed into the tooth cavity and there it solidifies to form the familiar silver-coloured filling. The term *amalgam alloy* is applied to the particles of alloy before they are mixed with Hg. They are really particles of an alloy which are suitable for amalgamation. The completed tooth restoration is called an 'amalgam filling' or more simply an 'amalgam'.

Amalgam is the most frequently used restorative material, being used for approximately three out of every four tooth restorations. Research and improvement have continued slowly over the last hundred years to maintain this pre-eminence. The main disadvantage of amalgam is that of appearance, which limits its use in the front of the mouth. Amalgam is relatively easy to manipulate but care must be taken to see that the technique used brings out the best properties. It is easy to handle amalgam in a careless manner and so produce a poor filling.

COMPOSITION OF SILVER AMALGAM ALLOYS

Dental amalgam alloys contain Ag, Sn, Cu and Zn, with the occasional addition of Hg, Au, Pt, Pd or In.

Silver and tin

The main ingredients are Ag and Sn. The equilibrium diagram of binary alloys between these two metals is a little complex and will not be dealt with in detail, as it has little practical significance for the dentist. All that need be known is that these two metals form two different solid solutions, a eutectic, and, most important of all, an intermetallic compound. The latter is Ag_3Sn and this phase is formed by a peritectic reaction when alloys containing between 25 and 27 per cent Sn are cooled slowly. This intermetallic compound has the precise composition of 73·15 per cent Ag and 26·85 per cent Sn, and alloys containing 25–27 per cent Sn consist almost entirely of this compound. It is usually referred to as the γ (gamma) phase.

High and low silver amalgam alloys

Most of the dental alloys available today are based upon Ag_3Sn with an Ag content of 72–73 per cent. A high silver amalgam sets more quickly, has a greater compressive strength and shows a greater expansion on setting. If the Ag content is reduced, i.e. if too much Sn is present, the amalgam is much slower to harden, it reaches a lower compressive strength and will probably contract on setting.

Despite these facts, some low silver amalgams are used, particularly in Europe. These consist essentially of equal proportions of Ag and Sn together with Cu, Zn, etc. Due to the free Sn, these alloys may take four or five times as long to harden as does a high silver amalgam. This may be considered an advantage by some, as it extends the working time. It leads, however, to probable damage to the filling by biting stresses applied during its long hardening period. Compressive strength at 24 hours is only just over half that of the high silver alloys, and the linear setting *contraction* may be as high as 0·6 per cent. Economically, these alloys may at first appear to be cheaper. But more alloy and less Hg is used for a mix of low silver amalgam. Since Hg is the cheaper constituent, the cost per mix or per filling shows little difference between high and low silver amalgams.

Copper

The incorporation of up to 5 per cent of Cu in the amalgam alloy increases the hardness and strength of the resultant filling. This forms

Cu_6Sn_5 in place of Ag_3Sn. Some amalgam alloys contain particles of an Ag–Cu alloy which raises the Cu percentage to a much higher level. With these additions, the alloy may not conform to the present specification requirements.

Zinc

Zinc is added for the same reason that it is included in the gold casting alloys. That is, it acts as a scavenger when melting the metals during manufacture of the amalgam alloy. In this way, the more important constituents of the alloy are protected from oxidation. Zinc can be omitted from the alloy and it will be seen later that a non-zinc alloy has some advantages. However, not only does the Zn maintain the composition of the alloy during manufacture, but it helps to 'iron out' slight variations in technique. The Zn also continues to act as a scavenger when the alloy is mixed with Hg and a 'cleaner' mix of amalgam is more easily obtained.

The main disadvantage of Zn is discussed under 'contamination'.

Mercury

Pre-amalgamated alloys contain up to 5 per cent of Hg, though 1–2 per cent is the more common. The inclusion of Hg in the alloy particles speeds the rate of amalgamation on adding further Hg and reduces the effect of moisture contamination.

Other metals

Platinum or Pd is sometimes added in small quantities. No pronounced benefit seems to be gained from their inclusion. However, alloys incorporating 10 per cent Au show better corrosion resistance and higher strength.

Gallium with a melting point of $29 \cdot 8°C$, has been used experimentally in place of Hg to produce a suitable 'filling alloy'. When mixed with face-centred cubic metals such as Au, Pd, Cu, Ni or with an intermetallic compound of Cu–Sn, the alloy hardens at mouth temperature. Gallium–copper–tin alloys have better strength, higher modulus of elasticity and similar expansion to Ag_3Sn amalgams. Gallium–palladium alloys show higher strength and a thermal expansion nearer to that of tooth structure. Gallium is expensive, however, and some of its alloys are toxic.

The addition of In either to the Hg or to the alloy gives a slight improvement in plasticity and in compressive strength, though it produces a slower setting material. Amalgamation is difficult when the In is incorporated in the alloy.

SETTING REACTIONS

The reaction between the two constituent materials is a rapid amalgamation of the outer layers of the alloy particles. When once this layer has formed, further amalgamation proceeds at a slower rate. This surface alloying is a solution of the amalgam alloy in Hg, and is accompanied by a reduction in the total volume of the metals.

While in solution, the Ag and Sn of the alloy form new intermetallic compounds with the Hg. These are not liquid at room temperature but possess higher melting-points. Therefore, they appear as solid metals.

In normal circumstances, the amalgamation or solution process does not involve the entire mass of each alloy particle, but is limited to its outer layer. Complete solution of very small particles takes place and rounding of others. The plastic mass at the stage when it is packed into the tooth cavity consists therefore of untouched 'cores' of alloy particles surrounded by a solution of alloy in Hg. In this soft mass of amalgam, crystallization of the new phases from the amalgamated solution soon commences, while at the same time solution continues inwards towards the centre of the alloy particles. These two conflicting processes of solution and crystallization continue until the formation of the new phases stifles the solution process. It is probable that on 'setting', the reactions do not cease, but merely slow down so that their effect is unnoticed; that is, they continue very slowly throughout the life of a filling.

Mechanism of setting

The determination of the mechanism of setting, and of the composition of the new crystalline phases, has been the subject of considerable investigation for many years. It is generally agreed that Hg reacts with Ag_3Sn particles to form a matrix consisting of a body-centred cubic phase Ag_2Hg_3 (or $Ag_{11}Hg_{15}$) called gamma–1 and a tin–mercury phase Sn_7Hg (or Sn_8Hg) gamma–2 which has a hexagonal space-lattice. Therefore the metallographic structure of set amalgam shows 'islands' of undissolved alloy particles, somewhat rounded in shape by solution, which are embedded in a matrix consisting of Ag_2Hg_3, and Sn_7Hg.

RELATION OF STRUCTURE AND PROPERTIES

The weakest and most easily corroded component of this composite structure is the Sn_7Hg gamma–2 phase. The gamma–1 phase, Ag_2Hg_3 and the original amalgam particles are both brittle alloys and probably have similar strength. A reduction in the amount of the gamma–2 phase or its elimination gives an amalgam both stronger and less easily corroded in the mouth.

Voids or empty spaces reduce the strength of the filling markedly. They are due to imperfect compaction or condensation of the amalgam. They may also arise from the fact that the gamma–1 phase possesses a less closely packed atomic structure than that of Ag_3Sn, that is, it is less dense. Crystallization of this phase, therefore, is accompanied by an expansion. On the other hand, the formation of the gamma–2 phase is accompanied by a contraction. These two occurring together lead to void formation even within a perfectly condensed filling. There is also evidence that a new phase AgHg, beta–1, may be found at mouth and hot food temperatures. At approximately 60°C, gamma–1 Ag_2Hg_3 decomposes. The Hg released reacts with Ag_3Sn particles to form further gamma–2 phase. That is, at this temperature the Hg may redistribute itself within the amalgam. This transition could also contribute to void formation during the life of a filling.

A reduction in the amount of gamma–2 phase is achieved by incorporating a 'dispersion strengthener' of Ag–Cu alloy, by incorporating Au, or by mixing particles of silver and copper amalgams.

An amalgam alloy may contain up to 30 per cent by weight of spherical particles of an Ag–Cu eutectic alloy. It is possible that during the setting reaction, the tin which would normally form gamma–2, diffuses into the surface of these Ag–Cu particles replacing Ag. A 'halo' of Cu_6Sn_5 appears round these spherical particles on metallographic sections. Thus the amount of gamma–2 is reduced or its presence may even be eliminated. The original intention of adding this dispersed phase was to act as a *dispersion strengthener*. It is probable, however, that the more important effect of this addition is the reduction of gamma–2, which in turn reduces corrosion and creep of the resultant filling.

The incorporation of ten per cent Au in the original alloy as a substitute for Ag, forming a ternary Ag–Au–Sn alloy also reduces or eliminates the gamma–2 phase, by replacing it with an Au–Sn phase.

Similar reductions in gamma–2 have been reported by mixing copper and silver amalgam alloy particles. The reduced flow was accompanied by an increase in tensile strength related to a reduction of the gamma–2 phase.

TECHNIQUE

The operator's aim in manipulating amalgam to produce a good filling is as follows:

> Ensure adequate wetting of the entire surface of each particle by Hg but with only a superficial attack on each particle. For good condensation or packing, arrange the particle size and shape distribution after amalgamation so that these particles can be packed together in as solid a structure as possible without the presence of voids and with as little matrix as possible between the particles. Eliminate as much Hg as possible during this activity, thus reducing the amount of solution taking place and the amount of gamma–2 phase formed.

Wetting of alloy particles

The wetting ability of Hg is poor, as indicated by its high contact angle on most surfaces. Apart from this, various factors influence the speed with which surface amalgamation of the alloy particles takes place. These are:

> Surface
> Shape and size
> Internal structure
> Proportion of alloy to mercury
> Method of trituration or mixing.

Surface

Particles with a clean surface are more readily attacked by Hg. Electrolytic polishing, treatment with an acid, or the incorporation of Hg in pre-amalgamated alloys, all increase the speed of surface attack. Dull, oxide-coated alloy particles require vigorous trituration to rub off the oxide film and thus allow amalgamation to take place.

Shape and size of particle

One method of making alloy particles is to cast an ingot of the alloy and to reduce this to small chippings or filings by turning or milling. Ag_3Sn is a brittle alloy and tends to break up into irregular-sized particles whose shape and size depend upon the method and the speed of machining the ingot.

Rounded alloy particles are manufactured by spraying a jet of molten alloy into an inert atmosphere or into a liquid.

Particle sizes range from 35μm for 'regular' alloys to 28μm for 'fine-cut'. Spherical alloys contain a range of sizes from 5-50μm.

Experimentally, thin platelets of amalgam alloy have been made by 'splat' cooling. A fine jet of molten alloy is directed against the inside of a highly polished rotating tube which moves downwards, thus forming a thin spiral ribbon. This can be broken up into thin platelets which are easily triturated and condensed. By using an alloy with the following atomic percentages Ag 60%, Sn 25%, Cu 15%, there appears to be rapid disappearance of the gamma-2 phase and its replacement by Cu_6Sn_5.

The particle size may be reduced by the method of mixing the alloy so that the original particle size and shape may not be the main factor in deciding the physical properties of the resulting mix. When using a method of mixing which does not alter the particle size, there are some advantages in selecting an alloy of fairly small rather rounded particles. This keeps the surface area constant for each mix and such an amalgam mixes quickly to a smooth mass and sets quickly. Some alloys consist of a mixture of spherical and irregular particles.

Internal structure

Particles with a homogeneous, unstressed crystal structure are attacked less rapidly and more superficially than those which are unhomogeneous or have been work hardened during manufacture. When irregular particles are to be manufactured by turning or by milling, the ingot of alloy is given a homogenizing anneal before it is cut up.

During cutting, the particles become work hardened and must be annealed (or aged) at 100–120°C. It is probable that when internal stress is present, contact with Hg leads to stress-corrosion cracking of the particles. This reveals fresh surfaces and accelerates the amalgamation process. As a result, too much solution of alloy and mercury takes place. Rounded particles are not work hardened during manufacture but they may not be homogeneous due to the different temperatures of crystallization of the various phases and they are usually homogenized after manufacture.

Proportion of alloy to mercury

When once sufficient Hg is present to wet all the surfaces, any more is unnecessary except as a lubricant to allow the alloy particles to move more freely into closer apposition during condensation. When excess Hg is present, however, solution continues for a longer period of time and therefore more matrix is produced. As soon as the particles are adequately wet, any excess Hg should be removed within a few minutes. When once solution has occurred, the situation cannot be reversed and when once Hg is combined with the alloy, it cannot be removed.

A slight excess of Hg is commonly used in order to ensure good wetting of particles and to give a smooth mix. The alloy:Hg ratio depends upon the surface area of the particles and the amount of lubrication necessary to promote movement of particles over each other. Alloy:Hg ratios vary between 5:8 (1:1·6) to 11:9 (1:0·8) parts by weight. The precise ratio varies with the particle size and it is advisable to follow the manufacturer's instructions as to proportioning. The amount of Hg required is also related to the vigour with which the alloy and Hg are mixed together.

The best method of measuring alloy and Hg is by purchasing separate portions of alloy of known weight. Ideally, these are capsulated together with the correct amount of Hg. Alternatively, preweighed alloy portions sometimes compressed to form a small pellet, are mixed with a known volume of Hg obtained from a dispenser. Another method is to use a dispenser which delivers a predetermined volume of both alloy and Hg. The dispenser must be used only with the alloy for which it was designed, as the weight of a given volume of alloy varies with its particle size. This method is not so satisfactory as alloys cannot be dispensed by volume as accurately as Hg can be. An older method is to proportion the alloy and Hg by weight using a small balance.

Storage of alloy and Hg in contact for any length of time before amalgamation is inadvisable since it usually results in a filling of poorer properties due to greater solution of particles. This effect is more marked when using compressed pellets of alloy.

In no circumstances should further Hg be added to a mixed amalgam as this reduces the strength of the filling markedly and also decreases its corrosion resistance by forming more gamma-2.

Methods employing unit mixes of which several may be used to fill a cavity are preferable since the manipulation of such unit mixes is constant. When a balance is used, the total volume of mix varies widely and it is difficult to control accurately the mixing and manipulation of the amalgam.

Method of trituration

When received from the manufacturers, the alloy particles generally have a light oxide film on their surface. If the alloy and Hg are simply mixed together by stirring, the particles may float on top of the Hg and amalgamate slowly. The Hg and alloy are rubbed together in order to remove any oxide film and speed up the process of amalgamation.

Mechanical amalgamation

For mechanical amalgamation, the alloy and Hg are placed in a small 'capsule' which may also contain a small ball-bearing or a 'lozenge-shaped' piece of steel. A clockwork or electric mechanism shakes the capsule backwards and forwards, thus forcing the steel ball through the amalgam alloy and Hg, and rubbing them together. Amalgamation is also achieved by simply shaking together alloy and Hg. A time-switch is incorporated in the machine to control the length of trituration time.

The mechanical amalgamator removes the 'personal factor' from the mixing of amalgams. Provided a constant alloy : Hg ratio, and volume and time of mix are maintained, the properties of the resulting mix will be constant. Also, mixing is very rapid and takes only a few seconds compared with one minute for hand trituration. With such a rapid mixing technique, it is possible to make one or two mixes of amalgam as required to complete a large filling. Usually the noise of the mix within the capsule changes when once a plastic mass has been produced, indicating that trituration is adequate. An alloy with a fairly small particle size is preferred for use with a mechanical amalgamator. Alloy in the form of a pellet may require longer, or more vigorous trituration to break it down to individual particles.

The slight rise in temperature due to vigorous mechanical mixing is of value in achieving easier wetting of the alloy particles.

Mortar and pestle

The mortar and pestle have been used for many years in triturating amalgam. The mixing force depends to a large extent upon the manner in which the operator holds the pestle. In a 'pen grip', the force is applied by the fingers to the side of the pestle. Such a grip will produce a force of approximately 8 N. If the pestle is gripped in the palm of the hand and the thumb pressed on the end of the pestle, this force may easily be doubled. A heavy pressure brings about quicker amalgamation, but more reduction in particle size.

During trituration, coarse particles are broken down to produce a smooth mix with suitable physical properties. A small particle size is not affected to the same extent by this method of mixing, though some decrease in size does take place. It is usual to stop mixing when the amalgam changes from a mixture of alloy and Hg to a smooth cohesive mass which tends to stick to the sides of the mortar. This change is fairly clearly defined and indicates the end of trituration.

Finger-stall mixing

Another method is to place the alloy and Hg in a rubber finger-stall and then mix them together by working the amalgam with the fingers through the rubber. This method avoids breaking up the alloy particles and ensures a more continuous apposition of alloy and Hg than occurs when using a pestle and mortar.

The alloy particles should be of only moderate size or some difficulty will be experienced in achieving a smooth mix. Usually a slightly lower alloy : Hg ratio of about 4 : 7 is used. This tends to make a weaker amalgam, as more Hg may remain in the completed filling.

Effect of mixing time

Under-trituration of an amalgam is to be avoided. The resulting mix is unsuitable for 'packing' into a cavity, and the filling will show poor strength and poor resistance to corrosion. It will also tend to be full of voids due to the difficulty of packing or condensing such a mix.

In a grossly over-triturated mix there is more solution of the particles and a greater reduction in their size. At the end of mixing, therefore, a greater initial contraction will be seen due to the greater solution of the particles, and this will be followed by a reduction in expansion since some crystallization has already taken place. The numerous crystal fragments which are present act as centres of further crystallization and the amalgam sets quickly. This reduces the time available for packing the amalgam.

CONDENSATION

An amalgam filling is built up from *small* portions of amalgam which are 'condensed' together to form a solid mass. At the same time further Hg may be removed.

Condensers may be hand or mechanical in operation. The condensing surface of the instrument should be shaped to fit the various corners of the cavity and should be about 2mm^2 in area. A smaller point penetrates the soft amalgam instead of condensing it, while a larger point may not condense adequately. Mechanical condensers condense the amalgam mainly by vibration and bring Hg to the surface of the filling. Generally, mechanical condensers are more efficient. After mechanical condensation the amalgam is applied more closely to the detail of the cavity wall than with hand condensation.

Removal of excess mercury

If the final filling contains more than 54 per cent Hg by weight, its compressive strength and corrosion resistance will be low, due to the presence of too much matrix. One should aim, therefore, for a maximum of about 50 per cent Hg in the mix when about to fill the cavity. When an excess of Hg, i.e. more than 50 per cent, has been used the mixed amalgam is squeezed either in a dental napkin or in a piece of chamois leather, or in a small press. The excess Hg appears on the surface and is removed, taking care to collect all droplets and not to spill them on the floor.

The removal of excess Hg reduces the rate of solution of the particles, and promotes conditions more favourable for crystallization. It also gives the amalgam sufficient 'body' to resist the packing force.

When filling a large cavity, it is possible to divide the mixed amalgam into several portions, and remove excess Hg from these in turn as they are required for the filling. Thus, one reason for using an excess of Hg in the mix is to prolong the working time. This method is limited by the fact that the later portions of amalgam will set if sufficient time elapses before they are required. Also, the longer the amalgam is left, less Hg can be removed from it. It is preferable, therefore, to use two or more mixes containing less Hg for completing a large filling, rather than to use one large mix containing an excess of Hg.

During condensation the surface layer of the amalgam becomes softer, due to the accumulation of Hg. This layer may be partly removed before packing further portions of amalgam into place. However, if too much Hg is removed from each portion of amalgam after condensation, the finished filling may not be a homogeneous mass, but will consist of layers of amalgam somewhat loosely joined together. In other techniques, Hg is gradually brought through successive additions of amalgam, until it appears on the surface. By this means the union between successive portions of amalgam is assured.

In either method, the cavity is overfilled so that the Hg is drawn into the additional material. This top layer is trimmed away leaving an amalgam surface with a lower Hg content. The superficial portions of an amalgam restoration nearly always contain more Hg than the deeper portions. This is due partly to the Hg expressed on condensing the first portions and also to a reduction in the vigour of condensation as the depth of amalgam increases. Since the strength and corrosion resistance of the edges of a restoration are crucial to its longevity, removal of any Hg-rich layer is essential.

As far as the properties of the resultant amalgam are concerned, no practical difference is noted between good hand condensation and mechanical condensation; but the latter method is quicker and less tiring to the operator.

Consistency

It is important to obtain a consistency appropriate for packing into the cavity. However, condensation is greatly facilitated if the particles of alloy are capable of packing together readily in a high density. Spherical particles in a suitable range of sizes will pack together more easily than irregular particles. If spherical particles are correctly graded for size, the smaller ones pack in the interstices between the larger ones. An alloy with a good size distribution of spherical particles, even at a high alloy : Hg ratio, may be sufficiently plastic to be puddled or patted gently into place rather than vigorously condensed. It then offers an opportunity for reducing the Hg content even further and so reducing the amount of gamma-2 phase. Many dentists, however, are used to condensing amalgam alloy vigorously into the cavity in order to remove excess Hg. Doubts arise in their minds about the properties of an amalgam which requires less condensation effort.

Force applied during condensation

When using a fine-cut alloy or a suitable spherical alloy, the work necessary to condense it adequately is greatly reduced. Nevertheless, the solidity and strength of a filling is always related to the amount of work put into condensing it and in addition, good condensation ensures closer adaptation of the restoration to the cavity walls.

Whilst the actual force applied varies between operators and depends upon the size of packer and the ease of access to the cavity, forces of 12–15 N are normally applied when condensing irregular-cut alloys whilst much lower forces of 5–8 N are adequate to condense a correctly designed spherical particle amalgam. A packing rate of 80–160 thrusts per minute is advisable. A slower rate of work usually achieves inadequate condensation.

CONTAMINATION

If amalgam is contaminated by moisture either during mixing or while it is being placed in the tooth cavity, a delayed but very considerable expansion may take place. The expansion is evident 3–5 days after mixing and continues for weeks or months, and may achieve the high figure of 4 per cent.

Contamination may occur at two stages of a filling technique. First, some operators place the already mixed amalgam in the palm of the hand, and then mix with the fingers of the other hand to produce a smooth mix. This is called *hand mulling* the amalgam. During this procedure any moisture and perspiration on the hands will be mixed with the amalgam. Secondly, while packing the amalgam into the cavity, care must be taken to isolate the tooth from the saliva or contamination will occur.

The delayed expansion is due to an electrolytic action within the amalgam, between the Zn and other metals and alloys anodic to it. The contaminating water acts as the electrolyte. Hydrogen is produced:- $H_2O + Zn \rightarrow ZnO + \uparrow H_2$, and this builds up internal pressure within the amalgam. To reduce this internal pressure the amalgam flows and expands externally. Blisters may also form on the surface of the filling.

An amalgam filling undergoing such expansion will press very hard against the tooth structure. Since the walls of an amalgam cavity usually diverge within the tooth to form an 'undercut' shape, a large expansion forces the filling further down into the tooth, and pressure will be applied to the floor of the cavity. The floor covers the sensitive tooth pulp, and the patient may experience severe toothache some 10 days after the insertion of a contaminated amalgam.

Delayed expansion from contamination is only seen in alloys which contain more than 0·01 per cent Zn. However, the regular use of non-zinc alloys may encourage one to become careless and allow contamination of all amalgam restorations, with consequent increase of their porosity and a reduction of strength. Pre-amalgamated alloys show a less marked expansion after moisture contamination.

No expansion occurs as the result of surface contamination of the filling after condensation, but before setting has taken place.

TRIMMING, CARVING AND
POLISHING THE FILLING

The surface layer containing excess Hg is removed from the filling and the amalgam left to harden. Within a few minutes, sufficient crystallization takes place to change the plastic amalgam into a somewhat harder material which can be carved to shape. If an attempt is made to carve the filling before it has reached this stage, the amalgam will be pulled away from the walls of the cavity. The closeness with which the amalgam is adapted against the cavity walls is of the greatest importance to the life of the restoration.

After 3–5 minutes, the amalgam may be carved with sharp instruments. Deep angular fissures should be avoided, as these predispose to fracture. Provided that the Hg-rich surface layer is removed, light burnishing after the filling has hardened assists in marginal adaptation and can reduce the Hg content of these important areas of the filling. Heavy burnishing expresses Hg on to the surface of the filling and this can lead to corrosion after a short period of time.

The surface of the amalgam should be smoothed by careful carving and the filling left for at least 24 hours before it is finally trimmed and polished. Despite every effort to produce a smooth surface, some roughening is apparent when the patient returns to have the filling polished. This surface roughness grows in time as crystallization of the new phases continues. It is less marked when an alloy of fine particle size is used.

Errors in carving can be rectified with carborundum stones or sharp 'finishing' burs. Then the surface is smoothed either by using finishing burs which have lost their sharp edges, or by applying fine pumice and glycerine on a bristle brush.

Trimming is followed by a polishing agent such as precipitated chalk applied moist with a bristle brush. Excessive heat during polishing must be avoided since this will bring Hg to the surface and cause early staining of the filling. Considerable heat may be generated by continuous polishing with rubber cup type instruments.

The filling must be polished over its entire surface in order to reduce corrosion. A highly polished surface has a continuous passive layer, and this reduces the possibility of further attack of the underlying alloy. A well-polished surface is simple to achieve in one-surface fillings, but presents difficulties in those fillings which contact adjacent teeth. If the side of such a filling is examined after a few years of wear, it will often show pitting on the surface. Unfortunately this defect is seldom seen until either the tooth containing the filling or the adjacent one is extracted. Pitting may also occur due to the liberation of H_2 from the surface of a contaminated amalgam.

CORROSION

In some mouths, due to lack of oral cleanliness, amalgam fillings blacken and tarnish. A passive layer forms, usually of sulphides, and this reduces further attack. Corrosion of amalgam is mainly by chemical attack on the gamma-2 phase and to a lesser extent on the gamma-1 phase. Decomposition products from breakdown of food debris attack the matrix and form Sn_2S_3, $SnCl_4$, and SnO_2. Breakdown of the filling is therefore more rapid when there is a continuous gamma-2 phase and where voids exist which cause differences in oxygen tension between various portions of the restoration and thus assist corrosive attack.

The structure of set amalgam is not homogeneous and some corrosion can be expected due to electrolytic action between dissimilar portions of the filling. Homogeneity can be improved by using a fine particle-sized alloy. A controlled condensation technique tends to remove inconsistencies in composition between different portions of the filling. Well-mixed and well-condensed fillings retain their polish if the patient is careful in oral hygiene.

MERCURY HYGIENE

It has been suggested that amalgam fillings may cause mercurial poisoning to the patient. This is extremely improbable as amalgams do not give off Hg vapour even at temperatures higher than those which occur in the mouth. The amount of filling material accidentally swallowed by the patient at the time of placing a filling is very small and has no toxic effect.

Mercury should be kept in unbreakable, sealed containers, away from sources of heat. The dentist and his chairside assistant must both be careful to prevent spillage of Hg either when measuring out a portion or when removing excess Hg from a mix. Working over a large tray is advised. Mercury gives off vapour to the atmosphere when not coated with saliva, etc. Spillage of Hg in the surgery can lead to fine droplets remaining in cracks or crevices of the floor and furniture, or in the pile of a carpet. This evaporates fairly rapidly if it lies near to a source of heat, such as a radiator, and can maintain a relatively high Hg vapour content in the atmosphere. The limit advised is $50\mu g/m^3$. Adequate ventilation or air conditioning helps to reduce the Hg vapour level. If Hg is spilled and cannot be cleaned up, it can be dusted with S (sulphur) or with a watery slurry of S and CaO.

At no time should the mixed amalgam be touched by hand. The technique of 'mulling' or 'palming' amalgam in the hand may produce symptoms of mercurial poisoning in a dentist or his assistant if it is used over á period of years. The free Hg in the mixed amalgam is absorbed by the skin. Since this technique also causes contamination, it should never be used.

Ultrasonic condensation can produce fine Hg droplets in the mouth which the patient then inhales. Normal mechanical condensation is therefore preferable.

Capsulated materials reduce the danger of mercury inhalation or absorption. Reusable capsules must, however, be leakproof during the vigorous agitation which is employed. The reloading of capsules designed for single use is not advised. Similarly if one uses a technique in which no excess of Hg is incorporated in the mix, the danger of losing Hg droplets when removing the excess is removed.

STRENGTH

Amalgam fillings are subjected to compressive, tensile, and torsion stresses when the patient chews. Their compressive strength is much less than that of the inlay casting golds, but is similar to that of dentine. But their tensile strength is only a fifth to a seventh of their compressive strength. An amalgam filling must be designed in relatively thick sections for adequate strength. It is highly desirable that an amalgam attains a high compressive strength as quickly as possible. A few hours after leaving the dentist's surgery, the patient will have a meal. If the amalgam has a low strength it will fracture when a biting force is applied. As a precaution, the patient should be advised not to chew on the new filling, and to take soft foods or liquids for the next meal.

Spherical and some fine-cut alloys attain a value near to their maximum strength very soon after hardening. High strength is achieved when there are no voids present in the filling, when the amount of gamma-2 phase is very low and when the mercury content is less than 54 per cent.

With good wetting and alloying of a clean particle surface, the fracture path goes through the gamma (Ag_3Sn) grains, the brittle component in the composite system. As already noted, strength is lowered markedly by the presence of voids.

Use of pins

Pins are sometimes incorporated into amalgam fillings in order to retain them and to 'strengthen' the filling. Unless bonding occurs between the surface of the pin and the amalgam restoration, it produces only a discontinuity in the structure and reduces the strength of the filling. Stainless steel is thus not advisable. Silver pins will bond but have poor mechanical properties themselves. Gold or silver plated base metal pins of suitable strength will bond if the conditions are suitable. Their surfaces must be clean and sufficient Hg must be available to wet the surface and so produce a bond. An amalgam mix of good plasticity is necessary to enable good condensation to take place in the restricted area round the pins. A spherical-particle alloy is preferred.

Flow and creep

Amalgam will flow under a load which is less than the value for its compressive strength. Flow of amalgams is due to the fact that they are not completely stable, and also have fairly low melting-points. During deformation very little strain hardening occurs and further alterations in shape are not resisted.

Flow is often measured by applying a static load to a small cylindrical specimen for 21 hours, starting 3 hours after amalgamation. This method of testing flow shows up the disadvantages of a slow-setting amalgam. With such a material, a great amount of flow takes place during the first 5 hours after mixing, as the amalgam has not completely set.

Creep of set amalgam is important in relation to the maintenance of shape of the restoration after setting. If an amalgam filling shows dynamic creep under chewing stresses, then the border of the restoration may flow over the enamel surface. This produces an apparent expansion of the filling out of the cavity. These thin margins will then fracture on further stress producing a 'ditched' amalgam. Creep is less in alloys modified to reduce the amount of gamma-2 formed, than in unmodified alloys.

A similar ditched appearance is produced by incorrect preparation of the cavity margins or by overfilling the cavity in the first place, both of which lead to fracture of the resulting thin enamel margins under masticatory stress.

Expansion of the filling as the result of contamination causes the filling to protrude above the level of the cavity margins. In addition, corrosion of the margins of the restoration can also lead to a ditched effect. It is suggested that corrosion of the gamma-2 phase liberates Hg which then reacts further with the gamma phase, producing expansion of the margins of the restoration. This effect is called *mercuro-*

scopic expansion. It occurs more readily when the margins of the restoration have been inadequately condensed and contain a large proportion of gamma-2 phase.

Breakdown of the margins of an amalgam restoration may therefore be due to incorrect preparation of enamel margins, overfilling, dynamic creep, contamination expansion, or mercuroscopic expansion.

EXPANSION AND CONTRACTION

At one time it was considered that an amalgam alloy must expand in order to seal the filling against the dentine of the tooth which is slightly elastic. It is now appreciated that a perfect seal is not obtained by this method and that a small linear expansion or contraction up to 0·2 per cent has little clinical significance.

Dimensional changes are governed by the amount of solution and crystallization which occurs after the filling has been placed. Generally, the finer cut and fine spherical alloys show a slight contraction whilst coarser alloys usually produce a slight expansion. Too much Hg in the filling leads to contraction and therefore for this and other reasons, should be avoided.

Figure 52 shows the typical contraction and expansion curve of an amalgam after mixing.

The first contraction is due to the solution of the alloy. This is

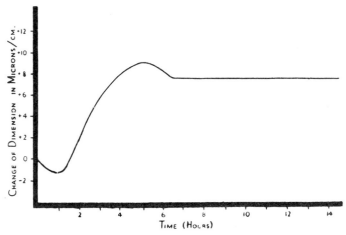

Fig. 52. Expansion curve of a silver–tin amalgam

followed by expansion from crystallization of the gamma-1 phase with finally, a small contraction due probably to the formation of a solid solution of Hg in Ag_3Sn.

All amalgam restorations show evidence of marginal leakage immediately after placement, but this leakage diminishes after some weeks. Metallic sulphides fill any small spaces between the filling and the tooth and so improve the seal. Marginal seal is also better when the cavity is lined with a cavity varnish, particularly one based on copal resin. The varnish should be applied over the entire surface including the margins.

Summary

Measure the amount of alloy and Hg.
Do not mix too much amalgam at once—use small unit mixes.
Do not undertriturate.
Remove any excess Hg by squeezing the mix.
Condense in small portions; do not use the mix after 4–5 minutes from trituration.
Overfill the cavity and remove the Hg-rich top layer.

Amalgams are relatively simple materials to use, and rightly have a very wide application in conservative dentistry. There is a large volume of literature available for study in order to complete the picture of which only the main outline has been drawn in this chapter. There are many variables in manipulation which are under the control of the dentist or his assistant and which affect the properties of the completed filling. The most satisfactory way of controlling these variables is to carry out a precise technique so that consistent results are obtained.

The filling must be well adapted against tooth substance so that little space exists between these two structures. In the case of a cavity which is surrounded by tooth substance adaptation during condensation is easy. But where a filling involves both the top and side of a tooth, some support must be made to prevent the amalgam falling sideways out of the cavity. A *matrix band* of stainless steel or sheet polymer is fitted, in order to make an open-topped cavity into which the amalgam can be adapted closely to the tooth substance.

Amalgam fillings sometimes fracture across their thinner portions when subjected to heavy biting pressure. Cavity outlines should be rounded and should not present sudden changes in cross-section of amalgam. Otherwise, stress concentration at narrow sections will predispose to fracture. This is particularly so when the restoration is resisting a heavy occlusal load from an opposing tooth or cusp.

Extensions to existing amalgam fillings after recurrent caries should have sufficient strength and retention themselves. Bonding or alloying between old and new amalgam is relatively weak unless the repair surface is effectively wetted with Hg before the new amalgam is placed in position. The initial bond strength is low but increases slowly with time. Reliance should not be placed upon this bond strength to retain the extension of the filling.

Due to the excellent thermal conductivity of amalgam, the restoration must have an adequate insulating layer between it and the pulp. This may be a layer of dentine if the cavity is shallow, or one of the cements in a deeper cavity.

Typical properties of high silver amalgams:

Composition	Ag	67–74 per cent
	Sn	25–27 per cent
	Cu	0–5 per cent
	Zn	0–1·5 per cent
	Hg	0–3 per cent
UCS	1 hour	50–150 N/mm²
	(the higher figure relates to spherical alloys)	
	6–8 hours	300–420 N/mm²
UTS	1 hour	15–20 N/mm²
	6–8 hours	50–65 N/mm²
Elongation		0·3–0·5 per cent
Mod. of elast.		300–370 × 10² N/mm²
Transverse strength is similar to tensile		
Linear dimensional change	24 hours	0 ± 0·2 per cent

COPPER AMALGAMS

Copper and Hg amalgamate to form an alloy consisting of a crystalline phase CuHg embedded in a solid solution of Cu and Hg. Unlike silver–tin amalgam, the copper amalgam is purchased ready mixed and usually contains 70 per cent Hg with 30 per cent Cu. A trace of Zn is sometimes present.

The pellets of amalgam are softened by heating them in an iron spoon until droplets of Hg form on their surface. They are then triturated to a smooth mass in a mortar and pestle, and remain plastic for quite a long time, setting slowly in 8–12 hours. On warming copper amalgam, Hg vapour is given off to the atmosphere and can raise the concentration locally well above the accepted limit. Due to the slow set, there is also some danger of absorption of Hg by the patient.

The hardness of the set amalgam is slightly greater than that of the silver–tin amalgam and it shows no flow. Unfortunately, the copper amalgams all contract on setting, no matter what technique is used. They are easily attacked by sulphides in the mouth, and their discoloration affects the tooth substance.

Copper is said to have a germicidal effect, and therefore its amalgam found a fairly wide use in filling deciduous teeth where all the decay could not be removed. More recently, however, the silver–tin amalgams have replaced those of copper, and are used in the conservation of children's teeth except where the filling is to be of only a very temporary nature. In mouths where the carious process is very active, however, there is less recurrence of decay round copper amalgam restorations than round those of silver amalgam.

Chapter 35
Non-metallic filling materials
Lining and luting cements

These materials are used mainly as temporary or semi-permanent fillings, and as a lute or cementing medium for inlays, crowns and bridges. They are used for lining the base of a cavity, to insulate the tooth pulp against undue thermal or chemical irritation which may be conveyed from other, and more durable filling materials which are placed on top of them. They are also used upon occasion to support weak tooth structure which must be left in place.

The various types of non-metallic lining, cementing and filling materials and their applications are shown in Table 6.

The silicate, silico-phosphate and glass ionomer cements are dealt with in Chapter 36 and the composite filling materials, fissure sealants and cavity primers in Chapter 37.

Many dental cements and filling materials contain chemicals which are very irritant to living tissues. The tooth pulp is a delicate organ and is readily damaged by any irritant which reaches it after permeating the dentinal tubules. In addition, the pulp can be damaged by excessive heat or cold. Where the dentine layer between filling and pulp is greater than approximately 0·40 mm, there is a greatly reduced possibility of damage to the pulp either by heat or by the placing of an irritant filling material in the cavity. However, there are occasions when the dentine barrier which remains is as thin as 0·01 mm; then protection of the pulp is essential. On occasions, the pulp may be entered during cavity preparation and then no irritant material can be placed in contact with it.

The packing of the filling on top of a lining frequently involves the application of moderate stresses to the lining. For example, when condensing a conventional amalgam alloy, stresses as high as 20 N/mm² may be applied, though the average stress is only about half of this value. Values for compressive strength have been recommended for

Table 6. Uses of non-metallic filling materials

Enamel (protection against caries)	Dentine (protection against penetration; possible bonding)	Lining (thermal and chemical insulation)	Lining (support and thermal insulation)	Anterior fillings	Posterior fillings	Luting
Fissure sealant (tooth varnish)	Cavity varnish	$Ca(OH)_2$	Zn phosphate	Silicate	Silico-phosphate	Zn polycarboxylate
Glass ionomer	Cavity primer	ZOE	Zn polycarboxylate	Composite	Composite?	Zn phosphate
Zn polycarboxylate			ZOE (fortified)	Glass ionomer		ZOE
			Glass ionomer	Acrylic		Silicophosphate
				Silicophosphate		Glass ionomer
						Composite cement
						Acrylic cement
						Cu phosphate?

lining materials which vary between 1-10 N/mm². It is of considerable importance that the lining achieves a high strength within a few minutes as the remainder of the filling may well be packed into place within 5 to 10 minutes of placing the lining. Whilst compressive strength of the lining is important, the modulus of elasticity of the material used for a lining should approximate to that of the restoration. Otherwise distortion of the restoration when subject to occlusal loading can occur, leading to marginal leakage.

For luting, the cement should flow readily to a layer as thin as 0·02 mm, though acceptable upper limits have been suggested as thick as 0·10 mm.

Cements must wet both tooth substance and the surface of the components being cemented into place, thus reducing the number of voids in the cementing medium. When placing a protective lining in position, a material of thick consistency is usually more workable. Indeed, a material with thixotropic properties would be ideal.

CAVITY VARNISHES

These are usually solutions of natural resins or synthetic polymers in acetone, chloroform, ether, or similar solvents. By evaporation of the solvent, a thin layer of varnish remains. Self-curing monomers may also be used to form a film. The purpose of such a film is to reduce, or preferably to prevent, the passage of any acid from cements into the dentine. To be effective, the layer of varnish must be continuous and impermeable. Most varnishes are semipermeable to acid, however, and only reduce the amount of acid which gets into the dentine. Those varnishes based on polystyrene appear to be more effective than those containing mainly cellulose or shellac. The permeability of cavity varnishes is related to their contact angle with water. The least permeable has a high contact angle.

A varnish film must be thin, otherwise it will aid marginal leakage of the restoration. If the varnish becomes viscous due to loss of solvent, a thick, irregular film will be formed. Such a varnish should be discarded or diluted. When used under a silicate restoration, the varnish must not cover the cavity margins, otherwise the anticariogenic effect of the fluorine in the cement is lost. A *thin* layer of copal varnish on the margins of a cavity filled with amalgam, however, improves early marginal seal.

In the thin layers in which they are employed, these varnishes are not effective thermal insulators.

The addition of $Ca(OH)_2$ or ZnO to varnishes makes a thicker film and improves their resistance to acid penetration. Colouring the varnish also assists in ensuring that it is correctly applied.

Whenever one of the 'acid' cements is placed against dentine in a cavity, it is preferable that a varnish layer be present. If a base of ZOE or $Ca(OH)_2$ cement is to be used, then this should be placed first, followed by a varnish. When Zn phosphate is used as the base, the varnish should be applied first.

CAVITY PRIMERS

Whilst cavity varnishes simply cover the surface of the dentine, a suitable monomer or comonomer could be applied to the dentine which bonded not only to the tooth but also to the restoration which was subsequently applied. These materials are designed to bond to composite fillings and are discussed in Chapter 37.

CALCIUM HYDROXIDE CEMENTS

These are suspensions of $Ca(OH)_2$ either in distilled water or in a solution of a polymer. They usually contain about 50 per cent $Ca(OH)_2$ by weight. The aqueous suspension is rather friable after drying with warm air. A solution of methyl cellulose in water or of a synthetic polymer in chloroform may be used instead of water. These give the cement more cohesion and improve its strength. However, the compressive strength of these materials may not be adequate to withstand the stress applied when condensing a material such as amalgam. Because of the low strength, the layer of $Ca(OH)_2$ cement may be protected by a thin layer of another cement. Any free acid from the second layer is neutralized by the hydroxide before it can reach the dentine and the pulp. The layer of $Ca(OH)_2$ cement should be at least 0·5 mm thick.

Calcium hydroxide cements are the least irritant materials and are placed as an initial layer in deep cavities where the dentine layer remaining over the pulp is less than 0·05 mm. These cements do not seal the cavity, however, since they shrink on hardening. Their pH varies between 11·5 and 13·0. Some materials set rather too slowly for an amalgam restoration to be condensed over them within a few minutes. In general, even when set, compressive strengths are only 7–9 N/mm². The force applied on packing an amalgam, particularly in the early stages, may be double this figure. On the other hand, a lining well supported by tooth substance will tolerate a force higher than its compressive strength value without displacement. Where such a lining is unsupported, however, it may fracture.

Two-component materials are available which show a higher compressive strength on setting with similar lack of any pulpal irritation. Indeed they are considered to stimulate the laying down of secondary dentine.

When accidental exposure of the pulp occurs during cavity preparation, the exposure may be 'capped' with this type of cement. Rapid deposition of secondary dentine occurs under the cement film. With the exception of ZOE, all other cements irritate the pulp tissue, and delay or inhibit secondary dentine formation. For 'pulp capping' the $Ca(OH)_2$ cement may be supported against pressure by placing it in a small cellophane cup. This is placed face downwards over the exposure.

Typical properties:

Compressive strength 24 hrs   7–9 N/mm²
Tensile strength   24 hrs   1–2 N/mm²
Solubility, H_2O, 1 week   25–30 per cent

A suspension of tricalcium phosphate ceramic has also been suggested as a suitable pulp capping material.

ZINC OXIDE-EUGENOL CEMENTS

Applicable specification: ISO 3107.

A mixture of eugenol, the main constituent of oil of cloves, with powdered ZnO will set slowly in the presence of moisture. The precise setting reaction varies with the method of manufacture of the oxide, its particle size and storage conditions. Speed of setting also varies with pH and the presence of moisture.

Setting occurs by an ionic acid–base reaction in which hydrogen ions in the eugenol are replaced by zinc ions to form zinc eugenolate. Attachment of the zinc ion to the eugenol is by chelation.

The hardened cement consists, therefore, of particles of ZnO in a matrix containing long crystals of zinc eugenolate. Both the oxide and eugenolate absorb additional eugenol.

It is probable that the setting process is initiated by a trace of H_2O:

$$ZnO + H_2O \longrightarrow Zn(OH)_2$$

$$Zn(OH)_2 + 2OHC_{10}H_{11}O_2 \longrightarrow Zn(OC_{10}H_{11}O_2)_2 + 2H_2O$$

(eugenol)   (zinc eugenolate)

Since the formation of zinc eugenolate liberates further H_2O, the reaction, when once started, continues. Hence these materials set more rapidly in a humid atmosphere.

A plain mix of ZnO and eugenol hardens in the mouth in about 12 hours, and there is a gradual leaching out of the eugenol from the surface layer of the filling into the saliva. For many purposes, a setting time of 12 hours is far too long, as it means that the dentist cannot complete a filling at one visit. He must see the patient again at a later appointment, when the cement has hardened sufficiently for an amalgam or other filling to be packed into place on top of it.

Setting time is reduced by the addition of 0·2–0·5 per cent of zinc acetate or other zinc salts. Rosin also accelerates the set and makes the hardened cement more cohesive and less liable to crumble when a further restorative material is packed on top of it. Working properties and strength of the cement are improved by the incorporation of fillers such as powdered quartz, alumina or spherical particles of polymers such as PMMA or polystyrene. The latter additions reduce the apparent viscosity of the mixed cement and may also strengthen the matrix by forming a composite. The incorporation of up to 10 per cent of polystyrene or methyl methacrylate polymer to the liquid also improves the mechanical properties of these cements. Other oils are added to the eugenol or oil of cloves to dilute its taste and to improve the viscosity of the mix.

Whilst these *modified* cements are suitable as a lining within a cavity, research has continued to improve the compressive strength of ZOE cements so that it is similar to that of phosphate cements. Other chelating agents have been substituted for eugenol, particularly o-ethoxybenzoic acid (EBA). These *fortified* types of cement consist of a liquid containing eugenol with approximately 40 per cent of EBA which is mixed with a ZnO powder containing 30 per cent alumina and 6 per cent hydrogenated resin. The strength of this fortified type of material approaches closely to that of the phosphate cements.

For use as a root-filling material, radiopacity of ZOE cements is improved by incorporating the carbonate or trioxide of bismuth. Some cements contain fluoride to reduce the incidence of secondary caries, though the clinical effectiveness of this has yet to be proved.

Cellulose acetate fibres are sometimes incorporated to increase the strength.

Zinc oxide will set when combined with several of the essential oils, though in some cases it does so very slowly. With thymol, however, setting is very rapid, as the thymol crystallizes. The resultant mass is thermoplastic, and when warmed slightly will flow over the floor of a cavity.

Solubility

In water, eugenol is first leached out followed by hydrolysis of the zinc eugenolate as the balance of the set cement is upset. A reversal of the original setting reaction then takes place. ZOE cements tend, therefore, to disintegrate after a period in the mouth.

Strength

Compressive strength varies widely depending upon the formulation. Strength increases rapidly over the first 15 minutes after mixing and only slowly thereafter. Mechanical properties are affected to a marked degree by powder : liquid ratio. A thick consistency should be used whenever possible.

Effect on the pulp

When set, the cement has a pH of 6·6 to 8·0 and so has little effect upon the vital tooth structures. ZOE and $Ca(OH)_2$ cements are the only ones which can be placed on the base of a cavity near the pulp of a tooth. All other cements cause irritation of this sensitive structure, and in some cases bring about its death. ZOE cements have only a slight transient effect upon the pulp. Eugenol dulls the sensitivity of the dentine, and its cement with zinc oxide acts as an 'obtundent'. In some cases where the living pulp has been exposed accidentally during cavity preparation, a mix of this cement can be placed over the pulp without causing its death. However, an initial film of $Ca(OH)_2$ cement is commonly applied.

Effect on bacteria

Zinc oxide–eugenol mixtures have a prolonged bactericidal effect, and will kill bacteria in or near the surface of the cavity, thus sterilizing the cavity to a limited degree.

Despite a setting contraction of approximately 1·0% by volume, they appear to seal the cavity better than Zn phosphate or silicate cements and thus reduce the incidence of further decay.

General clinical use

Because of their mild action on the pulp when placed in the cavity, their bacteriostatic effect and their capacity for sealing the cavity, ZOE cements are very good lining materials. The strength of the modified cements at 7–10 minutes is usually adequate to resist the stresses imposed when packing an amalgam into place. Due to the slow release of eugenol, however, neither silicate cements nor polymeric filling materials should be placed directly on a fresh ZOE base. The eugenol causes discoloration of silicate cements and retards polymerization of polymeric fillings. The continuous leaching out of eugenol is thought by some to be a source of discomfort to the patient and possible irritation to the surrounding soft tissues. Abrasion resistance of these cements is poor. Heavy masticatory load or vigorous tooth brushing causes rapid loss of shape. Thus they are only used as temporary filling materials for periods of up to 3 months.

As cementing media, ZOE cements offer advantages of minimal pulpal damage, particularly where only a thin layer of dentine remains. The fortified materials are more suitable for cementing and have the advantage that although a high powder : liquid ratio is necessary, the mix flows readily to a very thin layer. For temporary cementation of restorations, they find a wide use and when the area of cementation is relatively large and the stress which will be applied is moderate, fortified ZOE cements have been shown to be clinically satisfactory. One advantage is that a 'fixed' restoration may be removed for repair more easily if it is cemented with ZOE cement. However, the disintegration after a period of use in the mouth may require the re-cementing of the restoration at fairly frequent intervals.

Thermal diffusivity of ZOE cements is $3·5–4·3 \times 10^{-3}$ cm^2/sec[1]. This is higher than that of the Zn phosphate cements, and ZOE cements are therefore poorer thermal insulators.

There is a very wide variation in properties of these cements and it is difficult to give typical properties which represent those for the materials as used clinically.

ACID/BASE SETTING CEMENTS

All the rest of the dental cements set due to an acid–base reaction. This definition includes the chelation reaction such as that which occurs with ZOE and polycarboxylate cements. With the phosphate, silicate and glass ionomer cements, however, the acid–base reaction is more obvious. All these cements set to a composite type of structure consisting of an amorphous matrix surrounding relatively untouched particles of the base, to which the matrix is bonded. Only in the case of ZOE cements is there evidence of much crystallization of the matrix. Unlike the resin-bonded composite filling materials, however, there is no sharp interface between matrix and filler but a zone of transition between the two phases. Problems of adhesion and stress accumulation at the interface therefore are reduced.

Whilst compressive and tensile strength are quoted for many of the cements, an important property is that of toughness which is difficult to measure in dental materials. Toughness does not necessarily increase with strength. It is a measure of the total energy required to fracture the material. Unfortunately most dental cements, due to their structure, are brittle rather than tough.

ZINC POLYCARBOXYLATE CEMENTS

Applicable specification: Austral 1253.

Polycarbaxylate cements are based upon the reaction between an aqueous solution of a polymer of acrylic acid:

$$
\begin{array}{cc}
\mathrm{H} & \mathrm{H} \\
| & | \\
\mathrm{C} & = \mathrm{C} \\
| & | \\
\mathrm{H} & \mathrm{C} \\
& \diagup \diagdown \\
\mathrm{O} & \mathrm{OH}
\end{array}
$$

with ZnO. Hence the use also of the term *polyacrylate cement*. The polyacrylic acid is thought to chelate to metallic ions such as Z_n^{2+}, probably with cross-linking between chains:

$$
\begin{array}{c}
\overset{|}{\underset{|}{H}}\quad\overset{|}{\underset{|}{H}}\quad\overset{|}{\underset{|}{H}}\quad\cdots
\end{array}
$$

The reaction not only causes the cement to set, but the cement can bond by chelation to the Ca^{2+} ions in the hydroxyapatite crystal of enamel and dentine.

The polyacrylic acid and ZnO join together at many points to form a polymer network joining together untouched cores of zinc oxide. Other oxides such as MgO, $Ca(OH)_2$ or Al_2O_3 can be added to modify the properties and the reaction. Fluorides may be present so that F may be released and so reduce the solubility of neighbouring enamel. Polyacrylic acid granules of 15–18 μm, stainless steel or potassium titanite fibres may also be incorporated to improve the working properties and strength. The molecular weight of polyacrylic acid and its concentration in solution affect the consistency and the speed of setting. Molecular weights of 20–50 $\times$ 10^3, and concentrations of 30–45 per cent of polyacrylic acid are used. Thus a variety of cements of different viscosities can be made. Some cement liquids are dispensed in two consistencies, one grade for lining and a more fluid grade for luting.

The same powder is used with the different liquids. Some liquids contain copolymers of itaconic and acrylic acids.

Working qualities

In general, polycarboxylate cements can be worked at a moderately thick consistency without creating difficulties in pressing them out to a thin cement layer. Viscosity of the mix is greatly affected, however, if the cement liquid is left exposed to the air for any length of time. It loses H_2O rapidly to the atmosphere even within one minute. Mixing should be completed quickly within 45 seconds by incorporating the powder rapidly into the liquid. The cement handles well, being hydrophilic and thus tends to stick to and to flow over the tooth surface to which it is applied. Setting time varies with the powder : liquid ratio used, being less for thick mixes. The variation is much less than with Zn phosphate cements. A rise in temperature speeds up the setting reaction. Mixing on a cool glass slab is advised. The material adapts well to a cavity which has been simply surface dried. There is adhesion to stainless steel and instruments should be dipped in alcohol otherwise the cement is difficult to adapt to the cavity. Instruments should be cleaned immediately after use.

To obtain adhesion to enamel, the cement must be applied quickly, before it loses its gloss. Otherwise the possibility of bonding falls markedly.

Strength

Compressive strength varies with the consistency and with the molecular weight and concentration of polyacrylic acid present in the liquid. The luting materials are weaker than those designed for lining cavities.

The tensile strength is between that of the Zn phosphate and fortified ZOE cements. It would appear that the polycarboxylate cements are more resilient than the relatively brittle Zn phosphate cements. This would be anticipated from their structure. The setting reaction is rapid and the compressive strength attains 75 per cent of its 24-hour strength within 15 minutes, and 90 per cent of this strength within an hour.

Solubility and water uptake

The solubility in water and in acetic acid is about the same as that of Zn phosphate cements. Water absorption, which causes a decrease in strength, is higher than that of Zn phosphate cements. This is probably due to the presence of the hydrophilic group involved in the chelation reaction. If the patient mouth-breathes, the alternate drying and wetting of the cement causes it to break up rapidly. This is particularly so when the cement is used as a 'fissure sealant' to protect the surface of the enamel against carious attack.

Adhesion

Bonding is thought to occur to the calcium of the hydroxyapatite crystal in both dentine and enamel. Bond strengths of the order of 5–10 N/mm^2 have been quoted for enamel and 2–5 N/mm^2 for bonding to dentine. The values vary with the testing method employed. It is apparent, however, that bonding to enamel does take place under favourable conditions, since failure of cementation occurs more frequently within the cement than at the cement–enamel interface. Adhesion has also been explained by the presence of sulphate ions in the liquid. These are said to form gypsum with the calcium ions of the enamel. It is thought that the bonding to enamel improves in time in water. As already noted, the enamel surface must be clean, dry and free from debris. Light etching of the enamel surface by the poly-acrylic acid itself, cleans the surface and may roughen it slightly. Some reports indicate that treatment with 50 per cent H_3PO_4 may have a similar effect.

The cements bond well to the oxide surface on stainless steel. It is therefore useful to attach orthodontic appliances to teeth. With other cements, an orthodontic band has to encircle a tooth. With poly-carboxylate cement, a piece of sheet stainless steel can be attached to the labial or buccal surface of a tooth. The cement does not bond to por-celain or to PMMA. To gold alloys there is probably attachment rather than adhesion.

Effect on the pulp

Whilst the pH of a cement liquid is approximately 1·7, the effect on the pulp is much less than would be anticipated. The pH of the mixed cement is 3–4, and this rises to 5–6 after 24 hours. It is probable that the relatively large polyacrylic acid molecule cannot penetrate the dentinal tubules and that its reaction with the calcium of the dentine and perhaps with the protein, restricts its passage along the dentinal tubule. The clinical effect on the pulp when the polycarboxylate cements are used is similar to that when using ZOE cements.

The use of these cements as pulp-capping materials is of doubtful value in producing deposition of secondary dentine to repair the exposure.

In general clinical use, the pulpal reaction (and therefore the patient's discomfort) is less than that experienced with Zn phosphate cements. Typical properties:

P/L ratio	$1 \cdot 5 - 3 \cdot 5 : 1$ by weight	
Setting time	3–7 minutes	
UCS, N/mm² 24 hr	Lining	Luting
	50–80	40–70
UTS, N/mm² 24 hr	5–10	3–6
Film thickness		20–50μm
Solubility in water, 7 days	0·0–0·2 per cent	
pH, 2 hr	6·0–6·5	
24 hr	6·5–6·9	

ZINC PHOSPHATE CEMENTS

Applicable specifications: ISO R 1566; Brit 3364; Amer 8; Austral 1186, 1253.

Zinc phosphate (incorrectly called oxyphosphate) cement is supplied as a powder and a liquid, which set to a hard mass on mixing. The cement powder may be purchased in a variety of colours, or shades, so that the dentist can select a cement of similar colour to the tooth that he is treating.

Composition

Zinc phosphate cement powders consist mainly of ZnO, to which is added a little MgO. Various other metallic oxides are added by the manufacturer to improve the quality of the cement and to modify its colour. In addition, the powders may contain sodium or other fluorides. These are added with the purpose of reducing the solubility of enamel in contact with the set cement, and thus reducing the possibility of further carious attack.

The liquid is a solution of H_3PO_4 in water, which has been partly neutralized by the addition of $Al(OH)_3$ and ZnO. Cement liquid therefore consists of H_3PO_4, H_2O and metallic phosphates.

Water-settable cements have been developed based on varieties of tertiary zinc phosphate. These are mixed with water containing a retarder such as Rochelle salt. The powders, however, are hygroscopic and shelf life is not good. In addition, the properties of the resultant cement are less than those required by specification for the normal Zn phosphate cements.

Setting reaction

The cement powder and liquid are mixed together on a clean glass slab with a suitable spatula. The composition of the liquid makes it necessary to use mixing instruments which are not affected by the acid.

When mixed, the oxide and acid react to form first of all soluble acid zinc phosphate $Zn_3(H_2PO_4)_2$. Then this changes via $ZnHPO_4$ to insoluble phosphate, probably $Zn_3(PO_4)_2.4H_2O$ (hopeite). At the stage when the cement is placed in the tooth cavity, it consists of some free acid, soluble phosphate and the 'cores' of untouched powder particles. The cement then sets by the formation of an amorphous matrix of insoluble zinc phosphate binding together the ZnO grains. As a result of the chemical reaction, heat is released. The final volume of cement is less than that of the powder and liquid from which it arose.

The evolution of heat and shrinkage of the cement are considerable if pure oxide and unmodified acid are mixed together. The setting time is very short, and such a cement would be unsuitable for use in the mouth. For this reason, both the acid and the oxide are modified by the manufacturers to give a longer setting time. This is mainly achieved by reducing the available acid content of the liquid, by the addition of metallic oxides to form acid phosphates. The reactivity of the oxides is reduced by heating the mixed ingredients of the powder to 1000–1400°C when they partially fuse. After this treatment they are ground to a fine powder.

The setting time is also affected by:

> The surface area of the powder.
> The amount of water in the acid.

Particle size of the powder

The size of particles is limited when the cement is to be used as a lute, as large grains of powder will tend to form a thick layer of cement. The grains of powder are reduced in size by their partial solution in the acid, and it is possible to produce a layer of cement which is thinner than the diameter of the powder particles. Nevertheless, with an accurate casting technique, the space between the cast inlay and the tooth substance is very small. In order to fill this space with cement and yet allow the inlay to be placed in position, a fine powder must be used. The surface area of a fine powder is greater than that of a coarse one, and the cement will set more rapidly unless compensation is made by varying other factors such as the acidity or water content. The dentist cannot readily alter the size of the powder particles, but should select as a cementing material a cement which has a fine-grained powder.

Most full veneer crowns have a fitting surface which has a small degree of taper (Fig. 53). This should be 10° total, i.e. 5° either side.

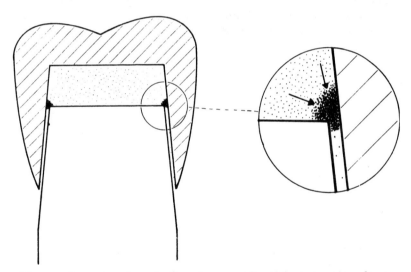

Fig. 53. Separation of powder from the cement liquid due to trapping of powder particles at the angle of the crown (see inset). Note also the difficulty of seating the crown correctly on the preparation

If this taper is too small or if the cement powder is too coarse, not only is there difficulty in seating the crown correctly, but separation of cement powder from the liquid occurs on seating the crown. The powder is trapped at the corners of the preparation and then acts as a filter for the cement which must be expressed from the upper part of the crown. As a result, the sides and edges of the crown are cemented mainly by cement liquid which washes away in the saliva. This effect is overcome by increasing the angle of taper, by using a superfine cement powder, or by providing an escape hole or vent in the occlusal or incisal surface of the crown. Alternatively, the 'fitting' surface of a metal crown may be etched electrolytically, except at the margins. This creates a larger space in which the cement can flow.

Water content of the liquid

The manufacturer adjusts the water content of the cement liquid so that maximum strength is obtained and a satisfactory working time is produced. The dentist must ensure that this concentration is maintained, by always replacing the stopper on a bottle of cement liquid immediately after it has been used. In a hot, dry atmosphere, evaporation is sufficient to cause crystallization of phosphates on the walls of the bottle of liquid. A bottle of cement liquid in this condition should be discarded. Even a small change of 1 per cent in the water content of the liquid produces a disproportionate drop in compressive and tensile strengths and an increase in solubility and abrasion.

Manufacturers should supply an excess of liquid so that changes in the water content are not as marked, particularly as the volume of liquid remaining becomes smaller. When all the powder has been used, the remaining liquid should be thrown away, and never used with a new bottle of powder. During its period of use, the contents of a bottle of liquid are open to the atmosphere for quite a long time, and changes in its water content are sufficient to make it unfit for further use.

The dentist can control the setting time of zinc phosphate cements by varying one of the following conditions:

> Temperature of the mixing slab.
> Powder : liquid ratio
> Rate of adding the powder to the liquid.

Temperature of mixing slab

Cements are usually mixed on a thick glass slab which is of sufficient bulk to maintain a constant temperature during mixing. The chemical reaction which takes place on setting proceeds at a faster rate when the temperature is raised, and is retarded at lower temperatures. Cement mixed on a cool slab will take longer to set outside the mouth than that mixed on a glass slab at room temperature. When cement is placed in the tooth cavity it is warmed to mouth temperature and setting then proceeds rapidly.

The glass slab and mixer can be cooled by immersing them in cold water for a few minutes before they are required for use. There are, however, two dangers which must be avoided in this method of cooling the slab. First, it must be carefully dried, as any H_2O which is left on its surface will be incorporated in the mix. Secondly, the atmosphere of a dental surgery may be very humid, particularly if hot water sterilizers are in use, and if the slab is cooled below the dewpoint of the atmosphere, moisture will condense on its surface and contaminate the mix.

Powder : liquid ratio

When a large amount of powder is added to the liquid, a high concentration of zinc phosphate is quickly produced, and the cement sets rapidly. More heat is produced when a thick mix of cement is used, but the resulting cement is stronger. The consistency of the mix is varied according to the purpose for which it is to be used. For cementing inlays, or crowns, a thinner mix is used, so that it does not resist the seating of the restoration. As thick a mix of cement as is practicable should always be used. The use of compressed tablets of cement powder has been suggested as a method of controlling the powder:liquid ratio.

Addition of powder to liquid

If the cement powder is added gradually in small portions to the liquid, setting is delayed, as the concentration of zinc phosphate produced at first is not great enough to cause setting. By this means, more time is available to achieve a smooth and homogeneous mix; but when all the powder is incorporated, the setting time is similar to that of a cement mixed all at once. Spatulation must not continue when once the cement has begun to set, or the phosphate matrix will be broken up and a weak cement will result. The powder should be added to the liquid in small portions over a definite short period of time in order to obtain a smooth mix of maximum strength.

Attachment

Retention by phosphate cements depends on the small surface roughness of the cavity wall, and of the surface of the inlay or crown. The effect of surface roughness in retention can be appreciated when cleaning hard cement from a glass slab. If the glass is new and smooth the cement will come away freely when the slab is placed in warm water. On the other hand, if the slab is scratched with use, greater difficulty is experienced in removing the set cement. All cast metal restorations have an irregular surface, and the fitting surface of a crown or inlay should be left in a clean 'as cast' condition and should not be smoothed. The quality of the retention achieved by a Zn phosphate cement lute, is probably due to the etching effect of H_3PO_4 on gold alloys and porcelains. This cleans and slightly roughens the surfaces to be cemented.

When the surface irregularities of the tooth and the filling are both filled with cement, numerous interlocking shapes are produced which join the two materials together. An inlay or crown is always made with slightly tapering fitting surfaces so that a shearing force is applied to the cement on trying to remove the filling. A strong cement resists this type of force better than when it is stressed in tension. A larger area of cement gives better retention.

If the layer of cement is thin, it will be more difficult to shear than a thick layer. A thin layer usually contains fewer air bubbles than a thick layer and is therefore stronger. Every attempt must be made to make an inlay or crown as accurate a fit as possible. It is doubtful whether the dentist can produce a cavity surface sufficiently smooth and an inlay of such perfect accuracy that there is not sufficient room between them for a fine cement powder. Ideally, the cement layer need only be one powder-grain thick, and this would represent the maximum strength of the cementing medium. Usually, the cement thickness is 20-50 μm and may be as great as 120 μm whilst still being clinically acceptable.

Pulp reaction

When first mixed and placed in the cavity, phosphate cements are very acid and show a pH of 2-3. As the setting reaction proceeds, the acid becomes partly neutralized, and after some hours the cement is only slightly acid. A thin mix of cement is more acid initially than a thick mix and remains at a lower pH value. It will affect the tooth pulp to a greater extent, particularly if it is placed in deep cavities. Similarly, when cementing splints or orthodontic bands in place on natural teeth, some decalcification of the enamel surface occurs if too thin a mix of cement is used.

A pulp reaction occurs under phosphate cement unless a thick barrier of dentine is still present between the cavity and the pulp. In deep cavities, only a thin layer of dentine remains, and the pulp should be protected by a layer of either ZOE or $Ca(OH)_2$ cement. The pulp reaction is probably due to the free acid present when the cement is placed in position.

Arsenic also causes a reaction, and oxides used for cements may contain only a very small amount of this impurity.

Strength

The compressive strength of phosphate cements increases with the powder:liquid ratio up to a maximum, after which no further increase takes place. Maximum strength of a cement is attained only with a very thick mix, and this cannot be used for cementing restorations in the mouth. As noted previously, cement should be mixed as thick as is practicable for the work to be carried out.

The strength of a cement reaches its greatest value 24 hours after mixing, although after 1 hour, three-quarters of this strength is attained.

Solubility

After a cement has been in contact with the saliva for some time, its strength falls quite markedly, due to solution and disintegration by the saliva. Cement shows a greater solubility in the mouth than it does when tested in distilled water under laboratory conditions. In acid media, Zn is leached out whilst in alkali, the phosphate is removed. Intra-oral failure could well therefore be due to the corrosive effect of acetic acid or lactic acid from the breakdown of food debris combined with the effect of saliva and foodstuffs.

The cement lute is the weakest part of an inlay, crown or bridge. If the cement washes out, further decay of the tooth will start. A thick mix of cement resists solution better than a thin mix as it has less matrix.

If saliva comes into contact with the cement before it has set, the strength will be reduced and the solubility increased, as mucin will be mixed with the cement. Saliva must, therefore, be excluded from any filling until the cement has set.

When the cement has set it must be kept moist and not allowed to dry out.

Shrinkage

All zinc phosphate cements contract on setting. If placed in water after setting, the linear contraction is 0·05 to 0·1 per cent, but if they are allowed to dry out, the shrinkage is much greater. When used as a cementing medium, 0·1 per cent shrinkage is negligible as it occurs in a very thin section. If the cement is used in thicker sections, for example as a temporary filling, the contraction is sufficient to cause leakage of the filling. Hence the unsuitability of Zn phosphate cements as temporary fillings where a perfect seal is required. Contraction after setting takes place mainly in 2 hours; after this time the cement is dimensionally stable if kept moist.

Effect on bacteria

The newly mixed cement is strongly bactericidal. This property is due to the low pH after mixing. Some time after setting, this effect is lost as the pH approaches neutrality. The Zn phosphate cements do not therefore inhibit further dental decay.

SUMMARY OF THE USE OF ZINC PHOSPHATE CEMENTS

Replace the stopper on the liquid bottle as soon as the amount of powder and liquid required have been measured. Do not use liquid which has gone cloudy. Discard any liquid remaining when the powder is finished.

Use the maximum amount of powder. This increases the strength, reduces the solubility and acidity, but speeds up the set.

Cool and dry the mixing slab and spatula. Do not chill too much or atmospheric moisture may condense on the slab. Cooling gives a longer mixing time and a smoother mix.

Add the powder in small portions to the liquid. This gives a longer mixing time.

Use a rapid rotary motion with a flat-bladed spatula.

Don't overmix. $1-1\frac{1}{2}$ minutes is usually sufficient.

Exclude all saliva, but do not dry out other cement fillings in adjacent teeth.

Apply cement to an inlay or crown first, then to the tooth.

Typical properties of zinc phosphate cements:

Setting time 37°C		5–8 minutes
Consistency		0·5 ml:1·1–1·8 g
UCS (N/mm²) 24 hours	Thick mix	100–170
	Thin mix	40–80
UTS (N/mm²) 24 hours	Thick mix	6·9
	Thin mix	3–5
Film thickness		30–40 μm
Solubility in water	7 days	0·1–0·2 per cent
pH	2 hours	6·0–6·2
	24 hours	6·4–6·8
Thermal diffusivity cm²/sec		2·0–2·5

COPPER PHOSPHATE CEMENTS

Applicable specification: Austral 1253.

These are similar to the Zn phosphate cements in their setting reactions, and the liquid is similar in composition. The cement powders contain various copper oxides in addition to ZnO, though in some cements copper oxides alone are used. In colour the cements do not resemble tooth structure, and their composition can be surmised from the colour of the powder as follows:

Red	Cuprous oxide	Cu_2O
Black	Cupric oxide	CuO
Green	Cupric silicate	$CuSiO_3$
White	Cuprous iodide	Cu_2I_2

Copper phosphate cements after mixing have the same bactericidal effect as Zn phosphate cements. There is some doubt as to the continuance of this effect after they have set. Some cements are called 'germicidal', that is 'bacteria destroying'. They should preferably contain a mercury salt such as phenylmercuric nitrate or mercuro-ammonium-chloride as these have more germicidal effect than a copper cement alone after setting. Copper-containing cements are therefore used to fill cavities in temporary teeth in circumstances where all the decay cannot be removed.

The addition of 2 per cent silver phosphate to Zn phosphate cements is also said to give germicidal properties. Silver salts darken to silver sulphide on exposure in the mouth. This type of 'silver' phosphate cement is therefore used only in posterior teeth.

The reaction of the pulp to copper cements is generally more severe than with the zinc phosphate cements due to their continuing low pH value. Deep cavities should be lined with ZOE cement. The copper cements have a compressive strength similar to that of Zn phosphate cements, but a higher solubility. They wash out of the cavity and must be replaced at fairly frequent intervals.

Some brands of black Cu cement set in the presence of saliva much better than the Zn phosphate cements do. Such a property is of value when cementing splints in place to control jaw fractures, or when fixing orthodontic appliances in the mouths of children. In such circumstances the saliva cannot be excluded entirely and black cupric oxide cement is used. The acid in Cu phosphate cements etches enamel and so improves attachment.

Chapter 36

Silicate, silicophosphate and ionomer cements

Applicable specifications for silicate cements: ISO R 1565; Brit 3365; Amer 9; Austral 1454. For silicophosphate cements: Brit 3365; Amer 21; Austral 1454.

SILICATE CEMENTS

Silicate cements are sometimes incorrectly called artificial or synthetic 'porcelains'. Although the cement powder has a similarity to that from which porcelain is fused, no similarity exists between the finished products either chemically or in their mechanical properties.

The life of a silicate filling depends to a large extent upon the care with which the material was used. The average life of such a filling is approximately 5 years though it may be as little as 8–12 months, or as great as 20 years. Frequently the initial excellent appearance is lost due to surface staining of the filling.

Composition

Powder

The powder consists essentially of an aluminosilicate glass containing F, Ca, Na, and phosphate. The glass has a three-dimensional structure made up from tetrahedra of (AlO_4) and (SiO_4). In each case the Al or Si atom is surrounded by four O^{2-} anions and occupies the interstitial space between them. The tetrahedra are joined to each other at the corners in a random manner by sharing an oxygen atom with another tetrahedron (see Fig. 38). In silicate cements, the ratio of Al:Si tetrahedra approaches unity. Fluorine is added at a relatively high ratio. This produces spherical droplets of a F-rich phase which causes the glass to be opalescent.

During manufacture the various ingredients are first carefully selected to eliminate impurities such as Fe, and after grinding are fused at about 1400°C. The resultant glass is pulverized until it has a suitable particle size distribution. The incorporation of up to 15 per cent by weight of F has advantages not only in improving the properties of the cement, but also in the effect of F which reduces caries of the surrounding tooth substance.

Liquid

The liquid supplied with silicate cements is similar to that for Zn phosphates, but there is less available acid. More of the H_3PO_4 has been neutralized by combination with oxides such as Al_2O_3 and ZnO to form soluble phosphates. Usually several different oxides are added to the cement liquid so that the percentage of any particular metallic phosphate in solution does not reach its saturation point. If the oxide of only one metal was added, its phosphate would tend to crystallize out of solution.

On no account should silicate powder be mixed with phosphate cement liquid, or vice versa, as the acidity and water content of the liquids differ. They are adjusted to give the correct setting time and optimum properties when mixed with their correct powders.

The incorporation of In in both powder and liquid is reported to improve the resistance of the resultant cement to attack by acid. The addition of diols renders the cement less prone to surface crazing on losing a little surface water.

Care of the liquid

Silicate cement liquid contains more H_2O than that for phosphate cements, and it will lose water readily to a warm, dry atmosphere. To prevent loss, the bottle of liquid must be stoppered immediately after use, and the measured amount of liquid should not be left on the slab before mixing. It has been estimated that a small bottle of liquid may be open to the atmosphere for a total time of 30 minutes while its contents are being used. As a further precaution a thin layer of liquid paraffin B.P. may be floated on top of the liquid to seal it from the air.

When crystals form on the walls of the glass bottle, loss of H_2O has taken place and the bottle should be thrown away. In any event, a bottle of liquid should be discarded when three-quarters of its contents have been used as its H_2O content will no longer be correct. As with phosphate cements, never use an old bottle of cement liquid with a fresh bottle of powder.

If an unstoppered bottle of cement liquid is left in a cupboard with other medicaments, the vapour of any essential oils present may contaminate the cement liquid and cause the cement to set very slowly.

Setting

The aluminosilicate glass carries a negative charge and functions as a base. The surface of the powder particles is attacked very rapidly by the H_3PO_4 in the liquid and liberates Al^{3+}, Ca^{2+}, Na^+ and F^- ions (Fig. 54).

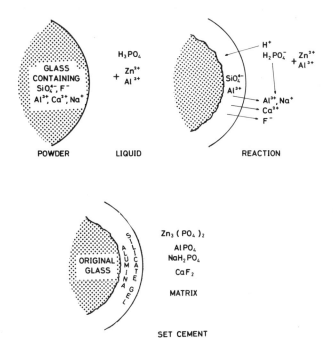

Fig. 54. Diagrammatic representation of the setting reactions of silicate cements.

These pass into the liquid and bring about a rise in pH. The surface of the particles is converted to a very thin layer of a gel either of silicic acid or of aluminosilica. This layer is only a few microns thick though in small particles which are less than 5 μm across, the effect will be complete throughout the particle. In larger particles, only the surface is affected. As the pH rises, polymerization of aluminium phosphates takes place forming eventually an insoluble $AlPO_4$ gel. This process occurs at the initial set. Other products formed are CaF_2, NaH_2PO_4 and $Zn_3(PO_4)_2$. Setting continues for several days after the initial polymerization process as shown by a gradual increase in the pH. The surface layer of gel on each particle acts as the bond between the original unaffected glass particles and the phosphatic matrix. The gel is probably bonded by means of ionic Si–O or Al–O bridges to the original glass and by hydrogen bonds to the phosphate matrix. Thus the final structure is a composite consisting of the original unaffected particles bonded together via a matrix to form an extremely strong but brittle material.

Amount of matrix

The strength, resistance to solution, and therefore the permanence of a silicate filling, depend to a considerable extent upon the amount of matrix which is present. It is only necessary to have sufficient matrix present to bind the powder particles together. It has been estimated that a correct silicate cement consists of 20–30 per cent of matrix, binding together 80–70 per cent of untouched powder particles. To achieve this proportion, as much powder as possible should be incorporated in the liquid.

Setting time

In order to achieve a good powder:liquid ratio, there must be sufficient time to incorporate the required amount of powder in the liquid. With a short setting time, the mix begins to set and thickens before all the powder has been added. In these circumstances the cement appears to be of the correct consistency, but the mix contains less powder. Silicate cements set more rapidly than Zn phosphate cements and shortening of the setting time by the accidental addition of H_2O or by mixing at a warm temperature must be avoided.

The reader will note that none of the following is given as a method of varying setting time.

> Ratio of powder to liquid.
> Rate of addition of powder to liquid.
> Time of spatulation.

Though alterations in these factors will affect the setting time, they should not be varied but should be determined by the manufacturer or the dentist, and when once a technique is established, no variation from the correct procedure should be made.

Mixing

Since the cement sets by the formation of bonds between the alumino-silica gel and the phosphate matrix, all manipulation of the cement must cease as soon as the mix begins to set, that is, when the pH become favourable for precipitation of the phosphates. If the mix is disturbed once it has begun to set, the bonding will be incomplete and the filling will be unsatisfactory. The powder is therefore added to the liquid in large portions so that reaction of the liquid with all the powder starts more or less at the same time.

In order to mix quickly, the cement powder and liquid may be placed in a capsule and oscillated on a mechanical amalgamator. This produces a mix in 10–20 seconds, compared with 60–75 seconds by hand spatulation. If the contents of the capsule are preweighed a correct powder:liquid ratio is also obtained. The ideal method is where the correct proportions of powder:liquid are dispensed in a capsule, separated by a thin membrane. This is ruptured before oscillation of the capsule, and a correct mix is obtained in a few seconds. However, the energy applied in mixing by this means decreases the setting time, since part of the energy appears as heat. The manufacturer makes due allowance for this when silicate cements are to be mixed in this manner.

Silicate cements are also mixed on a glass slab, with an agate, white plastic, or stellite spatula. It is essential to use a spatula made from a chemically inert material as the acid will attack many metals. In addition, the silicate powder is quite abrasive, and if particles are rubbed from a metal spatula, they discolour the filling. Agate has a similar colour to the cement and also resists abrasion quite well. Stellite spatulas are suitable, as the abrasion resistance of this alloy is very high. Contamination of the cement by metals or with dirt will discolour the filling, and detract from the appearance of the filling. Scrupulous cleanliness of the mixer and slab are obviously essential, and it is usual to keep a special glass slab for mixing silicates. Since the silica of the powder is hard, some scratching of the slab also occurs after a period of use, and these scratches will tend to hold the debris from the previous mixes of cement. The degree of scratching can be reduced by using a less vigorous mixing technique.

The glass slab and mixer should be cooled to a predetermined temperature, and after thorough drying, the powder is placed on the slab. Immediately before mixing, a volume of liquid less than that necessary to mix with all the powder is dispensed. Within a given space of time, depending on the temperature, the mix is completed, adding the powder as quickly as possible. The powder is folded into the liquid rather like mixing mortar, and not in a vigorous circular motion as with phosphate cements. If atmospheric conditions are such that cooling the glass will cause condensation of atmospheric vapour upon it, the filling should be postponed until a more suitable time when the relative humidity is less, or a capsulated material used.

Shade

Silicate cements darken slightly for some weeks after insertion due to an increase in translucency following water absorption. A restoration which is initially slightly light in colour will eventually match the tooth shade correctly. Compensation for this change is usually made in the manufacturers' shade guides.

Filling the cavity

A mass of cement sufficiently large to completely fill the cavity is packed into place and is then held in position by a thin nylon or celluloid strip. If the cement is packed into the cavity in small portions complete union between the portions of the cement does not take place, and the filling will not be as strong as one which is packed with one single mass of cement. The strip must not be removed until the cement has completely hardened, as any movement will break up the matrix and so weaken the filling.

Finishing

The retaining strip should conform as closely as possible to the finished shape of the filling, as polishing of silicate cements is impossible. The set cement consists of a heterogeneous mass of matrix and powder particles. Trimming with abrasives, and polishing of such a material will not give as good a surface as that produced when the cement sets against the smooth surface of the plastic strip.

Silicate cements increase in hardness rapidly over the first 3 hours and continue to harden slowly after this time for a further week. No attempt at polishing should be made until at least 3 hours have elapsed from the mixing of the filling, and preferably the procedure should be postponed for several days.

Shrinkage

All silicate cements contract on setting, and in theory there is always a slight space between filling and tooth substance. After a period of wear a dark line usually appears round the filling.

If the cement is allowed to dry out when once it has set, a further large shrinkage takes place and the filling will not return to its original dimensions when it is moistened once more.

Solubility and disintegration

Silicate cements show a relatively high solubility in water. But, since the permanence of silicate restoration, however carefully inserted, varies widely between patients, factors other than simple solubility of the cement in water must play an important part in the disintegration of a filling. Food remaining on stagnation areas in the mouth undergoes bacterial decomposition. The breakdown products, such as organic acids, attack the silicate cements. The matrix of the filling is gradually washed away so that the powder particles loosen and fall out of the filling. The initial stage of such a process is a staining of the filling due to the roughness of its surface when the matrix has dissolved away.

During the first 24 hours phosphates are washed out, followed later by a more prolonged washing out of various silicates.

In mouths where the environment is not particularly acid, silicate cement fillings have a long life. Where acid conditions prevail, however, the life is relatively short. It is difficult clinically to decide upon what is a suitable 'silicate mouth'.

Moisture contamination

Any moisture coming into contact with the cement before it has set washes some of the phosphate matrix out of the cement. The surface of the cement becomes opaque and rough and is soon eroded and stained. When placing a silicate filling, water must be excluded from the material until it has completely hardened. As soon as setting has taken place in the mouth and the contouring strip removed, the filling is coated with a varnish which remains in place until the patient returns to have the edges of the filling trimmed and polished. The filling should be protected from the saliva for at least 4 hours. Proprietary varnishes particularly those of copal resin or polyurethane, appear to be the most efficient in this respect. Greases and waxes do not remain in place long enough to protect the setting cement.

Drying out

If the filling is allowed to dry out during its life, it shrinks. The surface becomes opaque and chalky in appearance and it is rapidly washed away by the saliva. For this reason, silicate fillings are not advised in patients who respire entirely through their mouths (mouth-breathers). The warm air flowing past the teeth dries the saliva upon them, and causes drying of any cement fillings.

Similarly, when further fillings are being placed in a mouth in which silicate fillings are already present, care must be taken to prevent these drying out when the teeth are isolated from moisture.

Strength

The compressive strength of silicate cements is higher than that of the other cements, but is lower than any other restorative material except acrylic resin. Silicate cement is a brittle material, however, and though it may withstand a slow compressive stress, it can be fractured by sudden impact stress. This precludes their use in areas of high stress such as Class IV restorations.

Compressive strength increases with the amount of powder incorporated in the liquid up to a maximum, after which it reduces. One can assume that with too thick a mix there is insufficient bonding between the matrix and the particles. Usually, however, such a difficulty does not occur, but rather the opposite one of not being able to use sufficient powder. Capsulated materials ensure that the correct powder:liquid ratio is used for every filling.

Effect on the pulp

It has long been realized that when any of the dental cements which utilize H_3PO_4 in their setting reaction are used as a filling material in a deep cavity, damage to the tooth pulp will occur. Sometimes the irritation of the pulp is sufficiently severe to cause its death, though this may not happen until the filling has been in place for several months. Quite often the pulp dies without causing any pain to the patient, and it is only when the pulp subsequently becomes infected with blood-borne bacteria that an abscess is formed. In a deep cavity, the wall of dentine between the filling and the pulp is only thin, and it is possible for the acid to penetrate this layer of dentine and kill the pulp cells.

Death of the pulp under silicate cements has always been more frequent than with other materials and several theories have been advanced to explain this difference.

It has been shown that the acidity of silicate cement is high at the stage at which it is inserted into the cavity. Measurements give a pH of 2–4. The acidity reduces as the cement sets, but the cement always remains slightly acid and never reaches neutrality. The pH is highest initially when a thick mix is employed and attains its maximum in a shorter time, whereas a thin mix has a lower pH initially and takes much longer to approach neutrality.

A mix of silicate cement contains free acid which can enter the dentinal tubules, and may reach the pulp. In the case of silicate cements, penetration of the dentine by acid is assisted by the pressure from the strip which is placed round the filling.

The reaction of the pulp under silicate cements is more severe than under Zn phosphates, but not as severe as under Cu phosphate cements.

In deep cavities, and in young patients especially, a lining of ZOE or $Ca(OH)_2$ cement should always be used. This is followed by a layer of phosphate cement (Fig. 55). If silicate cement is placed directly over a

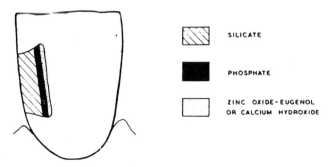

SILICATE

PHOSPHATE

ZINC OXIDE-EUGENOL
OR CALCIUM HYDROXIDE

Fig. 55. Silicate restoration in a deep cavity

ZOE lining, discolouration of the silicate cement may appear at a later date. This is probably due to penetration of oil from the lining into the silicate cement and occurs more frequently when a thin mix of ZOE cement is used. In shallower cavities a lining of phosphate cement may be employed, or a cavity varnish.

Effect on enamel

There is a low incidence of recurrent caries at the margins of silicate fillings. This is attributed to the passage of F from the filling to the enamel at the time of insertion of the filling and for some time afterwards. Fluorine replaces an OH^- ion in hydroxyapatite and so reduces its surface energy. Not only is the solubility reduced, but this change makes it more difficult for plaque to adhere to the enamel. Fluorine also acts as an enzyme inhibitor in the breakdown of carbohydrates, thus reducing the production of acid from this source.

SUMMARY

When using silicate cements:

Line the cavity to protect the pulp.
Isolate the tooth from the saliva.
Incorporate as much powder as possible in the mixing time.
Fill the cavity with one mass of cement. Trim away the excess.
Hold in place with a dry plastic strip to the contour required in the finished restoration. No movement at all while the cement is setting.
Varnish the surface of the filling after removing the strip.
Polish if necessary after at least 24 hours.
Never let the filling dry out during subsequent treatment.

Typical properties of silicate cements:

Powder:liquid	2·5:4·0 g/ml
Setting time at 37°C	3–7 minutes
Compressive strength	250–350 N/mm²
Tensile strength	8–18 N/mm²
Solubility in water, 24 hours	0·4–0·8 per cent
pH, 2 hours	4·0–5·0
24 hours	5·0–6·5
Thermal diffusivity	2·3–2·8 × 10⁻³ cm²/sec

SILICOPHOSPHATE CEMENTS
(STEIN-CEMENTS)

A mixture of zinc phosphate and silicate cement powder is sometimes used in an attempt to combine the lower solubility of the former with the aesthetic appearance of the latter. In some materials the powders are partly fused together, while others consist of simple mixtures. The liquids with which these powders are mixed are similar to those used for silicate cements.

The stein-cements are suggested for use as filling materials in cheek teeth, particularly for children. They are also used as semi-translucent cementing media.

Some materials are labelled 'germicidal' as they contain bactericidal mercury compounds.

The description silicophosphate cements covers a range of materials between those which resemble zinc phosphate and those which are mainly silicate cements. Their manipulation is the same as that of silicate cements.

By combining zinc phosphate and silicate cements, you do not necessarily get the best of both worlds.

As filling materials, silicophosphate cements show a compressive strength similar to that of silicate cements, that is higher than the phosphates. Their solubility also appears to be less than the silicates, but greater than the phosphates. Changes in pH on setting are similar to those of the silicate cements and protection of the pulp is equally necessary.

When used as a cementing medium, the film thickness tends to be rather great, due to the relatively large particle size. Their semi-translucent appearance, however, encourages one to use them for cementing porcelain jacket crowns. The space for cement in such a crown is greater than when cementing an inlay.

GLASS IONOMER CEMENTS

The setting reaction of silicate cements depends upon the release of ions from the surface of the glass particles on reaction with H_3PO_4. With this acid, there is a danger of pulp irritation. In addition, the phosphate matrix which is bonded to the glass particles by a silica hydrogel, is affected by the acid conditions which occur in the mouth either on drinking or eating acid foodstuffs or by the breakdown of sugars. In addition, there is no adhesion between silicate cements and tooth substance. On the other hand, silicate cements have excellent translucency and due to the release of fluorine ions, reduce the incidence of secondary caries round restorations.

With the advent of polyacrylic cements, developments proceeded in Great Britain to produce a cement based on the reaction of ion leachable glasses with polyacrylic acid.

Powder

The powder is finely divided aluminosilicate glass with a particle size usually less that 50 μm. The glass contains major amounts of Ca and F and small amounts of Na and phosphate. The proportion of alumina (which is the basic oxide) to silica (the acidic oxide), and the amount of fluxes in the glass is greater than in the case of silicate cement powders as polyacrylic acid is much weaker than H_3PO_4. In order that a reaction can take place at an appropriate speed, the glass must be of a more basic type otherwise the setting time is too long. Hence the use of a greater proportion of alumina in the melt.

As with the silicate cements, the opacity is due to the presence of F-rich droplets as a dispersed phase. The opacity is, however, greater in ionomer cements.

Liquid

The liquid is a solution of polyacryclic acid with a molecular weight distribution around 10^4. The viscosity of the solution is affected both by the molecular weight of the polyacrylic acid used and also by its concentration. The liquid may also contain certain hydroxy-carboxylic acids, probably tartaric acid.

Setting reaction

The reaction of polyacrylic acid with the surface of the glass produces Al and Ca polyacrylates. Setting occurs by the release of Al^{3+} and Ca^{2+} ions from the glass powder which cross-link the polymer chains of acrylic acid. As the ions are released from the surface of the glass, a hydrated silica gel is formed on the surface of the particles and this binds the matrix to the original particles as in silicate cements. Initially, Ca polyacrylate forms the matrix, joined at a later stage by Al polyacrylate.

With a high concentration of acrylic acid, cross-linking occurs more than chelation and this is better for cement formation. Unfortunately an increase in viscosity of the cement liquid accompanies an increase in molecular weight. This can be overcome by using lower molecular weight polymers in high concentration rather than vice versa. In addition, the shelf life of low molecular weight solutions is better than that of high molecular weight solutions. With high molecular weight acrylic acid, there is also a tendency to produce transient gelation during setting and this interferes with the setting reaction.

The rheological properties are affected by the addition of hydroxycarboxylic acids. These increase the speed of setting and the sharpness of the set point, while still allowing sufficient working time. Such acids presumably aid the extraction of ions but these are not immediately available for cross-linking as they react with the tartaric acid.

The structure of the fully set cement is therefore a composite of glass particles embedded in a matrix. Unlike the matrix in silicate cement, the matrix has a backbone of covalent bonds in the polymer chain with ionic cross-linking between the chains. It therefore presents a stronger and less soluble matrix than the metallic phosphate type of matrix in silicate cements.

MANIPULATION

The cement can be mixed to a thin consistency and so used as a lute without the danger of a large excess of strong acid. It can be used equally as a base in a cavity lining or as a restorative material. It is advisable however to place an initial layer of $Ca(OH)_2$ cement where the thickness of dentine between the cavity and the pulp is less than 150 μm.

The two stage setting reaction involving firstly Ca^{2+} and later Al^{3+} may account for the initial set of the material followed by a period of carvability before final hardening. The material thus passes through plastic, carvable and hard states.

The material may also be used as a fissure sealant. Under such a fissure sealant, the incidence of secondary caries is less and this may be due to the release of F ions. However, adhesive glass ionomer cements are only suitable as sealants where a pit or fissure orifice is larger than 100μm, that is, it can be detected with a sharp probe. Otherwise when the fissure is smaller than this or when it has been subjected to carious attack, minimum cavity preparation is necessary. It is suggested, however, that due to the relatively high water absorption of this type of cement, leakage of fermentable carbohydrates might occur, both through and round the cement, causing further caries.

Bonding to enamel and dentine

Adhesion is by the same mechanism described for polycarboxylate cement. Bond strength to enamel increases over a period of six months in water. The bond is probably both mechanical and chemical. The increase in bond strength can be attributed to the leaching of further polyacrylic acid from the cement which forms further bonds with the calcium of the hydroxyapatite crystal.

pH of the cement

The initial pH of this type of cement is said to be higher than that of silicate cements though the eventual pH is similar. In an acid environment, the erosion is approximately 1/10 that of silicate cement.

Typical properties:

P/L ratio (g/ml)	3–3·5
Setting time	4–5 minutes
UCS, N/mm², 24 hrs	190–210
UTS, N/mm², 24 hrs	15–17
Solubility in H_2O, 24 hrs	0·3 per cent
pH, 24 hrs	5·3

Chapter 37
Polymeric filling materials

Applicable specifications: Brit 5199; Austral 1278.

Until recent years, the restoration of teeth was achieved by placing in the cavity either metal fillings which did not resemble tooth structure, but which lasted many years, or cement fillings which were short-lived in some mouths but whose appearance could be excellent. No filling material yet combines the properties of durability and appearance. Various synthetic polymers have been used for fillings and have been found to be only partially suitable for the purpose.

Research continues to produce a durable, tooth-like restorative material.

SELF-CURING METHYL METHACRYLATE (DIRECT-FILLING ACRYLICS)

These materials first appeared in 1948 and are dispensed in the monomer-polymer form. They resemble in many respect the self-curing denture base materials already discussed. Usually the polymer is of a finer grain size than that used for denture base materials and it is pigmented with metallic oxides.

Polymerization

As described previously under the self-curing denture bases, polymerization at mouth temperature may be brought about by two types of reaction.

Peroxide type

In this type of reaction an activator, usually a tertiary aromatic amine, is present within the monomer, and the initiator, benzoyl peroxide, is incorporated in the polymer. Another possible activator is lauryl mercaptan which is more stable. Due to the fact that this activator works at a low pH, methacrylic acid is either added or present in the monomer. Although this activator finds little practical use today, it produces polymers with better colour stability than those whose polymerization is activated by an aromatic amine.

Sulphinic acid type

In other materials, however, an activator and initiator combined, such as p-toluene sulphinic acid or one of its salts, is used. This chemical acts directly on the monomeric molecules and each molecule of sulphinic acid starts a chain reaction. The resultant polymer is more colour stable than that formed when an amine is used. p-Toluene sulphinic acid is unstable and is usually present in the polymer together with a little benzoyl peroxide. Until the polymer is mixed with monomer, no reaction takes place.

Polymerization shrinkage

The difficulty which lies in the way of placing an accurate filling with these materials is the volume shrinkage of methyl methacrylate monomer. This may be 6–7 per cent by volume in the mixture of monomer and polymer used. Various methods of overcoming this shrinkage have been suggested. They include the use of pressure, building up the material in layers, or bonding an initial layer of polymer to the surface of the cavity. In the so called *cavity sealing technique*, a small proportion of methacrylic acid or glycerophosphoric acid dimethacrylate is incorporated in the monomer or is supplied as a separate liquid. This material is applied to the surface of the cavity where it penetrates and may react with calcium in the surface of the dentine. This initial layer may then join with the filling which is placed over it.

Defects of direct filling acrylics

With a careful technique, the initial fit of acrylic fillings at mouth temperature appears to be satisfactory. The coefficient of thermal expansion and contraction of methyl methacrylate is, however, 10–12 times that of dentine. Therefore a space appears between the filling and the tooth when cold foods or liquids are taken into the mouth. This space becomes filled with liquid which, when the filling warms up again, appears in the form of small droplets causing *marginal percolation*. The gap between the tooth and the filling becomes filled with debris after a period of time and shows as a dark line round the filling.

Polymerized methyl methacrylate has no effect upon bacteria. This, combined with a lack of fit due to thermal changes, is probably responsible for the tendency towards recurrent caries. The addition of fluorides may reduce the solubility of the enamel in contact with the filling though it is doubtful whether F is released to any great extent.

Phenol or eugenol plasticize the self-cure acrylic materials and retard their polymerization, as phenols are inhibitors of free radical polymerization. A recent lining of ZOE cement must be covered with a layer of another cement before inserting the acrylic filling.

Monomer may penetrate the dentinal tubules unless the cavity is lined. The cavity sealing materials have a very high acidity, with a pH of about 1·6. To prevent chemical irritation of the pulp, therefore, any cavity in which the layer of dentine remaining over the pulp is less than 1 mm should be lined. The long-term effect on the pulp, however, may be due more to continuous marginal leakage of the filling than to irritation from monomer.

Typical properties of acrylic filling materials:

Tensile strength	24 hr	25–30 N/mm^2
Compressive strength	24 hr	50–70 N/mm^2
Mod. of elast.	24 hr	2200 N/mm^2
KHN		10–16
Coefficient of thermal expansion		80–100 $\times 10^{-6}$/°C
Water absorption	24 hr	0·4–0·6 per cent

The direct filling acrylics have been largely replaced by the composite materials.

INJECTION OF THERMOPLASTIC POLYMERS

Various attempts have been made to inject into the tooth cavity thermoplastic polymers such as polystyrene, polyamide (nylon) and polycarbonates. These may be softened in a suitable small 'gun' and injected into the tooth cavity whilst molten, there to harden. When hard, they were trimmed and polished.

Polystyrene polymers soften at 140–190°C, depending upon their molecular weight. In use, they were too flexible under masticatory stress and thin sections at the cavity margins broke away. Marginal seal was therefore lost and pulp irritation and further caries followed.

Nylons soften within the same range of temperature but, due to their high water absorption, they soon showed distortion and lack of adaptation to the cavity.

Polycarbonates have a higher softening temperature of 250–340°C. There was some evidence that polycarbonates retained colour and marginal accuracy for longer periods than the other two thermoplastic materials. It was doubtful, however, whether any of these materials had better properties than the direct filling acrylic materials.

COMPOSITES

During the last two decades a large number of polymeric filling materials have appeared. Some have enjoyed only a short useful life, having had inadequate laboratory and clinical testing applied to them before they were offered to the dental profession. Materials have been found to be unsuitable due to faults such as excessive discoloration, abrasion, polymerization shrinkage and solubility.

The term composite is applied to a material in which two or more constituents are bonded together. The nature of the filler, of the matrix and of the bond between them, all affect the resultant properties of the composite.

The composite filling materials available in dentistry are basically room temperature polymerizing monomers, together with a filler. At one time the monomer used was methyl methacrylate but now other monomers or comonomers are used. The surface of the filler is treated to achieve bonding between the filler and the polymer. The filler reduces the coefficient of thermal expansion, water absorption, polymerization shrinkage and at the same time increases hardness, compressive strength, and modulus of elasticity of the composite.

Polymer matrix

Methyl methacrylate polymerized by a peroxide/tertiary amine (dimethyl-p-toluidine (DMPT) or dimethyl xylidine (DMSX)) system or a peroxide/mercaptan system has been used as the matrix for some materials. One material employed tributyl borane as an initiator. This reacts with water in the tooth to form free radicals. However, time has shown that plain methyl methacrylate is not the ideal choice for the polymer phase.

There are important advantages to be gained by using monomeric molecules which are larger than that of methyl methacrylate:

$$CH_2 = \overset{\displaystyle CH_3}{\underset{\displaystyle COOCH_3}{\overset{|}{\underset{|}{C}}}}$$

With larger molecules, polymerization shrinkage is less since there are fewer double bonds per unit volume. Larger monomeric molecules therefore produce a better starting point for the polymer matrix of composites. The monomers are also less volatile, and because of their large molecular size, are less likely to penetrate dentinal tubules.

The polymer phase of many composite filling materials today is based on the type of dimethacrylate monomer introduced by Bowen. This is an adduct of bisphenol A and glycidyl methacrylate. It can also be produced by the reaction of the diglycidyl ether of bisphenol A and methacrylic acid. The resultant monomer is derived from two molecules of glycidyl methacrylate and one of bisphenol A (see p. 392, upper two diagrams).

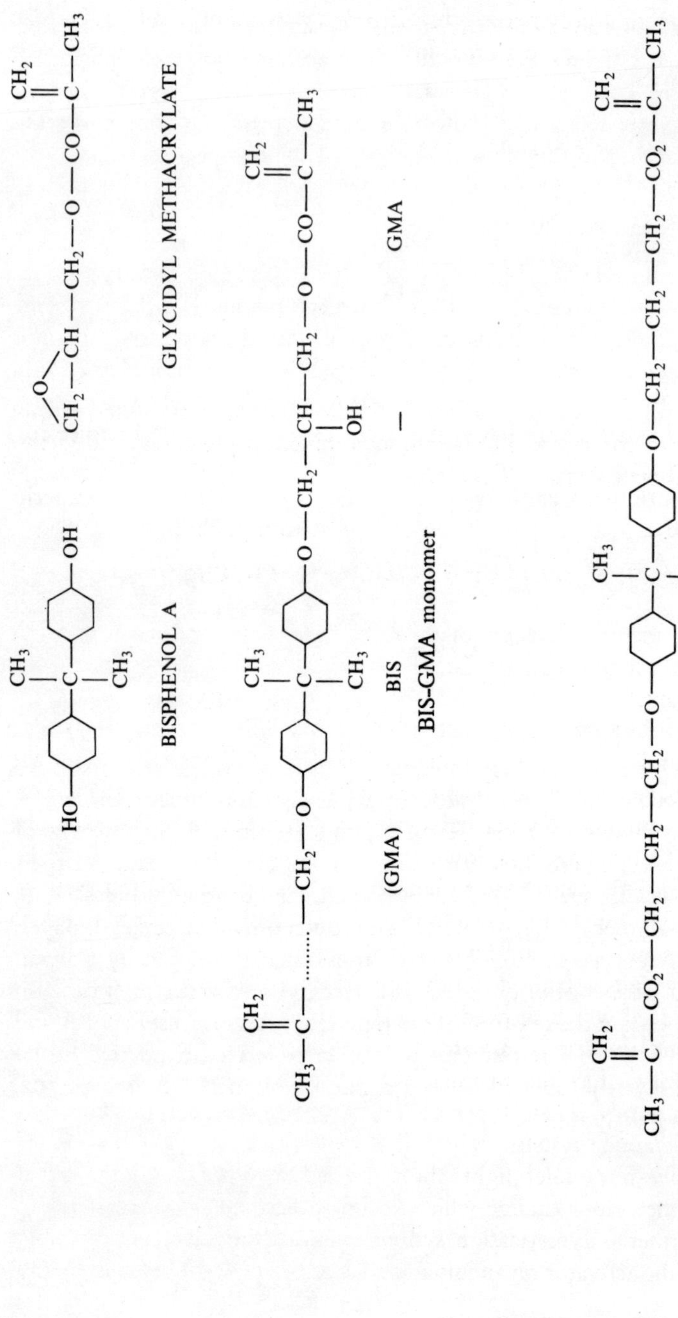

GLYCIDYL METHACRYLATE

GMA

BISPHENOL A

BIS

(GMA)

BIS-GMA monomer

BIS-EMA monomer

The monomer polymerizes through the double bonds at both ends of the chain, to produce a cross-linked structure (see p. 392, upper two diagrams).

Polymerization of BIS–GMA

Because of the viscosity of this pale yellow liquid, it is diluted with a di- or trimethacrylate. The commonest diluent at present is triethylene-glycol-dimethacrylate (TEDMA):

Methyl methacrylate or methacrylic acid have also been used as diluents. Methyl methacrylate, however, is volatile and both diluents are irritant.

Other dimethacrylates such as urethane dimethacrylate, have also been employed as the polymer matrix. The alternative monomers which have been, or are being developed, have fewer OH side chains and the resultant polymer has a lower water absorption. For example, BIS–EMA (see page 392, lower).

The materials also tend to be more colour stable. Some crystalline methacrylates have been produced experimentally which form eutectic mixtures and so remain fluid at room temperature whilst having low viscosity and volatility. In this way, a less viscous material could be produced which showed no change due to evaporation on storage or during the use of a batch of material. Also, the fact that they crystallize enables the manufacturing chemist to produce monomers of high purity. These types of monomer are also polymerized by a peroxide/amine system.

Usually ultraviolet light absorbers are incorporated in order to reduce the colour change which occurs in peroxide/amine systems.

A further polymerization system employs the effect of ultraviolet light as the activator on an initiator such as 1–2 per cent benzoin methyl ether. This initiator is normally added to the monomer shortly before use. Storage of monomer and initiator together is, however, satisfactory up to several days, dependent upon ambient temperature. Since polymerization does not start until the initiator is exposed to UV light, there is ample working time. After placement, the material is polymerized. However, the system is applicable only to layers of composite less than 1 mm thick as polymerization is very slow in thicker layers. Thus the filling has to be built up in successive layers, each of which is polymerized. The method allows, however, the use of a fluid mix.

Control of the wavelength of light emitted by the UV 'gun' is important and not always easy to maintain. The wavelength most suitable for activating benzoin methyl ether is about 365 nm. For some time it has been thought that tissue damage was only produced by radiations of wavelengths below 320 nm, but damage to the eye can follow exposure to radiations of 365 nm. It is wise, therefore, to handle the UV gun with care in case some unfiltered light of slightly lower wavelength escapes. Goggles for the patient or the operator are not necessary, but the end of the quartz rod which guides the light towards the tooth should never be viewed directly either by the operator or the patient.

Fillers

The fillers employed are taken from:

glasses	soda, barium, aluminosilicate
oxides	alumina, silica
synthetic materials	beta-eucryptite

These have varying coefficients of thermal expansion, all lower than polymethyl methacrylate. Beta-eucryptite has a negative coefficient. Fillers are incorporated in the composite from 60 to 80 per cent by weight, which is usually about 50 per cent by volume. The fillers may be in the form of irregular ground particles, or less frequently, as beads. Particle sizes range from 1–60 μm.

The use of barium-containing glasses overcomes to some extent the problem of radiopacity which arises when other fillers are used. When radiographing a restoration in a tooth, it is convenient if further decay shows up as a dark shadow on the X-ray as it does in relation to sound tooth structure. Thus the filling itself should have a radiopacity similar to tooth structure. Materials containing Al, Ta, La and Au as radiopaque fillers have also been developed experimentally.

To produce a strong composite, the filler and matrix must be bonded together. Then on stressing the filling, the more plastic or ductile matrix transfers stress to the stiffer filler which resists deformation. The surface of the filler may be treated with a silane coupling agent. Vinyl silanes were employed originally, but a stronger bond is achieved with γ-methacryloxypropyltrimethoxy silane. This bond is also more hydrolytically stable. Bonding of the matrix to this surface is then possible. The filler, after surface treatment, may also be coated with a thin layer of polymer. The latter method is said to produce better bonding between filler and matrix. Surface treatment of the filler also allows the use of a higher proportion of filler to polymer.

The working consistency, and the ease with which the material can be solidified within the cavity depends on the amount and the size, shape and size distribution of the filler particles. As in the case of amalgams, a correct selection of sizes makes the material easier to condense and reduces the amount of matrix.

Forms of presentation

Composite materials are available in two-paste, paste/liquid, single paste with initiator-impregnated pad, powder/liquid and capsulated forms. In the two-paste system, both pastes contain monomer and filler but one contains the activator and the other the initiator. The ratio of monomer to filler is therefore maintained although the initiator/activator ratio may vary. The peroxide-containing paste may have to be refrigerated because of its instability at warmer temperatures. Most paste materials should be stored below 25°C. In the paste/liquid systems, the liquid contains peroxide dissolved in glycol dimethacrylate. Dosing can be made with accuracy but it is difficult practically to incorporate a liquid with a stiff paste. Segregation of filler may occur on standing, but modern composites have additives to prevent this. However, if the material appears to change consistency on standing, it should be stirred.

One material, for the sake of convenience, is mixed on a pad impregnated with benzoyl peroxide but dosing of initiator by this method is not very accurate.

With the powder/liquid system, the shelf life is good, as the peroxide and filler are in the powder and therefore are not in contact with monomer. The peroxide itself can deteriorate, giving a slower set. The ratio of mixing, however, is variable and those properties affected by monomer/filler ratio can be changed. These are polymerization shrinkage, elastic modulus and coefficient of thermal expansion.

In the encapsulated form, the initiator and activator are each mixed with filler and are kept separate from each other and from the monomer until the capsule is broken or loaded. Some capsules can be converted to a syringe from which the mixed material is extruded. A high energy machine is necessary for mixing composites in capsules.

Consistency

The resultant consistency of mix in all methods of presentation depends upon the type of monomer system employed and the percentage of filler. Whilst stiff pastes can be handled more readily, there is a danger of non-cohesion of folded or added layers and the incorporation of air, creating voids. The more fluid mixes pack less easily but provide a more closely adapted and a more solid filling.

The rate of set of a composite material is of importance. It should have a pattern of setting similar to that recommended for alginates. That is, it should show an unchanging viscosity during its working time followed by a sudden snap set point. Materials which change viscosity and polymerize slowly are less easy to work since their consistency depends upon the time interval since mixing.

BIS-GMA systems set rapidly with an increase in viscosity as polymerization proceeds. Any delay will result in the application of a partially polymerized mix, which shows viscoelastic properties. Such a mix will recover partially on being packed into the cavity, and unless a matrix is applied which readapts it to the tooth, a space will be left between tooth and filling. The ease with which a cavity can be filled depends also on the way the material sticks to the packing instruments. Some materials pull away with the instrument, making it difficult to produce a solid restoration. Mechanical properties deteriorate to a considerable degree if the restoration contains air voids. This is particularly so if the voids are interconnected.

Rapid insertion of composites after mixing is necessary to obtain good adaptation, except for materials polymerized by UV light. However, with these materials, lack of bonding between successive layers may occur.

RETENTION TO TOOTH SUBSTANCE

Various suggestions for methods of attachment of polymeric materials to tooth dentine and enamel have been discussed in the literature. Both dentine and enamel consist largely of hydroxyapatite $Ca_{10}(PO_4)_6(OH)_2$. In dentine, this inorganic component comprises 75 per cent by weight. Whilst the presence of hydroxyapatite is confirmed by X-ray diffraction, evidence suggests that this is not the only mineral present. Calcium and magnesium carbonates have been detected, together with traces of sodium and chlorine. The remaining 25 per cent by weight of dentine is mainly collagen. Enamel, on the other hand, is almost entirely inorganic, only 0.25–0.45 per cent by weight being organic, mainly keratin. The organic component is least at the surface and increases towards the amelodentinal junction. The surface of enamel has been shown to contain F, Zn and Pb, while Mg and various carbonates are found in the deeper layers. Both dentine and enamel contain both loosely and firmly bound H_2O. Dentine is semipermeable and fluid seeps rapidly from cut dentinal tubules on to the surface of the cavity floor and walls.

The problem of obtaining adhesion is therefore one of dealing with wet surfaces, since it appears to be impossible to remove water entirely from tooth substance when the filling is being placed. In addition, it is impossible to maintain a dry environment for the completed filling not only at the mouth or occlusal surface of the cavity, but also where the restoration meets dentine on the cavity walls and floor. The need therefore is for an adhesive which has an affinity for the tooth surface greater than that of H_2O. It should be capable of displacing water molecules from the tooth surface and yet must be stable itself in a moist environment. It must not be affected by hydrolysis.

The various possibilities of bonding are therefore:

1. to hydroxyapatite by chelation or hydrogen bonds
2. to collagen via hydroxyl, carboxyl or amino groups
3. mechanical attachment.

Bonding to hydroxyapatite

Direct bonding of a restorative material to hydroxyapatite has shown little progress, though it is suggested that phosphonate-containing polymers could adhere to teeth by forming ionic bonds between hydroxyapatite and the phosphonate of the polymer. Suggestions have been made for *coupling agents* or *cavity primers*. These materials are designed to absorb on to and alter the surface of dentine or enamel and so enable a polymeric material in turn to be bonded to this initial layer. Perhaps the first coupling against was glycerophosphoric acid dimethacrylate incorporated in the cavity seal liquid used with an early direct filling resin. A surface active comonomer based upon a compound of N-phenyl glycine and glycidyl methacrylate (NPG-GMA) has been investigated, which is capable of chelating with the surface Ca^{2+} ions of tooth structure and which is potentially able to copolymerize with the monomers in composite materials. Another suggested method of adhesion is based on the use of a polyurethane which is a compound of polypropylene glycol and tolylene diisocyanate.

Interest has also been shown in the possible use of bioadhesives. The common sea mussel (*Mytilius edulis*) or the female lobster (*Homarus gammarus*) are able to attach themselves to almost any objects immersed in salt water including human enamel and dentine. Attempts have been made to analyse and reproduce the adhesive cement which these species form from their secretions since they are able to produce high adhesive forces in permanently wet conditions.

Bonding to collagen

The material which employs tributyl borane as a hardening agent can attach methyl methacrylate to collagen. Bonding is covalent by replacement of the hydrogen atom which is opposite the methyl group in collagen. After replacement of this atom by a suitable radical, this again is replaced by a radical from methyl methacrylate, thus achieving bonding.

However, although bonding has been proved experimentally, in a large number of cases it breaks down under moist conditions after a period of time. The most promising coupling agents or cavity primers appear to be those based on isocyanates.

Mechanical attachment

The main method of retention to enamel at present is mechanical, by the *acid etch technique*. Pre-treatment of the enamel surface with 30–60 per cent H_3PO_4 (3·5–7M) forms monocalcium phosphate monohydrate.

Sometimes 7 per cent of ZnO is added to reduce the acidity slightly. Higher concentrations of acid dissolve less apatite due to the formation of calcium phosphate hydrate. Citric acid is also used as an etchant and cleanser and has a similar effect to phosphoric acid. Lactic acid produces poor attachment. A thixotropic agent may be added to the acid to control the extent of its flow over the tooth.

This treatment of the enamel has several effects. It dissolves away both the prism cores and the interprismatic areas. Then, the monomeric composite matrix can penetrate into these irregular depressions creating 'tags' of polymer which offer numerous mechanical attachments. The tags formed are approximately 25 μm deep. They vary with the angulation of the enamel prisms at the surface and with the extent of the etching effect. The enamel margins may be bevelled to provide a larger area for etching and attachment. In various parts of the tooth there is prismless enamel and the tags are then inadequate to provide good mechanical retention. For this reason retention is poor on the surface enamel of deciduous teeth. Resistance to acid etching is probably related to the size of the crystallites of hydroxyapatite. Larger crystallites are more readily etched. The extent of acid etching is considered to be satisfactory when the enamel has a white chalky or frosted appearance. The quality of attachment of composites to enamel depends not only upon the depth and number of pits produced within the enamel, but also on the extent to which these are filled. In addition, the enamel must be dry and clean at the time the polymer is applied.

When using a colourless etching fluid, difficulties arise in seeing the precise area of application and in ensuring that no acid remains after etching is complete. To this end, one acid etch solution contains an indicator such as methyl violet which changes from green to violet as the pH increases. This indicates the extent of etching and in addition, enables one to see whether any etching solution remains on the tooth.

Etching increases the surface area available for attachment. It not only produces a pitted surface but also cleans the enamel surface removing debris and thus enabling the monomer to flow more readily over a debris-free surface. Acid etching also increases the surface energy of the enamel, thus increasing its wettability by the monomer base of the composite. A material of low viscosity flows more readily into the surface pits than one of high viscosity. With some materials, a preliminary coating of monomer, or a surface active copolymer in ethanol, is applied to the etched enamel surface to which the rest of the restoration bonds. With others, this is unnecessary.

Mechanical attachment to enamel prisms can be very effective. It is possible to attach an acrylic tooth between the enamel surfaces of the teeth on either side of a gap, and thus provide a 'bridge' to replace an anterior tooth, particularly in the lower jaw.

Acid etching techniques make the composites very useful for Class IV restorations with or without the use of pins. For example, in the treatment of a fractured incisor, the exposed dentine is protected by a $Ca(OH)_2$ cement. Then, the surrounding enamel is etched and a restoration attached to it, replacing the fractured portion of the tooth.

The use of composites to restore Class V abrasion cavities partly in dentine and cement is not advised as only one border of the restoration is of enamel. Attachment to dentine and cement even after acid etching is very poor. Normal cavity preparation giving retention for the restoration is therefore necessary. Acid treatment of dentine does not improve the attachment except by producing a clean debris-free surface, and since the acid is damaging to the pulp, it is not advised. In deep cavities particularly, it is advisable to protect the dentine with a layer of $Ca(OH)_2$ cement before etching the enamel. Then, if acid runs into the cavity, it will be prevented from entering the cut dentinal tubules on the floor of the cavity.

Care must be exercised in the use of 30–60 per cent H_3PO_4 to prevent damage to the patient's eyes, particularly when they are receiving treatment in the prone position. Open-necked bottles or the use of cotton wool pledglets is less safe than direct application from a plastic dispenser. If this has a small orifice and is flexible, the amount of acid released can be controlled.

Remineralization of the acid etched surface appears to take place within a few days of placing the restoration.

Attachment of composite fillings to the tooth can also be achieved by the use of pins inserted retentively into the dentine and round which the filling is polymerized. These pins do not strengthen, but weaken the restoration since there is no bonding between the pin and a composite material.

Mechanical properties

The modulus of elasticity and the strength of the PMMA-based materials is not as good as the newer materials based on aromatic dimethacrylates. However, lack of abrasion resistance, a property difficult to quantify, is a very important property in deciding the suitability of a composite, and the abrasion resistance of BIS-GMA-based composites appears to be less than that of PMMA-based materials. The BIS-GMA polymer matrix wears away leaving the filler particles standing proud and thus giving a rough surface. Eventually the filler particles fall out leaving pits in the surface of the restoration. Use of composites for Class I or Class II cavities is only advised where appearance is more important than longevity and even so, appearance deteriorates after a period of time.

On comparison with amalgam over a period of 2–3 years, composites have shown no higher incidence of fracture and marginal breakdown was slightly less.

Repair of composites by the replacement of a portion of their bulk generally produces a weaker restoration. If, however, care is taken to clean and dry the surface of the previous restoration and to apply a fluid consistency of new material in thin layers, the strength is adequate for clinical use.

Dimensional changes

There is no significant rise in temperature on polymerization but there is a volume shrinkage of approximately 0·7 per cent. Most materials polymerize in 4–5 minutes.

The linear coefficient of thermal expansion of composites is about a quarter of that of unfilled PMMA, but is still $2\frac{1}{2}$–3 times that of dentine. Accuracy of marginal fit is also affected by water absorption, which causes the materials to swell and so overcome polymerization contraction. With some materials water absorption is high and is accompanied by a moderately high solubility.

It has been shown that the strength of the enamel rods in tension is less than that of some composite materials. Thus, when composites are attached to enamel, damage to the enamel can occur when the composite material contracts on being cooled by food such as ice-cream. The polymer pulls away from the cavity margin taking with it broken fragments of enamel. Thus, unless the coefficient of expansion of tooth and filling are perfectly matched, tensile failure of the tooth substance could occur. On the other hand, it has been estimated that the tensile force that develops during polymerization is about 5 N/mm^2 and that the attachment should be of this order so that polymerization shrinkage goes towards the floor and walls of the cavity and not away from these surfaces. If such an initial attachment were produced, then it would ensure good filling of the cavity. Provided that the coefficients of expansion are matched and the cavity is retentive, then continuous adhesion after insertion of the filling may not be essential. It is usually suggested that water absorption with the accompanying expansion makes up for any initial marginal discrepancies. On the other hand, if one could create a slightly plastic or rubbery adhesive bond, then it would overcome slight dimensional changes and so maintain the bond by reducing the stresses set up at the interface. Cavity liners based on butyl or propyl methacrylate have been suggested.

Finishing

Finishing the filling must be left for at least 24 hours, otherwise a danger exists of pulling the partly polymerized material away from the cavity margins. Since most composites swell by water absorption, there are advantages in leaving the restoration unfinished for a week. By then, expansion will have closed any gaps between restoration and tooth, and finishing of the edge is possible. A smooth surface can only be produced by a matrix band of polyester or polythene, and it is extremely difficult to repolish the surface after trimming. The matrix and filler differ markedly in abrasive properties and difficulties exist in both producing and maintaining a smooth surface. Materials containing fine filler particles are easier to finish than those containing coarser particles. Air, which is often trapped within the more viscous mixes, produces voids which collect stain when they appear on the surface. In addition, unless care is taken in selecting the abrasive, an efficient abrasive will also trim the adjacent enamel surface. A 12-bladed tungsten carbide bur rotating at low speed under a water spray is probably preferable to a diamond abrasive as the bur leaves a smoother surface. Abrasives such as garnet for coarse finishing, followed by aluminium oxide and zirconium silicate are used on discs and polishing strips. Fine polishing with strips or discs coated with 1–5 μm diamond particles is also effective. An alternative method of producing a smooth surface is to revarnish the filling with a non-filled monomer polymerized by any of the methods including the use of ultraviolet light. However, surface roughness always occurs later when filler particles fall out from the surface. All composites attain a surface roughness characterized by the particle size of the filler, irrespective of the surface finish immediately after placement.

Effect on the pulp

Since many materials affect the pulp to a moderate degree, protection by $Ca(OH)_2$ cement is advised where only a thin layer of dentine remains over the pulp. Alternatively a phosphate or polycarboxylate cement can be used. Cavity varnishes can be used with some materials, but reduce the degree of polymerization of others. Whilst ZOE cement does not interfere with the polymerization of all materials, it produces an apparent darkening of colour in time, as well as a reduction in transverse strength of some materials. Recent ZOE cement linings should therefore be covered with a layer of a non-eugenol cement.

Appearance

The translucency and colour of composites depends on the optical properties of both matrix and filler. Some materials are available in one shade only, on the basis of their translucency. Others are available in several shades, or the basic shade can be combined with shaders. Colour stability is affected by the activator system used and by the presence of hydroquinone as a stabilizer for monomer. The replacement of hydroquinone by butylated hydroxytoluene has been suggested, as have other activator systems. Impurities in the BIS-GMA monomer may cause darkening. The incorporation of ultraviolet light absorbers reduces the rate of colour change.

Typical properties:

Tensile strength	24 hr	30–50 N/mm^2
Compressive strength	24 hr	200–400 N/mm^2
Transverse strength	24 hr	60–100 N/mm^2
Modulus of elasticity	24 hr	10–15 $\times$ 10^3 N/mm^2
KHN		40–50
Polymerization shrinkage, volume		1·5 $\pm$ 0·5%
Coefficient of thermal expansion		24 $\times$ 10^{-6}/°C
Water absorption	24 hr	0·5–0·4%

PRESENT SITUATION

There has been continuous development of composite materials over the last two decades. At present they are used mainly in Class III, IV and V restorations. Secondary decay is not reduced to the same extent as it is with silicate fillings though some composites have been shown to release F slowly. The possibility of excessive abrasion limits their use in Class I and II cavities in molar and premolar teeth though some materials are recommended by manufacturers for this purpose. Where people respire through their mouths, the life of silicate cement restorations is extremely short and composites are more suitable. Composites may also be used for changing the contours of tooth enamel buccally or lingually and so improve their shape for the retention of partial dentures by clasps.

The main difference between the presently available composites are their variations in shelf life, the viscosity of the mix (related to its capacity for wetting the surface detail of both enamel and dentine), the ease with which the material can be placed in position and its working time and simplicity of curing. Staining of the surface occurs with all materials in time due to the difficulty of maintaining a polished surface.

On comparison with amalgams, the composites appear to retain their finish at the cavity margins, but lose contour elsewhere.

'FISSURE SEALANTS' (TOOTH VARNISHES)

Decay usually starts in fissures on the occlusal surfaces of teeth or at contact points where plaque can remain unless oral hygiene is good. Various varnishes have been suggested based on polymeric systems similar to those employed both for composite filling materials and for coupling agents. Glass ionomer and polycarboxylate cements have also been used as fissure sealants.

To be effective, a fissure sealant should not only do what its name implies, but it should also be usable as a varnish on other caries-prone areas of the teeth, e.g. the interproximal contacts. To seal fissures and the enamel surface the varnish should adhere to enamel, it should have a cariostatic action and should be resistant to oral acids and abrasion, as well as being simple to use and non-toxic.

Cyanoacrylate adhesives appeared at first to be promising. These materials polymerize when spread to a thin film in the presence of water vapour. An autopolymerizing polyurethane material containing 10 per cent sodium monofluorophosphate has also been used. Attachment of this material was not good. However, it did offer the possibility of the slow release of F over a period of time. However, most of the present day polymeric 'fissure sealants' are made from monomers based on BIS-GMA. Usually for use as a fissure sealant, this monomer is diluted with methyl methacrylate. Synthetic hydroxyapatite and CaF_2 may be incorporated in the monomer. Polymerization is either by the amine/peroxide or the ultraviolet light/benzoin methyl ether system.

Acid etching, followed by drying of the enamel, is essential for the use of these varnishes and it appears that retention is again mainly by attachment. Whilst the materials show good attachment, they do not necessarily seal the surface against carious attack as there is no adhesion, only attachment, between the 'sealant' and the enamel. The sealer polymerized by a UV sensitive activator polymerizes further during its life though it absorbs water which plasticizes the film at the same time. The amine/peroxide polymerized materials appear to cure a little faster. The dimensional changes which follow water absorption and solubility affect the permanence of these varnishes. The water absorption may be reduced by the use of a monomer with a lower concentration of OH side chains.

Materials based on plain methyl methacrylate show in general a shorter clinical life than those based on BIS-GMA.

Films of sealant based on BIS-GMA appear to have a life of at least one year. In some cases they appear to wear away in 3–6 months. They have been shown, however, to be effective in reducing the amount of carious attack, particularly in the teeth of young persons. Success with the use of fissure sealants, however, appears to vary considerably between different operators. It is rather difficult to detect when the sealant remains or when it has been lost. In all cases the material is reduced in bulk within a year by abrasion of masticated foodstuffs. There is some evidence that the tags of polymer within the enamel surface may remain after the superficial layer has been abraded away. In addition, it appears that the $25\mu m$ layer of enamel into which the tags of polymer protrude is not subject to demineralization even when the surrounding untreated enamel is grossly etched again by an acid. Thus the protective effect of the tags may continue after the surface layer has been worn away and can no longer be readily detected. This difficulty probably accounts for the variations in success reported in the literature.

There is some evidence to support the argument that a small carious lesion at the base of a fissure could be arrested by the application of a sealant. Etching does not affect the enamel within the fissure, due to the presence of debris, but the sealant in this area could be retained (as is a composite restoration in the acid etching technique) by attachment to the surrounding enamel. Since the polymeric sealants are not bonded to the tooth surface, but only attached mechanically, there is, however, a possibility of leakage, particularly at the bottom of a fissure.

CYANOACRYLATE ADHESIVES

Cyanoacrylate adhesives have been used instead of suturing after surgery. A suitable medical grade cyanoacrylate is applied in a thin film where it polymerizes *in situ* holding the tissues together. It is important that there is no tension on the wound at the time. Biological degradation occurs in time as the tissues heal. The rate of degradation is related to the type of cyanocrylate which is employed. Methyl-2-cyanocrylate produces inflammation on degradation and the higher homologues are better. Isobutyl cyanoacrylate has a low biodegradability. The irritation from these materials is due to the fact that they liberate formaldehyde and cyanoacetate which are both toxic materials. Since these materials are biodegradable, it is understandable why their use as adhesives has only been short-lived in its application to the development of tooth restorative materials.

They have a limited use as lutes in the attachment of orthodontic appliances, as they fail in the moist oral environment. When used as pulp-capping agents, they fail to produce satisfactory dentine barriers. These adhesives have been used for retaining pins in dentine. Whilst they are convenient to use, the retention of the pin is less than that achieved by the use of Zn phosphate or polycarboxylate cements. Their use for denture repairs has already been discussed in Chapter 24.

POLYMERIC CEMENTS

These are either superfine acrylic polymers, a BIS-GMA comonomer mixed with a fine glass filler, or a powder/liquid composite of fluid consistency similar to those used for fillings. Polymerization is activated in the same manner as in the filling materials.

Their adhesion to acrylic restorations is good, and they may be used for cementing metal restorations in the mouth. In the thin sections of a cement layer, the dimensional changes of the material are not so important, while their solubility is less than that of the phosphate cements.

As with direct filling materials, the use of phenol and eugenol in the cavity is contra-indicated.

Usually these materials contain a high proportion of radiopaque filler which increases the strength of the resultant cement. It also prevents the appearance of apparent cavities at the edge of a restoration when an X-ray of an inlay or crown is taken.

Difficulties arise, however, in trimming away the excess cement at the edges of the restoration. Working time tends to be short with the acrylic cements and, since a crust readily forms on the mixed cement as monomer evaporates, wetting of the two surfaces to be cemented is poor. In addition, the crust on the surface creates difficulties of compressing the cement to a thin layer. Under ideal circumstances, a film of 10μm can be produced, but this is difficult to obtain in clinical practice. These cements have the advantage of relative insolubility. Thus if an inaccurately fitting restoration must be cemented into place, the large cement gap is filled more permanently by a composite cement than by other dental cements.

Pulpal irritation can be more severe than with Zn phosphate cements and in addition, water absorption into the acrylic cement occurs. Composite type cements are thus more suitable for cementation purposes in non-vital teeth.

Appendix

INTERNATIONAL SPECIFICATIONS AND RECOMMENDATIONS

ISO R 1559	Alloy for dental amalgam
ISO R 1560	Dental mercury
ISO R 1561	Dental inlay casting wax
ISO R 1562	Dental casting gold alloy
ISO R 1563	Alginate impression material
ISO R 1564	Agar impression material
ISO R 1565	Dental silicate cement
ISO R 1566	Dental zinc phosphate cement
ISO R 1567	Denture base polymer
ISO R 1795	Dental burs and cutters—fitting dimensions
ISO 1942	Dental vocabulary—List I, Basic terms
	List II, Dental materials
ISO 2157	Dental burs and cutters—nominal sizes and designation of working parts
ISO 3107	Dental zinc oxide/eugenol cementing materials

BRITISH STANDARD SPECIFICATIONS

2487	Denture base polymer
2585	Dimensions of dental X-ray films
2938	Dental amalgam alloy (silver–tin)
2965	Dental chisels, excavators, probes and scalers
2983	Hypodermic dental needles
3364	Dental zinc phosphate cement
3365	Dental silicate cement and dental silico–phosphate cement
	Part I. Silicate cements
	Part II. Silico-phosphate cements
3366	Dental cobalt chromium casting alloy
3384	Dental gold solders
3421	Performance of electrically heated sterilizing ovens
3507	Orthodontic wire and tape and dental ligature wire made of stainless steel

3508	Dental inlay casting wax
3520	Dental wrought precious metal alloy wire
3531	Metal surgical implants, drills and screwdrivers used for bone surgery
	Part. I. Materials for metal surgical implants
3886	Dental impression compound
3990	Acrylic resin teeth
4106	Surgical stainless steel monofilament wire. Fully softened
4178	Dental rotary instruments
	Part 1. Dimensions of shanks and chuck fittings
	Part 2. Shapes and sizes of heads of dental burs
4222	Dimensions of the transmission coupling (slip-joint) to dental handpieces
4227	Dental mercury
4269	Dental elastic impression materials
	Part 1. Elastomeric impression material
	Part 2. Alginate impression material
4284	Dental zinc oxide/eugenol impression material
4425	Dental casting gold alloy
4492	Glossary of terms relating to dentistry
4598	Dental impression plaster
4681	Mouth mirrors and mouth mirror handles
4722	Dental laboratory plaster
4750	Dental extracting forceps (performance requirements)
4796	Dental artificial stone
4824	Fibrelight cables and fittings for surgical equipment
5136	Toothpastes
5189	Dental casting investments
	Part 1. Gypsum-bonded investment materials
	Part 2. Phosphate–bonded dental casting invest ments
	Part 3. Ethyl silicate–bonded dental casting investment
5199	Resin-based dental filling materials
5211	Popular patterns of dental extracting forceps

AMERICAN DENTAL ASSOCIATION
SPECIFICATIONS

| 1. | Alloy for dental amalgam |
| 2. | Casting investment for dental gold alloy |

3.	Dental impression compound
4.	Dental inlay casting wax
5.	Dental casting gold alloy
6.	Dental mercury
7.	Dental wrought gold wire alloy
8.	Dental zinc phosphate cement
9.	Dental silicate cement
11.	Dental agar impression material
12.	Denture base polymer
13.	Denture self-curing repair resin
14.	Dental chromium–cobalt casting alloy
15.	Acrylic resin teeth
16.	Dental impression paste—zinc oxide-eugenol type
17.	Denture base temporary relining resin
18.	Alginate impression material
19.	Elastomeric impression material
20.	Dental duplicating material
21.	Dental zinc silico-phosphate cement
22.	Dental radiographic film
23.	Dental excavating burs
24.	Dental base plate wax
25.	Dental gypsum products
26.	Dental X-ray equipment

AUSTRALIAN STANDARDS

T2	Amalgam alloy
T6	Modelling compound
T16	Agar impression material
T18	Impression paste
T19	Local anaesthetics
T22	Casting investment
T24	Hypodermic needles
T28	Cobalt–chromium casting alloys
T31	Denture repair resin (cold-cure)
T32	Orthodontic wires
T36	Medical syringes
T42	Re-usable hypodermic needles
1022	Rubber dam

1032	Toothbrushes
1043	Denture base
1086	Chisels, excavators, probes and scalers
1093	Shanks and chuck fittings for rotary instruments
1097	Duplicating material
1139	Intra-oral X-ray films
1185	Elastomeric impression materials
1186	Zinc phosphate cement
1240	Latex elastic bands for orthodontic use
1241	Dental shellac baseplates
1253	Orthodontic band cements
1258	Gutta percha points
1264	Single-use hypodermic cartridge needles
1278	Direct filling composite material
1282	Alginate impression material
1453	Modelling wax
1454	Silicate (and silico-phosphate cements)
1581	Mercury
1582	Inlay casting wax
1583	Sticky wax
1616	Artificial stone
1620	Inlay casting gold. Denture casting golds
1622	Silver solder
1623	Gold solder
1625	Wrought golds
1626	Acrylic teeth
1651	Impression plaster
1652	Laboratory plaster

Conversion factors

in to mm	×	25·4
in² to mm²	×	645·16
in³ to m³	×	0·0164
oz to g	×	28·35
lb to kg	×	0·454
lb to N	×	4·45
psi to kg/mm²	×	0·0007
psi to N/mm²	×	0·00689
fl oz (Brit) to ml	×	28·41

mm to in	×	0.039
mm² to in²	×	0·00155
m³ to in³	×	60·98
g to oz	×	0·03527
kg to lb	×	2·205
N to lb	×	0·225
kg/mm² to psi	×	1422
N/mm³ to psi	×	145·04
ml to fl oz (Brit)	×	0·035

Prefixes to indicate multiples and submultiples of units

M	mega	10^6
k	kilo	10^3
m	milli	10^{-3}
μ	micro	10^{-6}

Elements

Ag	Silver	Mo	Molybdenum
Al	Aluminium	Mg	Magnesium
Au	Gold	Ni	Nickel
B	Boron	P	Phosphorus
Ba	Barium	Pb	Lead
Be	Beryllium	Pd	Palladium
Bi	Bismuth	Pt	Platinum
C	Carbon	Rh	Rhodium
Cd	Cadmium	Ru	Ruthenium
Co	Cobalt	S	Sulphur
Cr	Chromium	Sb	Antimony
Cu	Copper	Si	Silicon
Fe	Iron	Sn	Tin
Ga	Gallium	Ta	Tantalum
Hg	Mercury	Ti	Titanium
In	Indium	W	Tungsten
Ir	Iridium	Zn	Zinc
La	Lanthanum		

Compounds

Al_2O_3	Aluminium oxide
$AlPO_4$	Aluminium phosphate
$Al(OH)_3$	Aluminium hydroxide
BaF_2	Barium fluoride
$BaSO_4$	Barium sulphate
C_2H_5OH	Ethyl alcohol
$CaCl_2$	Calcium chloride
CaF_2	Calcium fluoride
CaO	Calcium oxide
CaS	Calcium sulphide
$CaSiO_3$	Calcium silicate
$CaSO_4$	Calcium sulphate
$Ca_{10}(PO_4)_6(OH)_2$	Hydroxyapatite
$Ca(OH)_2$	Calcium hydroxide
$Ca(PO_4)_2$	Calcium phosphate
CO	Carbon monoxide
Cr_2O_3	Chromium oxide
Cr_4C	Chromium carbide
$CuSO_4$	Copper sulphate
Fe_2O_3	Ferric oxide
H_2O_2	Hydrogen peroxide
H_2S	Hydrogen sulphide
H_2SO_4	Sulphuric acid
H_3BO_3	Boric acid
H_3PO_4	Phosphoric acid
HCl	Hydrochloric acid
HCN	Hydrocyanic acid
HF	Hydrofluoric acid
HNO_3	Nitric acid
K_2SO_4	Potassium sulphate
$K_2SO_4.Al_2(SO_4)_3$	Potassium aluminium sulphate (potash alum)
$KAg(CN)_2$	Potassium silver cyanide
$KAu(CN)_2$	Potassium aurocyanide
KCl	Potassium chloride
KCN	Potassium cyanide
KF	Potassium fluoride
KHF_2	Acid potassium fluoride

$KHSO_4$	Potassium hydrogen sulphate
MgO	Magnesium oxide
$NaCl$	Sodium chloride
$NaOH$	Sodium hydroxide
$Na_2B_4O_7$	Sodium borate (borax)
Na_2SO_4	Sodium sulphate
Na_3PO_4	Sodium phosphate
$NaHCO_3$	Sodium bicarbonate
NaH_2PO_4	Sodium hydrogen phosphate
NH_4Cl	Ammonium chloride
$NiCl_2$	Nickel chloride
$NiSO_4$	Nickel sulphate
$NH_4H_2PO_4$	Ammonium phosphate
PbO_2	Lead dioxide
SiO_2	Silica
SO_2	Sulphur dioxide
TiO_2	Titanium dioxide
WC	Tungsten carbide
$Zn_3(PO_4)_2$	Zinc phosphate
$ZnCl_2$	Zinc chloride
ZnO	Zinc oxide
ZnS	Zinc sulphide
$Zn(OH)_2$	Zinc hydroxide

Further reading

There has been a large volume of literature published on dental materials science since the last edition, and an adequate bibliography would extend to many pages, increasing the cost of this book. If similar activity continues during the next five or six years, many references would become out of date rather rapidly. No detailed bibliography is therefore given but the following texts and summary articles are a good source of references to previous work.

CHALIAN, V.A. and PHILIPS, R.W. (1974) Materials in maxillofacial prosthetics. *J. biomed. mat. Res. Symp*, **5**, 349.

COMBE, E.C. (1975) *Notes on dental materials*. 2nd ed. Churchill Press, London.

CRAIG, R.G. *and others* (1975) *Dental materials: properties and manipulation*. C.V. Mosby Co., St Louis.

CRAIG, R.G. and PEYTON, F.A. (1975) *Restorative dental materials*. 5th ed. C.V. Mosby Co., St Louis.

CRANIN, A.N. *and others* (1974) The present status of endosteal oral implants. *J. biomed. mat. Res. Symp*, **5**, 385

GREENER, E.H. *and others* (1972) *Materials science in dentistry*. Williams and Wilkins, Baltimore.

GUIDE TO DENTAL MATERIALS AND DEVICES (1974) Ed. 7. *Am. dent. Ass*, Chicago.

LAWRENCE, W.H. *and others* (1974) Development of a toxicity evaluation program for dental materials and products. *J. biomed. mat. Res*, **8**, 11.

PAFFENBARGER, G.C. (1972) Dental cements, direct filling resins, composite and adhesive restorative materials: a resumé. *J. biomed. mat. Res. Symp*, **2**, part **2**, 363.

PAFFENBARGER, G.C. and RUPP, N.W. (1974) Composite restorative materials in dental practice: a review. *Int. dent. J.*, **24**, 1.

PHILIPS, R.W. (1973) *Skinner's Science of dental materials*. 7th ed. W.B. Saunders, Philadelphia.

PROGRAM AND ABSTRACTS OF PAPERS (1975) *J. dent. Res.*, **54**, special issue A.

VON FRAUNHOFER, J.A. (1975) *Scientific aspects of dental materials*. Butterworth, London.

Index

Abrasion 291
  linear speed 293
  types of abrasive 296
  of acrylic teeth 285
Acid etch technique 398, 405
Acrylic cements 406
Acrylic crowns 287, 312
Acrylic denture base
  allergy 261
  copolymers 249, 266, 278
  crazing 262, 276
  dimensional changes 261, 272
  fluid resin 273
  injection moulding 254, 260
  mechanical properties 264, 272
  molecular weight 260
  mould seal, effects of 263, 282
  notch sensitivity 265
  plasticizer 249
  polymerization 255
  porosity 256
  processing cycle 259
  radiopacity 267
  rebasing 270, 275
  repairs 268, 274
  residual monomer 260, 273
  silicone-rubber mould 253
  strengthening 266
  surface treatment 268
Acrylic teeth 283
  bleaching and crazing 285
  union with denture base 273, 284, 286
Acrylamide gel 230
Addition polymerization 13

Adhesion (see also bonding) 34, 41, 107
Adhesives
  for alginates 223
  for denture repair 269
  for polysulphide rubber 235
  for silicone rubber 240
Age hardening 70
Airbrasive 294
Alginate impression materials 218
  adhesives 223
  cast surface 225, 226
  flow 220
  pH 226
  properties of 227
  storage 225
Allergic reaction 243, 261, 301
Alloplastic implant 318
Alloys 58
  eutectic 65
  fusible 126
  solid solution 62
  for implants 314
  for partial dentures 95
Alpha-hemihydrate 202
Alumina 297, 304
Alumina porcelain 308
Aluminium bronze 100
Amalgam (silver–tin) 329
  alloy: mercury ratio 336
  capsulated 336, 345
  condensation 339, 345
  contamination 341
  corrosion 343
  dies 321

dimensional changes 347
ditched filling 346
flow and creep 346
high and low silver 330
mercuroscopic expansion 346
non-zinc alloy 331, 342
pain under 342
particle size and shape 335
pins in 345
properties 349
setting reaction 332
spherical particles 335
splat-cooled 335
strength 345
trimming and polishing 342
Amalgam, copper 349
American Dental Association Speci-
    fications 410
Anelasticity 24
Annealing 56
    gold alloy 80, 88
    inlay wax 156
    stainless steel 117
Anodizing 152
Antiflux 130
Artificial stone 201
Atomic packing 9
Attachment (see also bonding) 34
    of implants 314
    of phosphate cement 367
Australian Standards 411
Autogenous welding 139

Back pressure effect 107, 185
Baseplate materials 157
Be in Co–Cr alloys 315
Beilby layer 50, 147, 299
Benzoyl peroxide 249, 255, 271
Binary alloy 58
Bioadhesives 398
Biochemical degradation of poly-
    mers 317, 406
Bioglass implant 314
BIS–GMA monomer 392, 393
Bismuth glass in PMMA 267
Blade-vent implant 315, 320
Blowpipe flame 131
Body-centred cubic 10, 12, 15
Bonding 34

glass ionomer cement 386
metal/ceramic 107
old and new amalgam 349
old and new gypsum 204
polycarboxylate cement 362
teeth and base 273, 284, 286
to collagen 398
to hydroxyapatite 397
Bonds
    covalent 7
    dipole 8
    directional 9, 10
    hydrogen 9
    ionic 7
    metallic 8
Brazilian tensile test 22
Brinell hardness 27
British Standard Specifications 409
Brittleness 23, 25
Bulk modulus 23
Burnishing 300, 343

Calcium hydroxide cement 354
Candida albicans 279
Carat 74
Carbon fibres 266, 317
Carbon steel 112
Cast iron 110
Casting
    asbestos liner 177
    compensation for shrinkage 175
    dimensions 97
    sprue reservoirs 186
    sprues 183
Casting defects 182
    back pressure 107, 185
    finning 181
    force 182
    porosity 185
Cathode 142
Cavity cleaning 327
Cavity finish 294
Cavity primer 354, 398
Cavity sealing technique 388
Cavity varnish 348, 353
Cement lute, thickness of 148, 310,
    363, 368, 383, 407
Chelation 210, 360
Chromium steel 113

Close-packed hexagon 10, 12, 15
Cobalt–chromium alloy 90
  compared with gold 96
  investments for 171
  soldering 138
  for implants 315
Coefficient of expansion 31
  of composite 401, 404
  of dentine, enamel 327
Cohesive gold foil 71
Cold work 54, 56
Colour temperatures 132
Composites 66, 317, 390
  consistency 396
  forms of presentation 395
  pins in 400
Compressive strength 24
  amalgam 349
  dentine and enamel 327
  glass ionomer cement 386
  gypsum 198, 201, 203
  investment 168, 170, 178
  lining cement 353
  phosphate cement 371
  polycarboxylate cement 363
  porcelain 308
  silicate cement 382
Condensation
  amalgam 339
  gold foil 72
  porcelain 305
Condensation polymerization 13
Constitutional diagram 61
Contact angle 34, 108, 179, 353
Conversion factors 413
Cooling curve
  alloy 59
  impression compound 208
  wax 155
Copolymerization 14, 249, 266, 278, 285
Copper amalgam 321, 349
Copper phosphate cement 371
Copper plating 145, 322
Coring 62
Corrosion 148
  crevicular 137
  electrolytic 148, 149
  intergranular 136

of amalgam 343
of instruments 112
of stainless steel 114, 136, 315
Coupling agents 398
Covalent bond 7, 108
Creep 30, 40, 102, 346
Cristobalite investment 131, 164, 177
Cross-linking 14
  in alginate 219, 221
  in denture bases 247, 263, 266, 271
  in polyether rubber 242
  in polysulphide rubber 233
  in silicone rubber 237
Crystal structure 12
Crystalline methacrylates 393
Current density 143
Current for spot welding 140
Cyanoacrylate adhesive 269, 404, 406

Decomposition of investment 169
Degassing 108
Delayed expansion 341
Dendritic growth 45
Densite 202, 323
Density 32, 40
Dental plaque 291
Dental porcelain 303
  changes on firing 306
  structure 308
  uranium compounds in 305
Dental vibrators 195
Dentifrice 300
Denture cleansers 300
Denture wax 157
Dermatitis 239, 252, 288
Devitrified glass 311
Dimensions of castings 97
Dipole bond 8
Direct filling acrylic 387
Direct pattern 159, 175
Dislocation 53
Dispersion strengthener 333
Ditched amalgam 346
Double-investment technique 180
Doughing time 251
Ductility 24, 39
Duplicating material 230

EBA (ethoxybenzoic acid) cement 356
Elastic bands 246
Elastic limit 21
Elasticity 22
Electrodeposition 142, 321
Electrolytic corrosion 148, 149
Electrolytic polishing 147
Elongation percentage 21
Epimine polymer 288
Etching of metals 50
Ethyl methacrylate 278
Ethyl silicate 171
Eutectic alloy 65
Eutectoid 68, 93
Expansion 31, 33
    of amalgam 347
    of gypsum 193
    of investment 176

Face-centred cubic 10, 12, 15
Fatigue strength 26, 39, 121, 264, 268, 272, 316
Filling materials
    desirable properties 326
    uses 352
Fineness 74
Fissure sealant 385, 404
Flame temperatures 131
Flexibility 23
Flow 30, 40
    alginate 220
    amalgam 346
    denture base 272
    impression compound 206
    impression paste 212
    tissue conditioner 214
    wax 156, 214
Fluid resin technique 273
Flux 129
Fortified ZOE cement 356
Functional impression material 215

Gallium 331
Galvanic current 99
Galvanic pain 150
Gaseous porosity of PMMA 256
Germicidal cement 383
Gillmore needles 192

Glass ionomer cement 383
    manipulation 385
    properties 386
Glaze, porcelain 305
Glycol dimethacrylate 248
Gold alloys 74
    carat or fineness 74
    compared with Co–Cr 96
    metal/ceramic 103
    white 86
    wrought 79
    yellow casting 80
Gold foil 71, 73
Gold plating 137, 146
Gold in amalgam alloy 334
Graft copolymer 14
Grain boundaries 45
    impurities in 54
Grain growth 57, 88
    on soldering 133
Grain structure 45
    deformation of 53
    dendrites 45
    size of 47, 187
Granularity 258
Graphite fibre 266, 317
Gutta-percha 288
Gypsum 190
    in alginate 219
    in investment 164, 167
Gypsum-bonded investment 163
    dies 323
    properties 170

Hardness 27, 29, 39
Heat generated by abrasives 295
Heat treatment
    hardening 68
    softening 56
    solder joints 135
    white gold 88
    yellow gold casting alloy 80
HEMA 266, 279
High frequency induction melting 92, 104
Homogenizing anneal 63, 81, 104, 335
Hydraulic forming of stainless steel 117

Hydrocal 202
Hydrocolloid impression material 216
  electroplating of 321
  irreversible 218
  reversible 227
  stress-relief 225, 229
  syneresis 217, 218, 225, 229
Hydrogen bond 9
Hydroxyapatite 319, 360, 398
Hygroscopic expansion 165, 180

Imbibition 217
Imino (aziridino) polymer 242
Impact strength 25, 39, 264
Impression compound 205
Impression paste, ZOE 209
  non-eugenol 211
Impression plaster 197
Impression wax 213
Indicators in alginate 220
Indirect inlay 321
  patterns 160, 175
Indium
  in amalgam 332
  in gold alloy 78
  in silicate cement 374
Initiation phase 255
Injection moulding 254
Injection of thermoplastic polymers 390
Inlay wax 158
  properties of 161
Intergranular corrosion of stainless steel 136
Intermetallic compound 66
  Ag_3Sn 330
International Specifications 409
Interpenetrating polymer networks 264, 272
Inversion change of silica 167, 169, 177
Investment soldering 130
Investment
  cristobalite 131, 167, 177
  decomposition of 169
  gypsum-bonded 106, 163, 177
  particle size and permeability 107, 169, 185
  phosphate-bonded 106, 173
  setting expansion 164, 173
  silica-bonded 171
  strength 170, 173
  thermal expansion 166, 177
Ionic bond 7, 103, 108

Knoop hardness 28

Laser beam 131, 132, 138, 139
Lead
  in alginate 219
  in polysulphide rubber 233
Lingual bar dimensions 97
Liquid state 6
Liquidus 61
Loads for spot welding 140
Low silver amalgam alloy 330

Malleability 24
Marginal percolation 389
Mat gold 71
Mechanical amalgamation 337
  condensation 339
Melting points of metals 32
Mercaptan rubber 232
Mercuroscopic expansion 346
Mercury hygiene 344, 350
Metal/ceramic bond 107
Metal spraying of dies 322
Metallic bond 8
Metallography 48
Metalloid 44
Microcharacter tester 30
Midline fracture of PMMA 265
Modified cutlery steel 115
Modulus of elasticity 22, 38
Moh's scale 29
Molecular weight
  acrylic polymer 260
  polyacrylic acid 360, 384

Newton—definition of 17
Ni sensitivity 91
Nickel-chromium
  casting alloy 99, 105
  wire 119
Nickel plating 145
Non-cohesive gold 72

Non-eugenol impression material 211
Non-zinc amalgam alloy 331, 342
Notch sensitivity of PMMA 265
Nystatin in tissue conditioning material 215

Occlusal rest dimension 97
Order hardening 64, 68, 75
Orthodontic elastic bands 246
Oxy-acetylene flame 92, 132

Palatal bar dimensions 97
Palladium
  alloys for metal/ceramic 105
  in white gold 86
  in yellow gold 77
Paraffin wax 154
Particle size of investment 107, 169
Passive layer 90, 116, 151
Peritectic reaction 67, 329
Permeability of investment 107, 169, 171, 185
pH of alginate 226
  calcium hydroxide cement 354
  glass ionomer cement 386
  silicate cement 381, 382
  zinc polycarboxylate cement 362
  ZOE cement 357
  zinc phosphate cement 368
Phosphate-bonded investment 104, 106, 173, 231
  for dies 323
Pigmentation of PMMA 249
Pin implant 320
Plaster 190
  expansion 193
  impression 197
  initial and final set 192
  joint between two mixes 204
  retarders and accelerators 198
  solubility 197
  soluble 200
  strength, wet and dry 196
  for casts 201
  in alginate 219
  in investment 164, 167
Plasticizer 249
Platinum

in gold alloy 77, 84
  in wrought wire 79
Poisson's ratio 24
Polarization 143, 144, 147, 151
Polishing 299
  amalgam 342
  composite 402
  electrolytic 147
  silicate cement 378
Polyacrylate cement 360
Polyester dies 324
Polyethyl methacrylate 288
Polyether rubber 242
  accuracy of 230, 243
  properties of 243
Polymeric cement 406
Polymerization
  addition, condensation 13
  degree of 272
  effect of eugenol on 270, 275, 389, 403
  inhibition of 248
  initiation of 255
  shrinkage during 256, 388, 391, 401
  temperature rise during 257, 272, 401
  under air pressure 273, 275
  under water pressure 275
Polymers 11
  thermo-hardening, thermo-set 15
  as implants 316, 320
Polystyrene
  copolymers 266
  in ZOE cement 356
Polysulphide rubber 232
  properties of 236
Polyurethane 280
Porcelain 303
  accuracy of fit of crowns 310
  alumina 308
  compared with acrylic 312
  fused to alloys 102, 107, 311
  glazes 305, 309
  properties 308, 309
  vacuum-firing 309
Porous implant 314, 316, 318, 320
Powdered gold 71
Pre-amalgamated alloy 331

Precipitation hardening 69, 70, 104
Primary pipe 48
Primary recrystallization 56
Propagation of polymerization 255
Proof strength 21
Properties of
  acrylic filling 389
  alginate 227
  aluminium bronze 100
  amalgam 349
  artificial stone 202
  calcium hydroxide cement 355
  cobalt-chromium alloy 92, 121
  composite 403
  dentine 327
  duplicating material 231
  enamel 327
  glass ionomer cement 386
  gold alloy 79, 83–87, 103
  gold solder 135
  gutta-percha 289
  heat-cure PMMA 265
  investment 170, 173, 324
  nickel-chromium alloy 99, 106, 120
  plaster (as an impression material) 197
    for general purposes 201
  polycarboxylate cement 363
  polyether rubber 243
  polysulphide rubber 236
  reversible hydrocolloid 230
  silicate cement 382
  silicone rubber 242
  stainless steel 116
  sticky wax 158
  tantalum, titanium 316
  temporary crown materials 288
  vitreous carbon 319
  wax 161
  zinc phosphate cement 371
Proportional limit 21, 37, 38
PTFE implant 317
Pulp reaction to
  copper phosphate cement 372
  polycarboxylate cement 362
  silicate cement 380
  ZOE cement 357
  zinc phosphate cement 368

Pumice 298
Pummy 298
Putty powder 300

Quartz
  in investment 177
  in porcelain 303

Radiopacity
  of composite 394
  of denture bases 267
  of ZOE cement 357
Rebasing 270, 275
Recrystallization 56, 119, 133, 141
Relining 270, 275
Remelting alloys
  Co–Cr 94
  precious metal 88
Repairs 268, 274
Reservoirs in casting 186
Residual monomer 260, 261, 272
Resilience 23
Reversible hydrocolloid 227, 229
Rhodium plating 146
Rockwell hardness 28
Root canal points 289
Rubber bands 246
Rubber base 232
Rupture strength 27

Scratch hardness 29
Secondary pipe in casting 48
Secondary recrystallization 57, 139
Self-cure PMMA 271, 288, 387
Setting reaction of
  alginate 218
  amalgam 332
  composite 393
  glass ionomer cement 384
  plaster 191
  polycarboxylate cement 360
  polysulphide rubber 232
  silicate cement 375
  silicone rubber 237
  ZOE cement and paste 210, 355
Shelf life
  of alginate 221
  of composite 395
  of polysulphide rubber 236

of silicone rubber 239
Silane coupling agent 310
    in composite 395
Silica
    forms of 164
    gel 171
    in porcelain 303
Silica-bonded investment 171, 231
Silicate cement 373
    acidity 381
    effect on pulp 380
    setting 375
    solubility 379
Silicone rubber 237
    accuracy of 230
    soft lining 278
Silicone-lined mould 253, 273
Silver plating 145, 322
Silver solder 120, 136
Size and number of sprues 183
Slip plane 52
Soft lining 277
    cleaning of 302
    fungus infection of 279
Soldering 128
    by passing an electric current 132,
        138
    cobalt–chromium alloy 138
    flame for 132
    gap between parts 130
    gold alloy 134
    nickel–chromium alloy 138
    stainless steel 136
    strength 134
Solid solution 62
    interstitial, substitutional 63
    ordered 64, 76
Solid state 7
Solidus 61
Solubility
    plaster 197
    polycarboxylate cement 361, 363
    silicate cement 379, 382
    ZOE cement 357
    zinc phosphate cement 369, 371
Solution hardening 64
Solution heat treatment 55
Space–lattice 12
Specific heat 32

Spherical amalgam 335
Splat-cooled amalgam 335
Sponge gold 71
Spot welding 139
Sprue
    reservoir 186
    size and number of 183
Stainless steel 114
    annealing 117
    austenitic 114, 116
    precipitation hardened 115
    soldering 136
    spot welding 139
    stabilized 118
    swaging 117
    for implants 315
Standard specifications 2
    American 410
    Australian 411
    British 409
    International 409
Stein-cement 383
Stellite 90
Sticky wax 158
Strain 17
    hardening 54
Strength
    compressive 24
    fatigue 26
    impact 25
    rupture 27
    tear 27
    tensile 20
    transverse 25
Strengthening
    of acrylic polymer 266
    of glass 311
    of porcelain 310
Stress 16
    compressive 18
    shear 18
    due to mould seals 282
    in acrylic polymer 262
    in wax 155
Stress-relief anneal 55, 119
Stress–strain curve 21
Stressed skin effect 309, 311
Sublingual bar dimensions 97
Superlattice 64

Swaging of stainless steel 117, 125
Sweating 139
Syneresis
  of duplicating material 231
  of irreversible hydrocolloid 217,
  225
  of reversible hydrocolloid 229
Synthetic waxes 154

Tack weld 140
Tantalum 316
Taper of crown 365
Tear strength 27
Temperature colours 132
Tempering of steel 112
Temporary stopping 289
Tensile test 20
  diametral (Brazilian) 22
Thermal conductivity 32
  dentine, enamel 327
Thermal diffusivity 33
  dentine, enamel 327
  ZOE cement 358
Thermal equilibrium diagram 58, 59
  Au–Cu 75
  eutectic alloy 65
  solid solution alloy 61
  steel 110
Thermal expansion 31, 41
Tin–nickel plating 101
Thiokol rubber 232
Tinfoil substitute 281
Tissue conditioning material 214
Titanium implant 314
Toothpaste 300
Toughness 23, 25
Toxicity testing 35
Transition point
  impression compound 208
  wax 155
Transplantation of teeth 313
Transverse strength 25, 39
Triaxiality 134, 137
Trituration of amalgam 337
Tungsten carbide 122, 296
Turbine solder 120, 137
Twinning 54

Type metal 126

Ultimate tensile strength 21, 38
Ultrasonic condensation 345
Ultrasonic vibration 294
U-V light activated polymer 393
U-V absorber in polymer 271, 393
Units, international system of 17

Vacuum investing 181
van der Waals' forces 8, 15, 103, 108
Varnishes
  cavity 353
  silicate cement 379
Vicat needle 192
Vickers hardness 28
Vinyl copolymer 277
Viscoelasticity 24, 215, 220, 234,
  243, 289, 396
Vitreous carbon implant 319
Vulcanite 246

Water-settable cement 364
Wax, properties 155
Weld-decay 117, 141
Welding 71, 128, 139
Wettability 34
Wire
  Cobalt–chromium 121
  nickel–chromium 119
  stainless steel 119
  titanium–nickel 121
  white gold 88
  wrought yellow gold 79
Work hardening 54

Young's modulus 22

ZOE cement 355
ZOE paste 209, 270, 275
Zinc phosphate cement 363
  acidity 368
  attachment 367
  particle size of powder 364
  properties 371
Zinc polycarboxylate cement 359
  properties 363